S0-ADG-033

Praise for

GLUTEN FREEDOM

"This tremendously valuable book provides clear and understandable information about the history of gluten sensitivity, autoimmunity in the gastrointestinal tract, and celiac disease, linked with best current knowledge about identification and treatment. Written by the acknowledged leader in the science of celiac disease and gluten-related disorders, the book gives clear guidance about the best ways to avoid and treat problems with gluten among affected individuals."

—JAMES M. PERRIN, MD, FAAP, PROFESSOR OF PEDIATRICS, HARVARD MEDICAL SCHOOL, MASSGENERAL HOSPITAL *FOR* CHILDREN

"Over the years, I've watched with great admiration and respect as Dr. Alessio Fasano's groundbreaking studies have literally changed the way the world looks at celiac disease. In *Gluten Freedom,* he cuts through the confusion and dispels the myths about gluten. An important work by one of the world's leading experts, this book is a must-read for anyone interested in the gluten-free diet."

—ALICIA WOODWARD, EDITOR-IN-CHIEF, LIVING WITHOUT'S *GLUTEN FREE & MORE*

"In an era when a gluten-free diet has become the panacea for relief of symptoms for a large number of clinical conditions (gastrointestinal, neurologic, and inflammatory), evidence-based information is sorely needed for both the public and the practicing physician to appropriately decide when gluten should be removed from the diet. This book, *Gluten Freedom,* by one of the world's experts on gluten and celiac disease, provides the appropriate objective evidence to make that decision."

—W. ALLAN WALKER, M.D., CONRAD TAFF PROFESSOR OF NUTRITION AND PEDIATRICS, DIRECTOR, DIVISION OF NUTRITION, HARVARD MEDICAL SCHOOL

"As a pioneer in the study of gluten-related disorders, Dr. Alessio Fasano is a hero. He has dedicated his life to shining light on the science behind these pervasive conditions, and the world is privileged that he has taken his time to share his insight in this remarkable book. Don't take a word of it lightly; he is one of the most credible experts there is."

—DANNA KORN, AUTHOR OF *LIVING GLUTEN-FREE FOR DUMMIES* AND *WHEAT-FREE, WORRY FREE,* FOUNDER OF R.O.C.K. (RAISING OUR CELIAC KIDS)

"Dr. Alessio Fasano knows more about the causes and symptoms of celiac disease and gluten sensitivity than almost any other physician practicing today. *Gluten Freedom* will help all those who have a problem with gluten understand the biological processes that underlie their health issues, plus what the latest research says about these conditions and how to treat them."

—JANE ANDERSON, ABOUT.COM SOURCE ON CELIAC DISEASE AND GLUTEN SENSITIVITY

"Everyone who is gluten free is lucky to have Dr. Alessio Fasano relentlessly pursuing answers to questions about celiac disease, gluten sensitivity, and other disorders triggered by gluten. He's never satisfied that we know enough. In his new book, *Gluten Freedom,* he's hot on the trail of what causes gluten sensitivity and might cure celiac disease, in addition to clearly explaining the science behind the role the gluten-free diet might play in some cases of autism and schizophrenia. Lest you think he's only about the science of gluten-related disorders, Dr. Fasano also offers a full gluten-free dinner menu with family recipes from his native Italy, as well as tips from experts including how to eat, cook, and travel on the gluten-free diet. If you're new to the gluten-free diet, this is the first book you should buy. If you already have a shelf full of gluten-free books, make room for *Gluten Freedom.*"

—AMY RATNER, EDITOR, *GLUTEN-FREE LIVING*

"An engaging, comprehensive, and easy read, *Gluten Freedom* is an excellent reference for those with gluten-related disorders, their caregivers, physicians, dietitians, and the general public as well. Dr. Alessio Fasano and Susie Flaherty are to be congratulated for this myth-dispelling, must-have work."

—MARILYN G. GELLER, CEO, CELIAC DISEASE FOUNDATION

"When faced with a diagnosis that requires someone to change their entire life, the questions become: 'Why' and 'How'? Not only does Dr. Fasano's new book *Gluten Freedom* provide a scientific explanation of why a gluten-free life can help you heal, but he also tells you how best to make this happen. *Gluten Freedom* contains in-depth information regarding not only celiac disease, but also other autoimmune diseases along with related disorders such as Hashimoto's disease and Autism Spectrum Disorder. Dr. Fasano walks the reader through the different manifestations of celiac disease, including non-responsive celiac disease, and then outlines a plan for living well on the gluten-free diet. With tips about navigating dining out and how to safely eat and cook for any age, from toddler to college through the golden years, and providing tempting recipes like 'Roast Lamb with Mint Chutney,' 'Super Bowl Chili,' and 'Chocolate Chip Cookies,' *Gluten Freedom* is an excellent resource for the newly diagnosed."

—KYRA BUSSANICH, AUTHOR OF *SWEET CRAVINGS:*
50 SEDUCTIVE DESSERTS FOR A GLUTEN-FREE LIFESTYLE (TEN SPEED PRESS)
AND THREE-TIME GLUTEN-FREE WINNER OF *CUPCAKE WARS*

"We are so grateful that this serious and complicated disease has been thoroughly researched by experts. They provide confirmation and guidance for those suffering from the effects of gluten and continue to educate the health-care professionals treating them. Thank you to Dr. Fasano and his staff."

—THE CENTRAL NEW YORK CELIAC SUPPORT GROUP

"As a lay person who has been active in celiac/gluten sensitivity support activities for over 20 years, I found this work, which is led by Dr. Fasano, to be immensely informative, on the cutting edge, and very, very readable."

—CLIFF HAUCK, CHAIR, WESTERN NEW YORK GLUTEN FREE DIET SUPPORT GROUP, INC. (CHAPTER # 33, CELIAC SOCIETY OF AMERICA)

"*Gluten Freedom* explains celiac disease in terms to be understood by the 'patient' as well as the professional. Dr. Fasano has been an expert in the world of celiac disease since his team at the Center for Celiac Research discovered in 2003 that the prevalence in the U.S. was at least one out of 133 individuals. You will enjoy reading the facts regarding celiac disease and learn practical suggestions for following the gluten-free lifestyle, including some of Dr. Fasano's own home Italian gluten-free recipes. Learn and enjoy!"

—JANET Y. RINEHART, FORMER PRESIDENT OF CELIAC SOCIETY OF AMERICA/USA; CHAIRMAN OF HOUSTON CELIAC SUPPORT GROUP

"*Gluten Freedom* is such an exciting resource for those diagnosed with celiac disease and others interested in gluten issues! Dr. Fasano provides a detailed description of what goes on in the gut (and other parts of the body that can be affected) of someone with celiac disease, and his explanations can be easily understood by everyone. I'm excited to see what new treatments are on the horizon for celiac disease, and the book's guide for maintaining a healthy gluten-free lifestyle is most helpful! I've read lots of literature about the diagnosis and treatment of celiac disease, but this book puts it

all together. If someone is looking for the best and most accurate source of information on celiac disease and living gluten free, *Gluten Freedom* is it!"
—Barb Huyette, RN, Chairperson, Central Iowa Celiac Connection, Des Moines, Iowa

"Gluten Freedom provides an in-depth look at the history of celiac disease, living gluten free, and promising research and treatment prospects. . . . The perspective of Dr. Fasano, a renowned pediatric gastroenterologist and researcher for celiac disease, is truly fascinating."
—Caitlin Sexton, RD, President, Greater Rochester Celiac Support Group

"This book provides a comprehensive understanding of celiac disease, gluten sensitivity, and gluten allergy. Dr. Fasano's insightful expertise and up-to-date research provides information that makes *Gluten Freedom* a must for every patient and practitioner."
—Elaine Monarch, Diagnosed Celiac and Founder, Celiac Disease Foundation

"When you are looking for answers for any questions, it's always best to go the experts! For this reason, we follow the science and developments of the Center for Celiac Research—the top authority in all things related to celiac disease and gluten intolerance—when conferring for our own individual health and making recommendations for reliable information to those seeking support through our group. We are happy to endorse the Center's new book with the confidence that you can find no better authority on gluten-related disorders."
—The Alabama Gluten Free & Celiac Community

"Gluten Freedom is an adventure into the newest research about celiac disease and non-celiac gluten sensitivity—easily understood, very readable, and very personal."
—Tri-County Celiac Support Group, Michigan

"Gluten Freedom celebrates the pioneers who are forging the way for the gluten-free community. From genetics and research to raising children and living with celiac disease and gluten sensitivity, Dr. Fasano and his contributors offer an engaging and easy-to-read guide. I highly recommend this book for readers in all stages of their gluten-free journey."
—Alice Bast, President and CEO, National Foundation for Celiac Awareness

"Gluten Freedom will provide patient and practitioner alike with the most current information on gluten-related disorders. This is indeed the information patients need to successfully live a gluten-free life."
—Anne Lee, EdD(c), RD, LD, Dr. Schär USA, Inc.

GLUTEN
FREEDOM

GLUTEN FREEDOM

*The Nation's Leading Expert Offers
the Essential Guide
to a Healthy, Gluten-Free Lifestyle*

ALESSIO FASANO, MD
WITH SUSIE FLAHERTY

WILEY

Wiley General Trade, an imprint of Turner Publishing Company
www.turnerpublishing.com

Gluten Freedom: The Nation's Leading Expert Offers the Essential Guide to a Healthy, Gluten-Free Lifestyle

Copyright © 2014 Alessio Fasano and Susie Flaherty. All rights reserved.

This book or any part thereof may not be reproduced or transmitted in any form or by any means, electronic or mechanical, including photocopying, recording, or by any information storage and retrieval system, without permission in writing from the publisher.

The information contained in this book is not intended to serve as a replacement for professional medical advice. Any use of the information in this book is at the reader's discretion. The author and the publisher specifically disclaim any information contained in this book. A health-care professional should be consulted regarding your specific situation.

Cover design and artwork: Maxwell Roth
Book design: Kym Whitley

Library of Congress Cataloging-in-Publication Data

Fasano, Alessio.
 Gluten freedom : the nation's leading expert offers the essential guide to a healthy, gluten-free lifestyle / Alessio Fasano, MD with Susie Flaherty.
    pages cm
  Includes bibliographical references and index.
 ISBN 978-1-118-42310-3 (hardback)

1. Gluten-free diet--Popular works. 2. Gluten-free diet--Recipes. 3. Self-care, Health--Popular works. I. Flaherty, Susie. II. Title.
 RM237.86.F37 2014
 641.5'638--dc23
                                      2014008601

ISBN 978-1-68162-051-0 (pbk.)

Printed in the United States of America

*To my sister Annamaria who, with her transcendent force,
has directed my path of science toward a destination simply
unimaginable when I started this wonderful journey.*
—AF

To my nephew, Martin.
—SMF

CONTENTS

PART ONE:
Gluten Enters the Picture

PART TWO:
Learning to Live Without Gluten

PART THREE
Gluten-Free for Life

PART FOUR
Going Beyond Gluten

EPILOGUE
Making Wishes Come True — 281

Contributors to

GLUTEN FREEDOM

Dr. Carlo Catassi

Pam Cureton

Jules Dowler Shepard

Shelley and Danielle Gannon

Meghan Harrington-Patton

Tom Hopper

Barbara Hudson

Sharone Jelden

Andrea Levario

Bob Levy

Dr. Mary McKenna

John M. Mink

Dr. Brian Morris and Rebecca Morris

Dr. Anna Quigg

Foreword

A Father's Dilemma
BY RICH GANNON

When you pick up this book, you may wonder why a former National Football League Most Valuable Player is writing the foreword to a book about gluten, celiac disease, and who should avoid wheat. Well, the answer is simple. While being a happily retired football player, I'm also a father, the most important position that I've ever played in my life. Early in parenthood, my wife and I found ourselves facing a situation that no parent ever wants to experience: my wife, Shelley, and I were fighting to save our young daughter's life.

It happened during my time with the Kansas City Chiefs late in the 1990s. Shelley and I had just moved to Kansas City, and Danielle was less than a year old. She was very fussy, and no matter what we fed her, she couldn't keep it down. She had been sick for a long time and was losing weight with no explanation for what was causing her distress. After many frustrating visits to doctors and countless medical tests, we were desperate for answers when we took her to a pediatric gastroenterologist at Children's Hospital in Minnesota in August 1998.

By then our daughter was very ill, and we were afraid that she might not survive this ordeal. Shelley called me one night in tears during training camp and was scared for Danielle. I immediately left training camp in Wisconsin and headed home to Minneapolis.

Back in Minneapolis, Danielle was finally diagnosed with the condition that had made her so sick; it was celiac disease. As you will learn in *Gluten Freedom,* celiac disease is an autoimmune disorder that damages the small intestine and prevents the proper absorption of nutrients. Gluten, found in wheat, rye, and barley, is the trigger for celiac disease, which affects approximately one in 133 people in the United States.

Finally, we had some answers about what was making Danielle so sick. I returned to training camp in Wisconsin, and Shelley put Danielle on a gluten-free diet, leading to our family's journey described by Shelley in Chapter Twelve. Danielle had lost a significant amount of weight. She was so sick by the time she was finally diagnosed that it took some time for her to recover and begin to act like a normal, healthy baby.

We found out about the work of Dr. Alessio Fasano and the Center for Celiac Research and took Danielle for an appointment to his clinic. I remember our first encounter with Dr. Fasano. I was struck by how friendly and down-to-earth he was. What was even more important was how knowledgeable he was about celiac disease. He was very easy to talk to, and we felt like he listened to our concerns and was really interested in what was best for our family.

Shelley and I didn't want other families to go through the nightmare that we had experienced prior to Danielle's diagnosis. I offered to become a spokesperson for the Center. In 2000, Danielle and I recorded a public service announcement (PSA) that was aired on national television to promote awareness of celiac disease.

If you happened to see the PSA, you know that by this time Danielle had gained weight and was running around like any normal three-year-old. Our efforts at outreach were amplified by the work of many other members of the celiac community. For example, the Gluten-Free Pantry in Glastonbury, Connecticut, sold a delicious gluten-free chocolate cake called "Danielle's Decadent Chocolate Cake" and donated proceeds to the Center. Our family still participates in the annual celiac walk/run that we helped to establish in Minneapolis, Minnesota, as part of the Center's annual national fund-raiser in May to mark Celiac Disease Awareness Month.

I hope that our work, supported by the Friends of Celiac Disease Research, and many other organizations and individuals, has kept some families from experiencing the anguish that Shelley and I felt in those terrible months before Danielle was diagnosed. I know that the collective efforts of so many other members of the celiac community kicked off a new level of awareness that led to greater recognition of celiac disease and other gluten-related disorders.

Several years later, when Shelley and our second daughter, Alexis, were both diagnosed with gluten sensitivity, we again turned to Dr. Fasano and the Center for Celiac Research for answers to our questions. He treated us with compassion and consideration as we learned to deal with this new condition called gluten sensitivity. Once again, we learned a great deal from Dr. Fasano and his team at the Center for Celiac Research.

During my eighteen years in the National Football League, I learned about passion, commitment, and excellence—those extra intangible qualities that make a team or an organization stand out and surpass the competition. Whether it's being the best football player, parent, or doctor, these qualities make a huge difference. Dr. Fasano's passionate commitment to improving the lives of people with gluten-related disorders is why this book is different from any other book about celiac disease and other gluten-related disorders. If you want the facts about your family and gluten, you will find them in *Gluten Freedom.*

Rich holding Danielle as a toddler, after her diagnosis

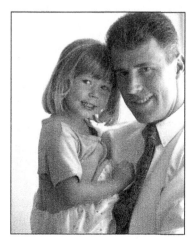

Preface

"It is often the failure who is the pioneer in new lands,
new undertakings, and new forms of expression."
—ERIC HOFFER

MAKING IT INTO THE LEXICON

I came to the United States in 1993 as a pediatric gastroenterologist and research scientist hoping to find a cure for childhood diarrhea. There's an old saying: "If you want to make
God laugh, tell God your plans." This has certainly been true
in my case.

I didn't achieve my goal of developing a vaccine for cholera; serendipity took me down a different path. And as I look
back over the last twenty years, I see the necessary failures and
many crossroads that led me to the work that I do today, which
is improving the lives of people with celiac disease and other
gluten-related disorders and unlocking the complex mechanisms of the autoimmune response.

As I look around my office, I see many reminders of the
patients and people who have made the entrepreneurial and
collaborative spirit of the Center for Celiac Research possible.
We've conducted research and made discoveries that have
changed the trajectory and treatment of celiac disease and gluten sensitivity in the United States and throughout the world.

I have a book in my office from 1994 that reminds me of
how far we've come in a very short time in the treatment of

gluten-related disorders. In May of that year, the U.S. Department of Health and Human Services and the National Institutes of Health's National Institute of Diabetes and Digestive and Kidney Diseases published an 800-page report on the epidemiology and impact of digestive diseases in the United States.

In great detail the book describes all the gastrointestinal diseases considered to be important in the United States, including rare and unusual diseases. The words "celiac disease" do not appear in this book. In 1994 the principal agency for protecting the health of the U.S. population was unaware that celiac disease existed in this country. The condition didn't even merit a footnote.

Thus, at the beginning of this journey, I had to explain constantly to my colleagues how to spell the word "celiac." When I started writing this book several years ago, I was using an older version of Microsoft Word. Every time I wrote the word "celiac," it was underlined in red, which is the symbol of a misspelled or unrecognized word.

Now I use a newer version of Microsoft Word that recognizes "celiac" in its spelling dictionary. The word celiac has finally made it into the popular lexicon. And although it might seem like a small thing, to me it's a fitting symbol of how the awareness of celiac disease and gluten-related disorders has grown so much in such a brief span of time.

As you will learn, the story of gluten and celiac disease is intimately tied to the development and research discoveries of the Center for Celiac Research. Operating on a shoestring budget with donations from volunteers, our small team has made a very large impact.

We changed the way the world looks at celiac disease, which is now identified as an autoimmune disorder, and other gluten-related conditions. The words gluten, celiac disease, and gluten sensitivity (also known as non-celiac gluten sensitivity) are now familiar not only to many people in the United States, but also throughout the world. Gluten-free alternatives abound in supermarkets and restaurants. In *Gluten Freedom,* we separate the facts from the fantasies to present the real story about celiac disease, gluten sensitivity, and the gluten-free diet.

Alessio Fasano, M.D.
Director
Center for Celiac Research
Massachusetts General Hospital *for* Children
Visiting Professor
Harvard Medical School
Boston, Massachusetts
April 29, 2014

Acknowledgments

In the creation of the Center for Celiac Research, and in the writing of this book, there are many people to thank. We acknowledge that we will no doubt fail to include everyone, so we extend our appreciation to all the people who have contributed not only to *Gluten Freedom* but also to the success of the Center. (You know who you are!) We extend a special thanks to our contributors (listed at front) and our colleagues whose names are included in *Gluten Freedom*.

We would like to acknowledge the people who were key in the establishment and growth of the Center for Celiac Research and the Mucosal Biology Research Center at the University of Maryland School of Medicine.

For their warm welcome and support in our new environment at the Massachusetts General Hospital in Boston, we would like to thank President Peter Slavin and Drs. Ronald Kleinman and Allan Walker, along with Joanne O'Brien, Suzzette McCarron, and Maureen Garron. We also thank the members of the Mucosal Immunology and Biology Research Center and the Department of Pediatric Gastroenterology and Nutrition at MassGeneral Hospital *for* Children.

We gratefully acknowledge our partners in the Celiac Program at Harvard Medical School, especially Drs. Ciarán Kelly, Alan Leichtner, Daniel Leffler, and Dascha Weir, along with dietitians Melinda Dennis and Karen Warman.

For their role in helping with administrative details and reading of the manuscript, we would like to thank Drs. Karen Lammers and Francesco Valitutti, Patricia Castillo, Pam King, and Elizabeth Shea. We would like to thank our tenacious agent, Marilyn Allen, and our patient editor at Turner Publishing, Christina Roth.

We most heartily thank the leaders and members of the international, national, and local celiac support groups who have given so generously of their time and knowledge to advance awareness of celiac disease and the mission of the Center to improve the quality of life for people with gluten-related disorders.

Finally and foremost—even though we have saved you for last—we would most especially like to thank all our patients and their families for their support and wish you health and happiness in all your endeavors.

Introduction

As an international expert on celiac disease and gluten-related disorders, I've treated thousands of children and adults for conditions
related to the consumption of gluten. The most fully understood
of these conditions is celiac disease, an autoimmune disorder that
results from eating products with gluten, which is mainly found
in wheat.

With today's emphasis on gluten-free foods in supermarkets
and restaurants, along with celebrities and athletes embracing the
gluten-free diet, it's hard to imagine how difficult it used to be for
people with celiac disease in the 1990s. In those early days, there
was very little commercially available gluten-free food. The old joke
was that you weren't sure if you were supposed to eat the product or
the box it came in because they both tasted about the same!

Before I founded the Center for Celiac Research in 1996, I
learned so much from the small group of patients I was already
treating for celiac disease in my clinical practice. During an early
meeting of support-group members, I decided to do an experiment
that would have a profound effect on both my professional future
and the mission priorities of the Center.

I passed out blank paper to the audience members and asked

them to treat it like "Aladdin's lamp" by writing their three top wishes in regard to their disease. I collected the papers at the end of the meeting and was not surprised by the results: Wish Number One: a treatment alternative to the gluten-free diet; Wish Number Two: improving their quality of life by educating physicians about celiac disease and by providing more palatable gluten-free food; and Wish Number Three: a way to avoid the cumbersome intestinal biopsy as a necessary step to diagnose celiac disease, especially for children.

I conducted this experiment with various groups around the country, and the answers were always the same. From that point on, activities at the Center were focused on these three goals. As I look back on our history and the explosive growth in the awareness and diagnosis of celiac disease, I can see now that all three of these wishes have nearly come true.

NAVIGATING *GLUTEN FREEDOM*

Is it really possible to eliminate celiac disease and other gluten-related disorders such as gluten sensitivity and wheat allergy? I believe this can become a reality for the next generation. But before we look at next steps for the global gluten-free community, let's see where we have come from, and where we presently stand on this journey to gluten freedom.

Gluten Freedom is presented in four parts. Part One opens with the story of how products with gluten traveled across the globe through the growth of agriculture. Now found on every continent where humans reside, celiac disease and other gluten-related disorders migrated along with the wheat, rye, and barley containing indigestible peptides.

Next I unravel the mystery of how these gluten peptides pose a danger to genetically susceptible individuals as I travel around the world to report on the growing global epidemic of celiac disease. Highlighted with the latest findings on gluten-related disorders, Chapter One features the unlikely story of how Center researchers uncovered the tip of the American celiac disease iceberg.

In Chapter Two, I dismantle the chemistry that makes gluten such an unusual and troublesome protein. Exploring the spectrum of reactions to gluten in Chapter Three, I define celiac disease and wheat allergy along with that new kid on the block: gluten sensitivity. We know that celiac disease is an autoimmune disorder, and I unravel some of the mystery about autoimmunity in Chapter Four. With gluten sensitivity, we're not quite sure what genetic or immune mechanisms trigger this condition. We do know that the number of individuals with gluten sensitivity is exploding. Center scientists are currently working on diagnostic tools for gluten sensitivity, which I also discuss in Chapter Four.

How can you tell if you or a family member has a problem with gluten? In Chapter Five, I focus on the diagnostic aspects of celiac disease and gluten-related disorders and include the "Fasano Diet" as a proved method for totally eliminating gluten. The effects of gluten on our brain and the supposed role of the gluten-free diet in Autism Spectrum Disorder and schizophrenia are highlighted in Chapter Six with the latest research from this controversial field.

Okay, now you've heard from me about gluten and the havoc it can create in certain humans. In Part Two, you'll get the perspective from the real experts: the patients who have found their way back to health by living the gluten-free lifestyle. With their expertise, I highlight stories, tips, recipes, cautionary tales, and more to help you achieve your own gluten freedom.

Successful treatment is the key to gluten freedom, and in Chapter Seven you'll learn the basic elements of the gluten-free diet along with vital nutritional considerations. Chapter Eight shows you and your family how to eat safely, whether at home in your own kitchen, in school, social or work settings, or traveling overseas. We'll travel to Southern Italy in Chapter Nine, where I teach you how to prepare a classic gluten-free full-course dinner, complete with delicious recipes.

As research shows, celiac disease and gluten-related disorders are not simply diseases of childhood, but they can develop at any age. Strategies on how to successfully live the gluten-free lifestyle are presented in Part Three with the help of the firsthand experience of my patients, friends, and colleagues.

Chapter Ten addresses the challenges that the diagnosis of a gluten-related disorder can present for a pregnant woman with celiac disease. In Chapter Eleven, we learn from an expert about how to advocate for your child in school settings.

Through a famous football family in Chapter Twelve, we learn how to keep the whole family happy on the gluten-free diet. Successfully meeting the challenges of the gluten-free diet while making the transition to college is featured in Chapter Thirteen.

Our research shows that the rate of celiac disease is rising among elderly people. In Chapter Fourteen, we learn what it's like to live with celiac disease from two elderly "experts": one who was diagnosed as an infant in the 1930s, and one who was diagnosed in his sixties.

The last section, Part Four, propels us into the future with the latest strategies for treatment, prevention, and a possible cure. The final chapter describes the latest and most exciting developments for the Center in our new phase at one of the world's top hospitals. Housed in the Mucosal Immunology and Biology Research Center at MassGeneral Hospital *for* Children (MGH*f*C) in Boston, Massachusetts, the Center for Celiac Research is also working in partnership with the Celiac Center at Beth Israel Deaconess Medical Center and Boston Children's Hospital to advance research and improve the quality of life for people with gluten-related disorders. And on the other side of the Atlantic with MGH*f*C's support of a visionary new research institute in my hometown of Salerno, Italy, I return to my Italian roots to create new synergies in international collaboration to search for clues to solve the puzzle of autoimmunity and other disorders.

In *Gluten Freedom,* my goal is to happily return people with gluten-related disorders to one of the most natural and joyous events in life: eating safely and eating well. Like most people, I take this for granted, but individuals with gluten-related disorders can't afford this luxury. They are constantly thinking: "Is this a safe meal for me to eat? Am I being contaminated with gluten? Should I take a chance on getting sick?"

For sufferers of gluten-related disorders, this book will bring back the joy of eating without worry. If you are newly diagnosed with a gluten-related disorder, you will want to add this book to your gluten-free resources. If you have lived with a gluten-related disorder for a long time, if you have a family member with a gluten-related disorder, or if you treat patients with gluten-related disorders in any health or community care setting, this book will become a valuable tool.

And finally, for the intellectually curious among you who simply wish to distinguish fact from fiction, this book will provide accurate "food for thought" about gluten and its role in your health. My hope is that like a good meal shared with close friends, you enjoy reading *Gluten Freedom* as much as I enjoyed writing it with my colleagues and friends. I extend my best wishes for your good health.

GLUTEN FREEDOM

PART ONE

Gluten Enters the Picture

CHAPTER ONE

Gluten Gets Into the Gut —and Other Places

"He was a wise man who invented beer."
—Plato

THE WORLD BEFORE GLUTEN

Once upon a time, there was no gluten. This complex and ancient protein, the main component of wheat, developed alongside humans throughout many thousands of years. A very strange and unique protein, gluten, and its close relatives secalin and hordein from barley and rye, are the only proteins we're not able to digest.

Let's put it in perspective. Every person has about 25,000 genes; wheat has five times as many. With more than 150,000 genes, wheat presents an extremely complicated genetic maze for scientists to untangle. Wheat and its protein components, including gluten, make us seem a lot less complicated than we might like to think we are.

The history of humans and the evolution of celiac disease are intertwined with the evolution of wheat and gluten: how they developed, how they continue to evolve, and how they affect humankind today around the world in a variety of gluten-related symptoms and disorders.

For the vast majority of our human evolution, we ate gluten-free diets. And then, approximately 10,000 years ago, the agricultural revolution was born. Humans stayed in one place to plant and harvest crops and gather animals into domestic herds.

The slow growth of agriculture led to larger societies and the development of creative pursuits. With stability and leisure time, our

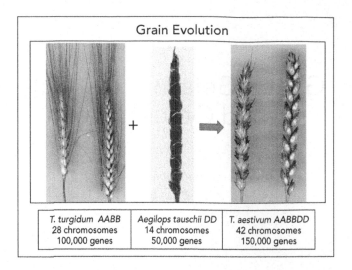

Grain Evolution

T. turgidum AABB	Aegilops tauschii DD	T. aestivum AABBDD
28 chromosomes	14 chromosomes	42 chromosomes
100,000 genes	50,000 genes	150,000 genes

ancestors began the slow journey from building cavelike structures to erecting the Colosseum in Rome and the Great Wall of China.

In stable agricultural societies wheat became one of the most precious and prestigious measures of wealth. The assets that defined wealth and security were viable and nonperishable merchandises of exchange. Wheat was one of the most valuable of those commodities. But for a very small number of people, the consumption of wheat came with an unexpected price.

EARLY CASES OF CELIAC DISEASE

Almost 2,000 years ago, one of the most celebrated early Greek physicians, Aretaeus from Cappadocia, reported what is believed to be the first recorded case of celiac disease. He described "koiliakos," from the Greek for pertaining to the abdomen as "suffering in the bowels."

After Aretaeus, it was approximately 1,800 years before celiac disease was mentioned again in medical literature. As a medical student in the 1980s, I spent a few months at the Hospital for Sick Children on Great Ormond Street in London. In the same location a century earlier, the British physician Samuel Gee gave a presentation describing celiac disease as a "kind of chronic indigestion which is met with in persons of all ages, yet is especially apt to affect children between one and five years old."

Following his medical intuition, Dr. Gee described celiac disease as a syndrome of malabsorption triggered by some unidentified foodstuff. He was right on target with his description of the condition, but missed the mark with his subsequent dietary intervention. Dr. Gee's recommendation was to feed patients bread that was "cut thin and well toasted on both sides."

Aside from his dietary recommendation, Dr. Gee's work represented a major breakthrough in the understanding of celiac disease. Unfortunately a similar breakthrough wouldn't appear for almost another century.

WHAT IS CELIAC DISEASE?

Celiac disease is a genetic disorder affecting children and adults. People with celiac disease are unable to eat foods that contain gluten, which is found in wheat and other grains. In people with celiac disease, gluten sets off an autoimmune reaction that can eventually lead to complete destruction of the villi, the tiny fingerlike projections lining the small intestine.

Healthy villi are vital to the proper digestion and absorption of food. People with celiac disease produce antibodies that, in combination with hormone-like substances called cytokines and the direct effect of immune cells, attack the intestine and flatten the villi, leading to malabsorption and illness.

Celiac disease is twice as common as Crohn's disease, ulcerative colitis, and cystic fibrosis combined. It affects one in 133 people in the United States. A panel of blood tests is now available to screen for the presence of specific antibodies. A biopsy of the intestine (before beginning a gluten-free diet) is usually needed to make a final diagnosis.

People with celiac disease are more likely to be afflicted with problems related to malabsorption, including diarrhea, bloating, weight loss, nausea, vomiting, anemia, osteoporosis, and tooth enamel defects. Celiac disease autoimmunity can also result in central and peripheral nervous system inflammation, pancreatic and other organ disorders including the gall bladder, liver, and spleen, and obstetrical and gynecological disorders such as miscarriage and inability to conceive.

Untreated celiac disease also has been linked (in extremely rare cases) to an increased risk of certain types of cancer, especially intestinal lymphoma. Currently, there are no drugs to treat celiac disease, and there is no cure. But people with celiac disease can lead normal, healthy lives by following a gluten-free diet. This means eliminating all products containing wheat, rye, and barley.

Celiac disease is not a food allergy. Food allergies, including wheat allergy, are conditions that an individual might outgrow (see Chapter Three). Celiac disease is an autoimmune disorder caused by the abnormal functioning of the immune system that unleashes an attack against your own tissue. If you have celiac disease, you have it for life.

DR. DICKE IDENTIFIES WHEAT AS THE TRIGGER

The real breakthrough that eventually led to the gluten-free diet as treatment was made by Dutch pediatrician Willem-Karel Dicke in an unlikely place: The Netherlands. As his research shows, for some time Dr. Dicke suspected that wheat might play a role in the symptoms and distress he witnessed in his young patients.

During World War II when wheat flour was difficult to obtain, the mortality rate of Dutch children with celiac disease dropped dramatically. Dr. Dicke followed his earlier hunch that this dramatic swing in mortality was associated with the use of potato starch. With the resumption of wheat flour in children's diets following World War II, the rate of celiac disease returned to rates seen before World War II. This reinforced Dr. Dicke's earlier suspicion that wheat flour was responsible for the symptoms endured by the children known as "celiacs."

In the decades before Dr. Dicke's discoveries, many children thought to have celiac disease were fed bananas almost exclusively for three to six months. A pediatrician from New York City named Sidney Haas developed the diet in the 1920s. It remained the guiding therapy until 1950, when Dr. Dicke published his thesis with a meticulous dietary study that documented gluten as the dietary trigger of celiac disease.

GLUTEN GOES GLOBAL

After Samuel Gee defined celiac disease in the nineteenth century and Willem-Karel Dicke explained how to treat it in the twentieth century, we began to take a closer look at the condition. Based on Dr. Dicke's clinical and research work in the 1950s, celiac disease was considered a gastrointestinal problem that exclusively affected children mainly of Caucasian origin. The typical child with celiac disease was described as fair-skinned, with blue eyes and blond hair, and with Northern European ancestry.

Early in the 1970s, the first diagnostic tools were developed and epidemiological studies were performed. These studies showed that celiac disease was a condition confined mainly to northern Europe, but not present on other continents. Scientists were asking why celiac disease had such a peculiar distribution.

A famous Italian geneticist named Dr. Luigi Cavalli-Sforza came up with an interesting, but ultimately flawed, theory a decade later. He suggested that agricultural practices born in the Tigris and Euphrates river valley (an area corresponding to today's Turkey) moved from south to north and from east to west at the speed of approximately one kilometer a year. According to his theory, agriculture and gluten-containing grains reached northern Europe much later than in other parts of the developed world.

Because people with celiac disease had a high mortality rate in the ancient world, Dr. Cavalli-Sforza reasoned that in regions where agriculture developed first, people with celiac disease had been eliminated by natural selection. He argued that although the disease (and its predisposing genes) had already disappeared in much of the areas where agriculture originated, it was still present in places like northern Europe where gluten-containing grains were introduced much later. It seemed like a plausible explanation, but careful epidemiological research mainly performed by Center for Celiac Research scientists would prove otherwise.

HUNTING FOR CELIAC DISEASE

Since Dr. Cavalli-Sforza's theory was put forth in 1984, several investigators have implemented well-designed and systematic epidemiological studies to measure accurately the prevalence of celiac disease around the world. Dr. Carlo Catassi, co-director of the Center and a close friend of mine, is a pioneer and leading authority in the field of celiac disease epidemiology.

His breakthrough studies, which began in Italy, helped us recognize that celiac disease affects many more people than previously thought. Using blood samples from 17,201 healthy Italian students in 1996, he showed that celiac disease occurred in one in 184 subjects. Dr. Catassi's results also showed that most atypical cases (patients without the classic gastrointestinal symptoms associated with celiac disease) remain undiagnosed unless clinicians actively search for celiac disease as the cause of these extraintestinal symptoms.

Under Dr. Catassi's leadership, and in collaboration with many other colleagues worldwide, the Center embarked on epidemiological studies in places where Dr. Cavalli-Sforza had questioned the existence of celiac disease, including the Middle East, North Africa, South America, and Asia. These studies overturned Dr. Cavalli-Sforza's theory and placed celiac disease on the map in Libya, Egypt, North Africa, India, and most recently, China.

HIGH MORTALITY IN THE DESERT

The case of the Saharawi people in Western Sahara provides a very dramatic example of what gluten can do to the susceptible part of a population. Living in the Sahara Desert, the Saharawi people have been confined to refugee camps since the late 1970s as a result of civil war in North Africa. When this nomadic population became displaced, famine and mortality from malnutrition became a major concern for international human rights agencies.

To save the Saharawi, interventions that included food relief were implemented. International relief agencies asked, "What kind of food can we send that is multipurpose and nonperishable?" Wheat was the obvious choice.

A nomadic population that for thousands of years had based its diet on fruits, vegetables, camel milk, and camel meat was exposed to gluten-containing grains for the first time. The result was the highest rate of celiac disease described in the world thus far, affecting nearly 6 percent of the general population. Most Saharawi children with the condition still remain undiagnosed and run the risk of an early death because of chronic diarrhea and malnutrition.

The unfortunate experience of the Saharawi people gives us a snapshot of the early interplay between humans and gluten. It takes us back 10,000 years in time when all the susceptible individuals were alive and celiac disease made its deadly selection. Over millennia, only those with a milder form of celiac disease would have survived. Without intervention, we could predict that the prevalence of celiac disease would ultimately drop to 1 percent in the Saharawi population. It would eventually reflect the same rate for most of the world, after this negative selection had occurred.

In North Africa, the Saharawi people are an exceptional case. Although celiac disease is more common in Egypt, Libya, and other areas of North Africa, Dr. Catassi tells us that celiac disease is not common in Sub-Saharan Africa. The staple cereals, including millet and rice, are mostly gluten-free, and the genes related to celiac disease are much less frequent than in Western countries.

CELIAC DISEASE IN THE DEVELOPING WORLD

Through Dr. Catassi's studies, we know we've underestimated the burden caused by celiac disease in developing countries. Clinicians might assume that celiac disease doesn't exist in developing countries or might not realize its many clinical manifestations. Combine this with scarce diagnostic facilities and an emphasis on other causes of small intestinal damage, and the suffering of vulnerable populations increases.

In developing countries, a child with celiac disease often presents with the distended belly and emaciated limbs associated with chronic protein-energy malnutrition (e.g. stunting, kwashiorkor, and marasmus). We often see chronic diarrhea, abdominal distention, stunting, and anemia. This severe stunting increases the risk of death, especially among children with chronic diarrhea. The risks of developing severe diarrhea and dying from dehydration are greatest among the youngest children, especially during the summer months.

In most developed countries, it's easy to replace cereals that don't contain gluten (for example, rice and corn), and there are many palatable gluten-free, commercially available products made for patients with celiac disease. This isn't the case in most developing countries. Providers have to take local dietary habits into account by using naturally gluten-free products that are locally available, such as millet, manioc, and rice, and use separate, dedicated machinery for milling.

In both industrialized and less-developed nations, physicians, nurses, dieticians, school personnel, affected families, and the general population need to be taught about treatment and the gluten-free diet. Creating support groups for patients and families can help affected individuals cope with the daily difficulties of treatment.

Whether it's a ten-year-old boy with celiac disease in India or a fifty-four-year old woman with gluten sensitivity in California, education and support groups can make an enormous difference in sticking with the gluten-free diet.

A CHANGE FROM RICE TO WHEAT

From epidemiological studies, we now know that no region in the world is spared from the celiac disease epidemic. Another intriguing and troubling scenario is unfolding in China, a country inhabited by 1.3 billion people. China has always been considered immune from celiac disease. The most obvious explanation is that, with the exception of some northern regions, the Chinese diet is mainly based on rice.

China's economy continues to grow at a fast rate, with an increasing Western influence on diet and lifestyle. Kentucky Fried Chicken opened its first restaurant in China in 1987 and was followed by the first McDonald's at the edge of Tiananmen Square in 1992. The growing economy is paralleled by a growing number of Chinese moving from the "tu" (rustic or backward) lifestyle to the "yan" (foreign or progressive) lifestyle.

In China, consuming Western-style food, and thereby eating increasing amounts of gluten, has become a sign of climbing the social ladder of the Chinese economy. The predictable byproduct has been increased reports of celiac disease in China. My pessimistic prediction is that along with expanding its economic boundaries, China will also expand its boundaries for celiac disease and other gluten-related disorders.

NORTH AMERICA: THE NEW FRONTIER OF CELIAC DISEASE

Unlike the relocated Saharawi people or the growing Chinese middle class, we thought that people in North America had a different relationship to gluten and celiac disease. Until the very recent past, we thought that celiac disease didn't exist in North America. It was as if nature, or some undetermined force, was sitting in the middle of the Atlantic Ocean and redirecting all the celiac disease eastward to Europe and sending all the other cases of gastrointestinal disease, such as inflammatory bowel disease, westward to North America.

Of course, this makes no sense. And neither did the idea that celiac disease didn't exist in North America. For the few people accurately diagnosed with celiac disease twenty years ago, the selection of gluten-free products was sorely lacking in both quality and quantity.

FINDING THE AMERICAN "CELIACS"

This was the scenario when I came to the United States from Naples, Italy, in 1993 to become chief of the new Division of Pediatric Gastroenterology at the University of Maryland School of Medicine.

In my viewpoint, the perception of celiac disease in North

America had not changed much in the four decades since Dr. Dicke's discoveries. It was still considered by most physicians—if they had even heard of it at all—to be extremely rare. Their typical view was that it only affected children, and the only clinical presentation was gastrointestinal distress.

The environment in Naples had been quite different. In Europe in the 1990s, it was estimated that one in 300 people had been affected by celiac disease. As a pediatric gastroenterologist in Italy, I was accustomed to seeing 15 to 20 children a week with celiac disease.

This was the result of an awareness campaign among Italian health-care professionals that led to large screening campaigns in school-age children. Progressive policies were developed that included general screening of all children attending elementary school, which has now been abandoned as not cost-effective. Government subsidies of gluten-free products for individuals with celiac disease, however, are still in effect in Italy.

During my early days in the United States, where the disease was considered extremely rare, I didn't expect to encounter many clinical cases. But after weeks, and then months, and finally a year of not seeing a single case of celiac disease, I began to wonder what was happening. At that time, we believed that the recipe for celiac disease called for two ingredients: genes and the ingestion of grains containing gluten.

If this was true, why was there such a huge discrepancy between the rate of celiac disease in Europe and the United States? After all, many immigrants had ancestors from Europe. We shared their genes and were eating the same grains. In 1996, my curiosity led me to write the paper "Where have all the American celiacs gone?" as I tried to find the answer to this puzzling question.

GOING AGAINST THE GRAIN

There seemed to be only two possible explanations to justify the difference in the rate of celiac disease between the two continents. Either there was a third factor in the United States that prevented the interplay of factors that caused the development of celiac disease, or the disease was overlooked.

The second scenario turned out to be the correct one. But it would be many years working against stiff opposition to our research before Center researchers would prove conclusively that celiac disease affects the general population in the United States at the same rate as the general population in Europe.

We founded the Center for Celiac Research in 1996 at the University of Maryland School of Medicine, the same year we organized the first scientific meeting in North America on celiac disease. We then began screening blood donors for the most cost-effective and rapid approach to answer our question.

This turned out to be an uphill battle, since we faced what was almost an impossible mission. Along with the widespread skepticism of the scientific community, we also had to face the fact that there were no U.S. labs to perform large-scale numbers of diagnostic tests for celiac disease. Under the leadership of our Hungarian colleague, Dr. Karoly Horvath, we set up our own Clinical Laboratory Improvement Amendments (CLIA)-certified laboratory to obtain certified diagnostic results from blood samples.

With no commercial labs available, no economic support because celiac disease was of no interest to industry or federal agencies, and with the premise that we were targeting an extremely rare condition, we embarked on what some of my colleagues defined as "professional suicide."

Our first approach was to screen blood donors for the most cost-effective and rapid approach for an answer to our question. We were looking for high levels of autoantibodies in blood samples that indicated celiac disease. Since similar studies had already been performed in Europe, I decided to use the same strategy I had used in Naples. I went to the Baltimore office of the American Red Cross and explained our goal, with the hope of obtaining unused blood to be used in the original screening of donors.

The officer listened politely to my request. He gave me some paperwork to fill out and a bill for six dollars per sample. Since the blood samples from the Red Cross in Naples had been free, I asked for the same consideration. He explained that there were many costs: costs associated with processing the samples, costs associated with labeling the samples, and costs associated with delivering the samples.

My Neapolitan nature, which is "always negotiate," jumped to the fore, and I offered him a fraction of the requested price. The Red Cross officer looked at me as if I came from another planet, and I was sure I would soon be asked to leave his office. But sure enough, we engaged in a contractual discussion worthy of an Italian marketplace before finally settling on the midway price.

We shook hands, smiled, and had a good laugh about the whole experience. Neither one of us knew, that with this handshake, we had started a movement toward awareness of gluten-related disorders that would grow exponentially in the United States. Indeed, the direct outcome of this purchase would be the proof that celiac disease was not rare at all in the United States.

CELIAC DISEASE "ARRIVES" IN THE U.S.

We purchased 2,000 blood samples from the Red Cross. And in a matter of a few weeks, the generally accepted statement that celiac disease was extremely rare in the United States (affecting approximately one in 10,000 people) was replaced with a prevalence rate of one in 250 among our blood donors.

The response from the scientific and medical community was cold, at best. Our friends told us we were wasting our time. Our harshest critics once again pointed out that celiac disease did not exist in the United States. I knew that the only way to conclusively prove our hypothesis was with a large epidemiological study.

I've heard epidemiology, which is the incidence, distribution, and control of diseases, called the "long division of science" because it has so many factors–literally! It took more than five years, two million dollars, exhaustive paperwork, and hundreds of volunteers and students to complete our epidemiological study. With screenings from more than 13,000 people from across the United States, we definitively placed celiac disease on the U.S. medical map in

2003. That year "Prevalence of celiac disease in at-risk and not-at-risk groups in the United States" was published in the *Archives of Internal Medicine.*

The results of the largest epidemiological study of celiac disease in the United States opened the first chapter of the modern history of celiac disease outside Europe. It proved conclusively that celiac disease affects as many as one in 133 people in the general U.S. population. The figure parallels the statistics reported in Europe at the time. The results from our massive screening demonstrated that celiac disease had been overlooked for a very long time in my newly adopted country.

The prevalence rate in our 2003 study actually parallels European figures. In Canada, Australia, and New Zealand, which are industrialized nations with high populations of people with European ancestry, we see similar rates of celiac disease. In South America, many countries with high populations of people of European origin show roughly the same prevalence of celiac disease as Europe and North America.

In North America, more testing is needed to establish the rate of celiac disease among African Americans. Unpublished data from the Center on a limited number of subjects shows that the prevalence rate for celiac disease in African Americans is one in every 200. And just as with race and gender, celiac disease is found in people of all ages.

We also saw that for many patients, gastrointestinal symptoms were not the predominant symptoms, and intestinal damage was generally milder than in previous decades. In other words, this was the beginning of our understanding that classic gastrointestinal symptoms and celiac disease were only one part of the panoply of possible reactions on the spectrum of gluten-related disorders.

SPREADING THE WORD ABOUT CELIAC DISEASE

Once other studies confirmed our findings on the prevalence of celiac disease, it was only a matter of time before the medical establishment began to acknowledge that this was indeed an accurate picture of the condition in the United States. In other words, there were a lot of people with undiagnosed celiac disease. They hadn't "gone" anywhere!

WHAT IS GLUTEN SENSITIVITY?

As the word "sensitive" suggests, non-celiac gluten sensitivity or gluten sensitivity, as I refer to it, is a reaction to ingesting gluten-containing grains. Although symptoms (particularly gastrointestinal) are often similar to those of celiac disease, the overall clinical picture is less severe. Just as in celiac disease, gluten sensitivity can affect all body systems and generate a wide variety of symptoms.

Gastrointestinal symptoms can include diarrhea, bloating, cramping, abdominal pain, and constipation. Behavioral symptoms can include foggy mind, depression, and Attention Deficit Hyperactivity Disorder (ADHD)–like behavior. Other symptoms include anemia, eczema, joint pain, osteoporosis, and leg numbness.

Recent research at the Center for Celiac Research shows that gluten sensitivity is a different clinical entity from celiac disease. It doesn't result in the intestinal inflammation that leads to a flattening of the villi of the small intestine that characterizes celiac disease. The development of tissue transglutaminase (tTG) autoantibodies, used to diagnose celiac disease, is not present in gluten sensitivity. Preliminary research data from the Center for Celiac Research indicates that it affects approximately 18 million people, or 6 percent of the U.S. population.

A different immune mechanism, the innate immune response, comes into play in reactions of gluten sensitivity, as opposed to the long-term adaptive immune response that arises in celiac disease. Researchers believe that "gluten-sensitive" reactions do not cause the same long-term damage to the intestine that untreated celiac disease can cause (see Chapter Three).

We began an aggressive awareness campaign, which we continue to this day, to educate health-care professionals and the general public about celiac disease and other gluten-related disorders. We partnered with support groups and supported government initiatives to disseminate accurate information about food labeling and gluten-free products.

When our seminal epidemiological study was published in 2003, the estimated number of people diagnosed with celiac disease was approximately 45,000. Our study projected that 2.5 to 3 million people are affected in the United States, meaning that at that time only 2 percent of affected individuals were diagnosed. This statistic suggests that celiac disease is humankind's most prevalent genetically linked disease. It occurs much more frequently than type 1 diabetes, cystic fibrosis, or Crohn's disease.

FINDING THE UNDIAGNOSED PATIENTS

Placing celiac disease on the U.S. map created a lot of questions. How do we find the remaining individuals affected by celiac disease? Do we screen the entire U.S. population of 300-plus million? Or do we target people specifically at risk for the disease? We embarked on another major project at the Center to do the latter.

With a network of primary care physicians both in the United States and in Canada, we began screening people on a case-finding basis by testing the relatives of people with celiac disease or other factors that put them at risk. In only one year of screenings in 2006, we were able to diagnose 43 times more cases of celiac disease compared with the diagnosis rate before our case-finding study.

We achieved three main goals with this project to find and treat undiagnosed celiac disease patients. The first was to alleviate the discomfort of people who had suffered with symptoms for years, sometimes as long as ten to twelve years before receiving an accurate diagnosis. The second was to limit health-care expenses through prompt diagnosis and remove patients from the health-care pipeline of unnecessary tests and procedures. And the third was to successfully educate health-care providers about celiac disease.

Before the study results were published, some of the participating physicians were convinced that there was "no such thing" as celiac disease in North America. After the study came out, they became some of the strongest advocates for early screening when celiac disease was suspected.

In 2004, the National Institutes of Health organized a consensus conference on celiac disease to review the many facets of the disease and its related conditions. With increased awareness and our case-finding study (see Chapter Five), the number of people diagnosed with celiac disease rose steadily and is now approximately 320,000.

Gluten Under the Microscope

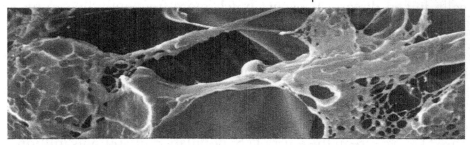

THE REST OF THE CELIAC STORY

The history of celiac disease has entered a new phase. As we learn more about how gluten affects different individuals, we've learned that celiac disease is only part of the story. The full spectrum of gluten-related disorders, including wheat allergy and gluten sensitivity, contains many pieces that have yet to be uncovered as we search for the missing parts about how gluten peptides affect humankind.

With our groundbreaking study in 2003, we only opened a little wider the Pandora's Box of gluten reactions and its attendant complications. Recent research at the Center has uncovered molecular differences in celiac disease and gluten sensitivity, opening the door for the development of diagnostic tools for gluten sensitivity. With this discovery, we shifted the paradigm to create new definitions of celiac disease, gluten sensitivity, and wheat allergy on a new spectrum of gluten-related disorders.

CHAPTER TWO

New Clinical Faces of Gluten Freedom

"All disease begins in the gut."
—Hippocrates

LIFE BEGINS WITH THE GUT

Do you remember the earthworm you dissected in high school biology class? Basically a giant intestine, that earthworm is an exquisite example of the evolution of the gut.

More than two billion years ago, as oxygen accumulated in the oceans, the evolution of single cells began. Approximately 800 million years ago some single-celled organisms learned that by joining forces, they would become more efficient at metabolizing nutrients. This evolutionary discovery led to the development of the first multicellular organism, which was basically a gut.

As cells divide and form organs in the human embryo, they first differentiate into the gut, immediately followed by the heart, the brain, and the spinal cord. This gives credence to Hippocrates's assertion of the gut as the origin of disease. It's also the origin of life. At the gross anatomical level, whether it's an earthworm or a human, an intestine in good working order exhibits a beautiful simplicity that belies its complexity.

The digestive tract is only one of the areas in the body that produces mucus, that slimy stuff that helps to protect our tissues. Mucosal immunology is the study of the immune system in mucus membranes throughout the human body.

At the molecular level, the human gut becomes a complex battlefield with many different "soldiers." There is no neutral zone, as the immune system recognizes and differentiates dissimilar invaders as "friends" or "foes" and strives to find the correct response of surrender or attack, or tolerance and immune response.

When gluten arrives on the intestinal mucosal battlefield of a person predisposed to a gluten-related disorder, what should be recognized as a friend becomes coded as a foe, for reasons that we are only now beginning to understand.

IS GLUTEN FRIEND OR FOE?

In celiac disease, the reaction to gluten is orchestrated by specialized soldiers of the highly specific adaptive immune system called "T-cells." These immune cells become armed at the forefront of the battlefield where the gluten invader needs to be attacked: the gut mucosa, our largest interface with the external world. (Chapter Four details the exquisite mechanisms of our adaptive and innate immune response.) In wheat allergy reactions, the presence of specific gluten peptides activates the recruitment of other soldiers called B cells. These cells mature into plasma cells that produce specialized weapons (antibodies) called immunoglobulin E (IgE).

IgE is a class of antibodies that targets and neutralizes invaders such as bacteria and viruses. The production of IgE triggers the release of chemical mediators such as histamine from other immune cells called basophils and mast cells, thus triggering the variety of symptoms that characterize wheat allergy (see Chapter Three).

In contrast, celiac disease, which affects approximately 1 percent of the general population, is an autoimmune disorder in which the immunological response goes haywire as the immune system attacks its own cells. Celiac disease is identified by three factors: 1) the presence of specific markers in blood serum, most notably serum anti-tissue transglutaminase (tTG) autoantibodies; 2) the autoimmune damage in the intestine that characterizes this condition; and 3) the onset of signs and/or symptoms typical of celiac disease, including co-morbidities (the presence of two more disorders) with other autoimmune diseases, including type 1 diabetes and Hashimoto's thyroiditis.

Besides celiac disease and wheat allergy, there are cases of gluten reactions in which neither allergic nor autoimmune mechanisms are involved. As previously described, these are generally defined as gluten sensitivity (or non-celiac gluten sensitivity). Some individuals who experience distress when eating gluten-containing products and show improvement when following a gluten-free diet may have gluten sensitivity instead of celiac disease. Research conducted recently through the Center indicates that gluten sensitivity is controlled by the oldest immune reaction, which is our innate immune response.

Unable to tolerate gluten, patients with gluten sensitivity develop an adverse reaction when eating gluten that does not usually lead to small intestinal damage, which is a marked difference from celiac disease. While the gastrointestinal symptoms in gluten sensitivity may resemble those associated with celiac disease, the overall clinical picture is generally less severe and is not accompanied by the concurrence of anti-tTG autoantibodies or autoimmune disease.

Typically the diagnosis is made by exclusion. An elimination diet and "open challenge," the monitored reintroduction of gluten-containing foods, are most often used to evaluate whether health improves with the elimination or reduction of gluten from the diet.

DISMANTLING THE GLUTEN PEARL NECKLACE

Although a majority of people can tolerate and safely eliminate gluten, no one is able to completely digest it. Studies on the disordered physiological functions of celiac disease show that gluten proteins are not completely metabolized by the intestine. The principal components of wheat gluten that are toxic for people with gluten-related disorders are a family of closely related proteins called gliadins, which are extremely rich in two amino acids: proline and glutamine. To make use of the food we eat, complex molecules like proteins need to be broken down into their basic building blocks. In proteins, these building blocks are called amino acids.

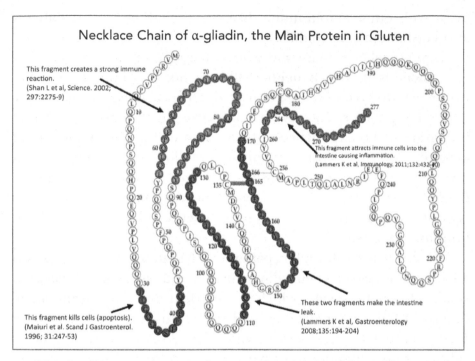

Necklace Chain of α-gliadin, the Main Protein in Gluten

This fragment creates a strong immune reaction.
(Shan L et al, Science. 2002; 297:2275-9)

This fragment attracts immune cells into the intestine causing inflammation.
(Lammers K et al, Immunology. 2011;132:432-40)

This fragment kills cells (apoptosis).
(Maiuri et al. Scand J Gastroenterol. 1996; 31:247-53)

These two fragments make the intestine leak.
(Lammers K et al, Gastroenterology 2008;135:194-204)

Think of a protein strand as similar to a pearl necklace with a single "pearl" as the protein's amino acid components. Each necklace has multiple pearls of twenty different "colors," the number of amino acids present in nature. The sequence of the colors, or amino acids, changes from necklace to necklace or from protein to protein.

Our digestive enzymes break the necklace into pieces called peptides, which are then "peeled" off the strand one at a time. They can then be absorbed by the intestine and transported to various sites in our body to be used as fuel for energy or as building blocks to construct our own proteins. All of the proteins we ingest can be completely dismantled with the exception of one strange, unusual protein. Yes, you guessed it. That protein is gluten and, more specifically, its components gliadins and glutenins.

Indeed, treatment of these proteins with our digestive enzymes in a laboratory beaker leaves large undigested fragments (a piece of unbroken necklace), or peptides. While any ordinary peptide from a foodstuff other than gluten can be dismantled by intestinal enzymes within sixty minutes, those derived from gluten can resist digestion for as long as twenty hours!

Unfortunately, we're still a long way from unraveling the complexity of the gluten peptides. Indeed, gluten contains a large variety of indigestible peptides that can stimulate a strong immunological response of both an adaptive and innate nature in genetically susceptible people. More than fifty different gluten peptides that can trigger a specific T-cell response have been identified, although only three of these seem to be the dominant triggers.

One of these three peptides, called a 33-mer (a peptide with 33 amino acids), is considered a celiac super-instigator. It contains six partially overlapping sequences, which can instigate the aggressive response by specialized immune cells (soldiers of the immune army) called T-cells. Other gluten peptides are able to elicit an innate immune response in antigen-presenting cells, which are cells that recognize proteins. Antigen is a substance that is capable of instigating the immune system to produce antibodies, which are weapons produced by "B" cells to fight enemies.

The presence of these undigested gluten peptides in the upper small intestine is perceived by our gut immune surveillance system as the presence of a potential enemy. Based on studies from the Center for Celiac Research and colleagues worldwide, I am now convinced that our immune system mistakenly interprets gluten as a component of a dangerous bacterium or bacteria. When this happens, it unleashes an immune response similar to that triggered by bacteria to rid the body of the attackers.

This response is elicited in everyone. It is not exclusive to people affected by gluten-related disorders. Consequently, I have colleagues who support the notion that gluten is toxic for humankind and, therefore, everybody should embrace a gluten-free diet.

Although I have contributed to the discoveries of some of these inappropriate immune responses elicited by gluten in humans, I do not share the position of the proponents of a "gluten-free world," who often cite my work to support their position. We engage daily in a war with many dangerous bacteria but rarely do we lose this battle, which is an event that leads to infection. We are also engaged in a daily confrontation with gluten, but only a minority of us will lose this battle. These are the genetically susceptible individuals who will develop gluten-related disorders.

HOW CAN I TELL IF MY SYMPTOMS ARE RELATED TO GLUTEN?

If you think you have health issues related to gluten consumption, the first thing to do is to talk to your family physician or health-care provider. Tell him or her about your symptoms and make sure to include both gastrointestinal and other symptoms, such as fatigue, migraines, "foggy mind," depression, joint pain, and others. Many other conditions can masquerade as gluten-related disorders. It's important to get a complete evaluation, including testing.

If your blood tests come back positive for antibodies that are biomarkers of celiac disease (see Chapter Five), then the next step is an endoscopy. This nonsurgical procedure is used to examine your digestive tract to take tissue samples that will show if you have the damage to your intestinal villi that is typical of celiac disease.

If the results of all tests for celiac disease are negative, and once other conditions, including irritable bowel syndrome (IBS), Crohn's disease, arthritis, neurological conditions, and others have been ruled out, talk to your health-care professional about undertaking a gluten-free diet. This is the only current treatment for celiac disease and gluten sensitivity.

Please do not undertake the gluten-free diet as treatment without the supervision of health-care professionals. Nutritional considerations as well as health considerations must be taken into account with this treatment.

Wheat allergy is more straightforward in its presentation. A person who is allergic to wheat has typical reactions of a food allergy, which include respiratory and skin reactions. People who are allergic to wheat must be vigilant about avoiding cross-contamination.

CHAPTER THREE

The Spectrum of Gluten-Related Disorders

"Man lives for science as well as bread."
—WILLIAM JAMES

THE WORLD IS A GIANT BREAD BASKET

What do people eat the most of? Around the globe, wheat, rice, and maize are the most widely consumed food grains. Among these grains, wheat, an immensely diverse crop, is the most widely grown. Plant breeders worldwide have produced more than 25,000 plant varieties developed specifically for certain characteristics such as high crop yield.

Humans eat most of the world's production of wheat in the form of bread, other baked goods, and pasta and noodles, along with bulgur and couscous in the Middle East and North Africa. Wheat flour and its sticky component, gluten, are found everywhere. The functional properties of gluten, especially its elasticity and ability to trap air, make it a very popular ingredient in food processing.

Indeed, we can almost surely assume that every one of the nearly 7 billion people on earth will sooner or later ingest gluten-containing grains. Nevertheless, as predicted by epidemiological research, only a minuscule fraction (approximately 70 million) of the world's population would react to the ingestion of gluten by developing celiac disease. Indeed, one common assumption about reactions triggered by gluten exposure is that celiac disease is the only culprit.

Wait a minute—not so fast! In the complex world of gluten proteins, there is plenty of blame to go around. As you know by now, the spectrum of gluten-related disorders includes wheat allergy and gluten sensitivity as well as celiac disease.

SO WHAT IS GLUTEN GOOD FOR?

Why is this dietary protein potentially harmful for so many people around the world? One reason could be plant breeders selecting wheat varieties with higher gluten content. This gradual development of wheat strains with higher gluten content has been dictated by technological factors in food processing rather than by nutritional factors.

According to the most recent research, however, the genetics of wheat has not changed during the past few decades. Therefore, the recent surge of gluten-related disorders cannot be accounted for by the introduction of the genetically modified organism technique, as some bloggers claim.

Because of its low content of lysine, an amino acid important for our daily activities, gluten is of limited nutritional value. Its unique visco-elasticity in dough formed from wheat flour assures gluten a pivotal role in the production of bread, other baked goods, pasta, and noodles. The complex plant storage protein plays a supporting role in many dishes such as gravies, soups, and sauces, and is widely used in many processed foods.

The functional properties of gluten, along with its elasticity, stickiness, and ability to trap air, depend on the structures and interactions of the gluten proteins. When mixed with water and yeast, gluten prolamins (those gliadins and glutenins we mentioned before) interact to form a protein network that traps starch and gases during dough fermentation. These characteristics make gluten-containing grains unique in the quality and quantity of foodstuffs that can be produced.

Imagine the aroma emanating from a wonderful pizza or crusty loaf of bread. Picture the crunchy pizza crust or soft interior of the bread. Now try to make bread or pizza using rice instead of wheat flour. With only rice flour, you won't get soft, light, or crunchy. Instead, your efforts will be rewarded with flat, uninspiring, and less than palatable results.

Luckily for people who must follow a gluten-free diet, alternative flour blends have been developed that very closely mimic the properties of gluten. But most patients tell me that one of the things they miss the most is the light texture that gluten gives to baked goods.

Nowadays gluten is one of our most abundant and diffuse dietary components, particularly if you have European ancestors. In Europe the mean consumption of gluten is 10 to 20 grams per day, with segments of the general population consuming as much as 50 grams of daily gluten or more. In the United States, the mean consumption is 10 to 40 grams per day. Keep in mind that a slice of whole wheat bread contains 4.8 grams of gluten and a serving of pasta contains 6.4 grams of gluten.

Together with meat and milk proteins, gluten makes up the most largely consumed protein group by most people worldwide. Because gluten is so pervasive, everyone who is potentially prone to a gluten-related disorder, even people with a low degree of susceptibility, are likely to be affected by some form of gluten reaction during their life span.

WHO'S EATING ALL THAT GLUTEN-FREE STUFF?

In the last five years, the gluten-free market has grown exponentially. Even during our work on this book we've witnessed a remarkable growth in the number of gluten-free products in supermarkets and restaurants.

Who are all these people who are now eating "gluten-free?" Why have they embraced this expensive and quite challenging diet? Some interesting analyses from an unlikely source, Google Trends, sheds some light on who is eating all that gluten-free food.

In the early 2000s the low-carb diet was very popular and the low-fat diet was less so, but it was still in use by a large number of people. According to statistics from Google Trends, the gluten-free diet didn't appear in U.S. populations until 2005, two years after the publication of our findings showing a prevalence of celiac disease of one in 133 people in the United States.

Since then, according to my Google Trends data, there has been a steady increase in the consumption of gluten-free products. In 2008 the gluten-free diet surpassed both the low-fat and the low-carb diet in popularity. For the U.S. population in general, adopting a gluten-free diet is becoming an increasingly popular dietary choice. The gluten-free market has moved from niche products to mainstream.

With U.S. consumers fueling demand, the market for gluten-free food and beverage products grew at a compound annual rate of 28 percent from 2008 to 2012, according to the consumer research company, Packaged Facts. The market finished with almost $4.2 billion in retail sales in 2012 and is expected to exceed $6.6 billion in sales by 2017.

Approximately 3 million Americans suffer from celiac disease, and only a fraction of these patients have been diagnosed. This implies that people suffering from other forms of proven gluten reaction, including gluten sensitivity and wheat allergy, are contributing to this market growth.

Data from our Center suggest that approximately 0.1 to 0.3 percent, or 900,000 people in the U.S. suffer from wheat allergy. We estimate that 6 percent, or almost 20 million, are affected by gluten sensitivity. Without a specific diagnostic test to detect gluten sensitivity, at the moment we can only estimate the magnitude of the problem from our clinical data.

The remaining consumers of gluten-free products (approximately 37 million) are people who choose the diet to lose weight. Now that's a tough proposition! Or they choose it because it's perceived to be healthy, or for other personal or medical reasons. Some of these people think the gluten-free diet "cleanses" their body by going back to how our ancestors ate before the agricultural revolution.

"THE NEW KID ON THE BLOCK"

By now, it may be apparent that teasing apart the various human reactions to gluten presents a complicated puzzle for scientists and clinicians. Following our epidemiological study that first placed the celiac disease flag on the North American continent, it became obvious that our top priority was to increase awareness among health-care professionals and the public.

When I look back, I see that our prevalence study was like a tidal wave. It started quietly and came without warning signals. And it generated consequences that not even I was able to appreciate at the time. I would never have predicted that I would go from seeing one patient a year with celiac disease in the early 1990s to currently treating more than a thousand patients each year in our clinic for various gluten-related complaints.

In the early years our initial task was to tell people how to spell "celiac" and the second was to explain what gluten was all about. Now we're facing a totally different reality. The pendulum has swung from oblivious ignorance about celiac disease to a topic that is constantly in the spotlight of media, talk shows, and professional meetings.

DO I HAVE CELIAC DISEASE?

Consequently, I haven't been surprised to see a crowd of people with a variety of complaints come to our clinic. After many years of suffering, these people came with the hope that a diagnosis of celiac disease would explain the cause of their symptoms.

Thus, the number of people claiming to have problems with gluten grew exponentially during the few years following the publication of our study in 2003. But the problem was, they didn't meet the criteria for celiac disease.

Our typical response in situations like this is to search for other causes. Once we ruled out celiac disease, we thought gluten had nothing to do with their clinical troubles. We sent the patients home and told them they could eat gluten. Nevertheless, a growing number of patients returned to our clinic claiming they had followed our advice. Their symptoms hadn't improved, and they were at the "end of their ropes." They decided to undertake a gluten-free diet against our advice. And magically, their symptoms went away.

My interpretation of this outcome was that these people were enjoying the typical placebo effect. I thought the elimination of gluten was a purely incidental intervention with no clear mechanism explaining the improvement. It took one of my former medical postdoctoral fellows, Dr. Anna Sapone, to point out that there was more to this than we realized.

GLUTEN CREATES A DIFFERENT RESPONSE

Dr. Sapone, who completed her PhD at the University of Maryland while working at the Center, has done a lot of traveling back and forth from her native Naples. Approximately five or six years ago, Dr. Sapone told me that she was seeing a similar phenomenon in the patients she treated at her clinic in Naples.

She insisted that this was an as yet unrecognized reaction to gluten that had already been described by the alternative medicine community as gluten intolerance or gluten sensitivity. I explained to my young colleague that such a thing didn't exist. I told her we had no evidence that these people indeed were responding to gluten in a way similar to our wheat allergy or celiac disease patients.

Nevertheless, the stubborn Dr. Sapone insisted that we study these patients in more detail. Together, with other colleagues at the Center, she was able to demonstrate that yes, gluten was indeed inducing yet another response. This time, however, the response engaged the most ancient branch of the immune system, the innate immune response, as we've previously described. These collaborative studies led to a work published in 2010 that stated, for the first time, that gluten sensitivity was a clinical condition distinct from celiac disease.

Other studies followed, both from our Center and other researchers confirming the data. This created a whirlwind of interest and confusion that reminds me of what we experienced with celiac disease twenty years ago. We are once again surrounded by skepticism and criticism from our nonbeliever colleagues, a déjà vu for sure.

What kind of symptoms does a patient with gluten sensitivity experience? How do you distinguish gluten sensitivity from other forms such as celiac disease or wheat allergy? And most important, how can you diagnose these individuals?

These are indeed some of the key questions researchers are addressing to better understand what gluten sensitivity is all about. Research scientists from the Center are getting closer to finding biomarkers for gluten sensitivity. A biomarker is a compound in the blood or tissue that we can use for diagnostic measurement.

In the meantime, the stories of these two patients exemplify the diagnostic challenges and the rewarding results we can obtain in identifying and treating people who fulfill the criteria for gluten sensitivity. (For patient confidentiality reasons, the identifying characteristics of all patients in *Gluten Freedom* have been changed.)

JOSEPHINE AND JENNIFER

Josephine came to our clinic six months after she started experiencing heartburn and acid reflux symptoms, which were sometimes accompanied by a stomachache. The forty-year-old mother of two had previously been treated for acid reflux with no relief of her symptoms. Her situation had become much more alarming with the onset of dizziness, headaches, numbness of the fingertips, and persistent parasthesia (a tingling sensation of the skin or "pins and needles").

Her internist immediately considered the possibility of multiple sclerosis and performed the appropriate tests to rule out this condition. Other diseases that can present with similar symptoms include Lyme disease, Epstein-Barr virus, and many more. But tests for these came back negative as well.

Because her gastrointestinal symptoms persisted, she was referred to a gastroenterologist. He tested her for celiac disease and also performed an endoscopy. Her results were normal. After searching for an answer for six months, she was left with the recommendation to visit a psychiatrist to treat what was defined as anxiety and depression as a result of her gastrointestinal problems.

Despite that recommendation, she decided to undertake a gluten-free diet instead. Within a week, her neurological symptoms improved. Three weeks later, her heartburn and acid reflux had disappeared.

Even more remarkable was the case of Jennifer, a young woman in her thirties who came to our clinic in a wheelchair. She had been examined by a variety of specialists. None of them could explain why a previously active runner was now reduced to using a wheelchair. She couldn't walk for more than a few steps, and her situation was deteriorating. Because she showed some antibodies against gliadin, she was referred to our clinic as the last possible place to find an answer to the puzzle of her reduced mobility.

We evaluated the situation, concluded that gluten sensitivity might indeed be at least part of the problem, and placed her on a gluten-free diet. We asked her to come back in three months. For her follow-up visit, she came into the clinic with the aid of a cane. At her six-month visit, she walked in unaided.

With her improvement, it seems possible that the nerve inflammation (what we define as gluten-induced peripheral neuropathy) that most likely caused the loss of muscular strength in her legs was indeed due to gluten sensitivity. When we saw her almost one year after her initial visit, we were both shocked, and indeed very pleased, to hear that she had recently run in a marathon.

Jennifer and Josephine are two extreme examples that by no means represent the ordinary experience of most of our clinic patients with gluten sensitivity. Nevertheless, their stories exemplify the complex challenges we face in managing what still remains mostly a "black box" in the spectrum of gluten-related disorders.

THE CONSENSUS ON GLUTEN-RELATED DISORDERS

So, what is gluten sensitivity? Because of the tremendous confusion about the condition, I called for a consensus conference with 14 other experts to discuss the matter. In February 2011, we gathered in London at the first international consensus conference on gluten-related disorders. I co-chaired the conference along with Dr. Carlo Catassi and Dr. Anna Sapone.

We spent two days brainstorming around a table in a small room close to Heathrow Airport in London. At the end we emerged with a new classification of gluten-related disorders, a new way of naming these disorders, and a definition of gluten sensitivity. But without biomarkers to identify this disorder, we had to agree on a diagnosis of exclusion. The proceedings from that meeting were published the following year in the journal *BMC Medicine.* The article, which is still one of the most-often-viewed pieces in the journal, caused turmoil in a scientific community divided into "believers" and "nonbelievers."

Even more interesting is that some of the skeptics have now accepted the existence of this new clinical entity (again, a déjà vu similar to our experience with celiac disease years ago). For this reason, after only one year, we reconvened a much larger panel of experts in Munich, Germany, which led to another manuscript being published in the journal *Nutrients.* This article spelled out the great progress made in such a short period of time in our knowledge about gluten sensitivity.

Until we find and validate specific biomarkers, gluten sensitivity remains defined as the clinical condition in which wheat allergy has been ruled out using specific tests, and celiac disease has been ruled out by both the absence of specific autoantibodies and also by an endoscopy showing normal intestinal mucosa. Unlike celiac disease, this condition is not linked to the genetic components that indicate celiac disease, Human Leukocyte Antigen (HLA)-DQ2 and -D8. In other words, if you have the genes for celiac disease, they are not necessarily linked to gluten sensitivity.

And finally, if symptoms are triggered by exposure to gluten and relieved by their elimination of gluten-containing grains from their diet, then it's gluten sensitivity. But there's a catch: the gluten challenges must be double-blind studies. The patient doesn't know and the medical operator doesn't know about the gluten content in the diet. This approach rules out the possible placebo effect of the diet.

Based on this definition, we reviewed the clinical history of almost 6,000 patients from our Center from 2004 to 2010. Our review revealed that abdominal pain is at the top of the list of symptoms, as it's experienced by almost 70 percent of gluten sensitivity patients. It's followed by eczema, (40 percent) and/or rash, migraine headaches (35 percent), "foggy mind" (34 percent), chronic fatigue (33 percent), diarrhea (33 percent), depression (22 percent), anemia (20 percent), tingling of fingertips (20 percent), and joint pain (11 percent).

Based on the same review, we estimate that approximately 6 percent of the American population may be affected by gluten sensitivity. Of course, these are only estimates in lieu of identifying biomarkers for a direct diagnosis of gluten sensitivity.

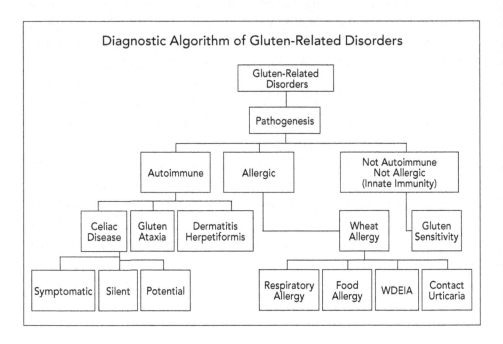

WHY JUST GIVING UP GLUTEN CAN BE A BAD IDEA

There is no doubt in my mind that there are people who are adversely affected by gluten. The type of their reaction depends on the specific genetic predisposition that dictates the type of immune response that can be either allergic (wheat allergy), autoimmune (celiac disease), or yet another type of immune response, probably an innate immune response as described in gluten sensitivity.

Many people who come to our clinic, especially those who already practice a gluten-free diet, simply want to get an answer that resolves their symptoms. Often they question why it's so important to establish in which part of this spectrum of gluten-related disorders they belong.

They want to know why they need to undergo a gluten challenge, which can be pretty uncomfortable. That means they have to eat foods containing gluten again for several weeks to build up the antibodies that are used to determine the diagnosis of celiac disease. These patients reason that no matter in which part of the spectrum they fall, they still need to follow a gluten-free diet. So what difference will it make? Why is it important to establish which form of gluten-related disorder they belong to?

The simple answer is that although all these patients need to be on a gluten-free diet, the way it needs to be implemented and the long-term consequences are extremely different, depending on which disorder affects them. We know that in celiac disease there is a genetic component that increases the risk in other family members. And we know that a mistake in the diet can not only have immediate consequences, but it can also cause cumulative problems that can be devastating over time. And most important, we know that celiac disease will never go away.

Conversely, we don't know if gluten sensitivity has a genetic component. We do know that both gluten sensitivity and wheat allergy may have different thresholds of gluten reaction. These conditions can change in the same person over time. We know that a mistake in diet can result in immediate consequences, but we don't know whether there are long-term consequences.

The table on the following page summarizes the major characteristics of each gluten-related disorder. The time interval between gluten exposure and onset of symptoms can go from a few minutes, as in wheat allergy, to days as in gluten sensitivity, to many years as in celiac disease.

Characteristics of Gluten-Related Disorders from *BMC Medicine*

	Celiac Disease (CD)	Gluten Sensitivity (GA)	Wheat Allergy (WA)
Time interval between gluten exposure and onset of symptoms	Weeks — Years	Hours — Days	Minutes — Hours
Pathogenesis	Autoimmunity (Innate and Adaptive Immunity)	Immunity? (Innate Immunity?)	Allergic Immune Response
HLA	HLA DQ2/8 restricted (~97% positive cases)	Not HLA DQ2/8 restricted (50% DQ2/8 positive cases)	Not HLA DQ2/8 restricted (35–40% positive cases as in the general pop.)
Autoantibodies	Almost Always Present	Always Absent	Always Absent
Enteropathy	Almost Always Present	Always Absent (slight increase in intraepithelial lymphocytes)	Always Absent (eosinophils in the lamina propria)
Symptoms	Both intestinal and extraintestinal (indistinguishable from GS and WA with GI symptoms)	Both intestinal and extraintestinal (indistinguishable from CD and WA with GI symptoms)	Both intestinal and extraintestinal (indistinguishable from CD and GS when presenting with GI symptoms)

The origin and development of the three conditions is very different. We know that the genetic predisposition markers, HLA-DQ2 or -DQ8, must almost always be present in people with celiac disease. This is not the case with wheat allergy and gluten sensitivity

By definition, autoantibodies like tTG are present only in celiac disease as the autoimmune reaction to gluten, but they are always absent in the other two. And similarly, the autoimmune mechanism leading to intestinal damage is almost always present in celiac disease, but absent in gluten sensitivity and wheat allergy.

But the trickiest part is the symptoms. In gluten reactions, the symptoms overlap each other and can't be easily distinguished. That makes it impossible to establish which part of the gluten-related disorder spectrum the patient belongs to based solely on clinical judgment.

Finally, we are well aware of the comorbidities and complications associated with celiac disease. So far, we haven't identified any of these comorbidities in the other two forms of gluten-related disorders. The story of a family from Oregon illustrates what can happen when a gluten-related disorder exists with other conditions.

PICKY EATERS, GLUTEN SENSITIVITY, AND THYROID DISORDERS

Many parents know what it's like to try to get a picky child to eat new things. Who hasn't hovered over their toddler trying to get the child to taste a new fruit or vegetable? But for Hope's parents, the eating habits of their daughter were especially troubling. It took them years to find out that Hope's health issues, including a limited appetite, were related to an autoimmune thyroid disorder that seemed to be affected by her consumption of gluten.

Always short for her age, Hope had urinary tract complications in her early years and underwent bladder surgery at the age of three. Her parents thought her eating habits might improve after the surgery, but she remained a very picky eater, sticking to limited portions of basic food choices of mainly crackers, hot dogs, apples, banana, cheese, and milk.

"She was three and half before she would eat pasta and five years old before she would even try chicken nuggets," said Hope's mother. "She was always much shorter than other kids," said her father, "and she didn't want to sit still to eat. Even as a baby, we'd have to trick her to get her to open her mouth to eat."

Hope was seven years old when she was taken to a well-respected pediatric endocrinologist looking for some answers to her short stature and limited appetite. The pediatric endocrinologist gave Hope "a battery of blood tests," said her father, "but couldn't find anything wrong. We were strongly urged to give her growth hormones, but like most parents, we had some reservations about that treatment.

"We had decided not to give her growth hormones and let nature take its course," said her father. "But at our last appointment with the endocrinologist, they checked one more set of blood tests just to see if anything unusual showed up," recalled her father.

"Hope had elevated levels of thyroid stimulating hormone (TSH), a hormone produced in the brain that stimulates the thyroid to produce its hormones. This was something we hadn't seen previously."

The endocrinologist initially thought it might be a lab error, but the results from tests repeated three days later were even more startling: Hope's TSH levels had increased to four times higher than normal. She was diagnosed with Hashimoto's disease.

In Hashimoto's disease, also known as chronic lymphocytic thyroiditis or Hashimoto's thyroiditis, the immune system attacks the thyroid gland. The resulting inflammation can eventually lead to an underactive thyroid, or hypothyroidism.

Hashimoto's disease is the most common cause of hypothyroidism in the United States. Research studies have linked celiac disease to an increased risk of autoimmune thyroid disorders like Hashimoto's.

The endocrinologist told Hope's parents that there wasn't anything they could do for Hope except to wait until her thyroid wore itself out, which could "take up to twenty or thirty years" said her father, and "then treat her with thyroid medication."

"We thought that there must be more that we could do for our daughter. We wanted to keep looking for answers, so I started to see what I could find out about Hashimoto's disease," said her father.

After learning about a possible connection between an autoimmune thyroid disorder like Hashimoto's and gluten-related disorders, Hope's father called the endocrinologist to see if gluten or wheat might be causing a problem for Hope.

The endocrinologist told the family that there was no association, but her father's research was suggesting otherwise. The specialist told the family that it probably wouldn't be worth taking gluten out of Hope's diet, recalled her father.

"I was reading all the time, every chance I got, about thyroid disorders," said her father. "I read many of Dr. Fasano's articles and wondered if Hope might have celiac disease or whether gluten was playing a role in her thyroid problem."

"I went to Dr. Fasano's website and eventually contacted him to learn more about his ideas about autoimmunity," said Hope's father. "Dr. Fasano told me that although we don't know for sure that gluten and wheat can trigger autoimmune thyroid disorders, he suspects that this might be the case for some patients."

Despite the fact that Hope tested negative for celiac disease, her family was so convinced that Hope was sensitive to gluten that they placed her on a gluten-free diet. In only a few weeks, her TSH levels decreased dramatically. They returned to normal after several weeks on a rigorous gluten-free diet.

"The most amazing thing was that for the first time in her life, Hope began to have a normal appetite for food. Not only did she begin to finish everything on her plate, but she started to ask for seconds and thirds," said her father. "She began to eat like she'd never eaten before. It was like she had just gotten rescued off of an island."

Hope also had been suffering from an extremely itchy rash on her arms and neck for many months. The family was amazed to see that the rash completely resolved two weeks after being on a gluten-free diet. The family's research suggested that removing dairy could be beneficial for some people with gluten intolerance because casein, a protein found in dairy, can sometimes have a similar effect on the thyroid as does gluten.

Accordingly, the entire family implemented a gluten-free and dairy-free diet, which meant some major changes for Hope's mother, the cook in the family. "Initially, I had no idea what my husband was talking about as far as removing gluten from our diet," she said.

The dietary changes came about right after the family was undergoing another change. They were moving their household to a new location, which made for a chaotic few months.

"We were extremely busy, so it was especially challenging. My other children also had experienced some health challenges such as gastrointestinal and respiratory issues, and our youngest child suffered from repeated ear infections," said Hope's mother. "I was hoping that these changes might also help the other children."

The move to the new diet resulted not only in an increased appetite for Hope, but also a growth of more than a 1/2 inch in the first three months. The family also noticed a dramatic improvement in their five-year-old son's health and behavior after implementing the diet. He stopped having ear infections, and his parents noticed that his ability to focus and concentrate at school was markedly better with the dietary changes.

One unexpected benefit of the family's dietary changes was that Hope's mother noticed that her chronic knee and foot pain dramatically improved after going on the gluten-free diet. "I was supposed to have foot surgery, and I've been getting hydrocortisone shots and taking ibuprofen for years," she said. "But I'm not in pain anymore. Compared to having foot surgery, this very simple lifestyle change has made it so I can run and play with my kids."

The family wanted to share their story so that other families might pursue an assessment for gluten-related disorders when answers for persistent health problems aren't forthcoming. "To see how the change in diet has turned our daughter's life around has been amazing. We are so grateful to Dr. Fasano for helping us to restore our daughter to good health after so many years of health problems," said Hope's parents.

Note from Dr. Fasano: Years of work and research have provided a clearer understanding of some of the mechanisms of celiac disease and wheat allergy. There are still very few facts, a lot of fantasies, and many concerns, however, that await clarification in the broader health implications of gluten-related disorders. These include particularly devastating conditions such as Autism Spectrum Disorder and schizophrenia that are examined in Chapter Six. But for now, let's take a look at wheat allergy.

SEARCHING FOR CLUES TO WHEAT ALLERGY

My hometown of Salerno, Italy, is at the crossroads of many beautiful spots in the Mediterranean. Drive fifteen miles south, and you come to Paestum, one of the most magnificent settlements of the Magna Graecia, with temples that are more beautifully preserved than the Parthenon or the Acropolis in Athens.

Drive twenty miles north, and you're in Naples, a melting pot of political, geographic, and culinary cultures. Drive fifteen miles west, and you come to Capri, one of the pearls of the Mediterranean and a favorite spot of Roman emperors with its famous "Blue Grotto." South of Naples, you can drive along the Amalfi Coast from Positano to Salerno. The winding road, where you are suspended between steep, rocky mountains above and the emerald sea below, brings you to places like Amalfi, Ravello, and Vietri sul Mare.

But the place that has intrigued me the most since childhood is Pompeii. Fifteen miles north of my hometown, it has always been one of my favorite destinations. It's not the beauty that draws me to Pompeii. It's not the landscape or the cuisine that makes this place so special.

It's the fact that visiting Pompeii is like jumping into a time machine that projects you almost 2,000 years into the past. You can walk back in time as you step into the snapshot of an ordinary day now forever crystallized in time. In AD 79, Mount Vesuvius erupted, and all in its path perished. The rapid surge of hot ash, pumice, and volcanic gas that killed humans and animals also preserved them for history to witness the traumatic destruction. At Pompeii and Herculaneum in the still-preserved Roman "pistrinas" or bakeries, we find clues to an occupational hazard that is still with us today.

ONLY ONE FORM OF WHEAT REACTION

At the time of the major eruption of Mount Vesuvius in AD 79, there were more than 30 bakeries in the area around Pompeii. The Romans enjoyed bread, pastries, and other confections, and bread was the staple food of the lower classes.

Slaves, who made up more than a third of the Roman population by the first century BC, worked in the bakeries, pulling the grinding wheels along with the mules. Archaeological evidence suggests that Roman bakery workers wore masks to protect them from the flour dust.

An allergic reaction to inhaling wheat flour is a common form of occupational asthma. Centuries after the Roman bakeries lay in ruins, Italian physician Bernardo Ramazzini described respiratory symptoms shared by bakers exposed to flour dust in the 1700s. The father of occupational medicine reported that shortness of breath and urticaria, an itchy skin rash characterized by pale red and raised bumps, was common among the bakery workers in Italy.

Whether wheat allergy is caused by inhaling flour dust or by eating products with some form of wheat in the ingredients, it's a completely different entity from celiac disease or gluten sensitivity.

JUST THE FACTS

True or False: Celiac disease is an allergic reaction to wheat.

By now, I hope most readers will realize that the above statement is false. Celiac disease is an autoimmune disorder, not an allergic reaction. In celiac disease, the immune system is unable to distinguish between self and nonself components. The body mounts an immune response against its own healthy tissue, damaging the villi of the small intestine leading to the malabsorption of nutrients.

True or False: Wheat allergy is a food allergy triggered by gluten.

The above statement is true: wheat allergy is defined as a food allergy triggered by the protein in gluten. Food allergies trigger a different immunological response, which is usually more immediate than the response resulting from celiac disease or gluten sensitivity. That allergic reaction will vary based on whether the wheat is inhaled or eaten. People with wheat allergies may also be allergic to grains such as barley, rye, and oats that have similar proteins.

If you view the spectrum of the body's reaction to gluten as a railway line with celiac disease and gluten sensitivity as the main offenders, wheat allergy is a sidetrack off the main line. Wheat allergy is rarer than celiac disease, occurring in approximately 0.1 to 0.3 percent of the U.S. general population, or ten times less often than celiac disease. Wheat allergy is defined as an adverse immunologic reaction to wheat. That means it can do a lot more than just make you sneeze when you inhale flour or eat a hamburger bun.

Depending on how wheat enters your system and the underlying immunologic mechanisms, the allergic reaction can affect your skin, your gut, and/or your lungs. Along with baker's asthma, allergic reactions to wheat range from annoying itchy skin and hives to fatal anaphylaxis (see below).

In allergic reactions to wheat, the immunologic culprits are the IgE antibodies, which play a central role in the pathogenesis of allergic diseases. IgE antibodies differ from the autoantibodies produced in the gut during active celiac disease and follow a different immunological mechanism. Celiac disease autoantibodies are mainly of the class IgA.

A true food allergy causes an overproduction of the IgE antibody in reaction to a protein. In the case of wheat, it's the complex proteins found in gluten. On the other hand, food sensitivity (not food allergy) can trigger similar symptoms, but there is no increased production of IgE antibodies.

THE IMPACT OF WHEAT ALLERGY

How widespread is wheat allergy? Although research is limited, recent studies from Europe and North America provide some data on the prevalence of food allergy and food sensitization, including wheat allergy.

A population-based birth cohort study follows a representative sample from a select population from birth. In one such study from Stockholm, 4 percent of a group of 2,336 four-year-olds showed a sensitization to wheat, which decreased over time. Another study that analyzed the blood samples of 273 children from the age of two to ten years reached the opposite conclusion. This study showed that the prevalence of IgE in response to wheat progressively increased from 2 to 9 percent as the children aged.

The investigators speculated that IgE sensitization to wheat occurs primarily in early infancy, whereas pollen sensitization becomes the primary allergic reaction when children reach school age. In a systematic review by Zuidmeer et al., two population-based studies from the United Kingdom and one from Germany reported positive wheat challenge tests in children, with a prevalence rate as high as 5 percent.

Part of an ongoing family-based food allergy cohort study in the United States revealed that the estimated heritability of food-specific IgE was statistically significant for nine tested food allergens, including wheat. This means that if there is a family member affected by wheat allergy, the likelihood that other members of the family may develop wheat allergy is higher when compared to the general population. In addition, significant positive associations between parents and their children were observed for IgE specific to wheat.

The bottom line is that there are conflicting data in the literature on the real impact of wheat allergy and how it has changed over time. The general trend, however, is that wheat allergy is more frequent in children with a prevalence rate of 3 to 5 percent. It decreases in adolescence and adulthood to reach a rate of approximately 0.3–0.4 percent in the general population.

RESPIRATORY REACTIONS IN WHEAT ALLERGY

Much of the research on adverse allergic reactions to wheat has focused on respiratory allergy (the baker's asthma found in Roman bakeries), which is a common occupational allergy found throughout the world. In Poland, respiratory symptoms ascribed to occupational asthma were observed in 4.2 percent of baker's apprentices after only one year; the rate doubled to 8.6 percent after two years.

An allergy to wheat in the diet is probably less widespread in the general population. The proteins responsible for dietary allergy in wheat are also less clearly defined than those contributing to the respiratory allergy. Recent studies indicate that there are intriguing similarities and differences between the two conditions.

Scientists knew little about the proteins responsible for baker's asthma until studies in the 1970s showed that multiple allergens were present. Water-soluble proteins from wheat were particularly reactive with the IgE antibodies (specialized weapons that trigger the release of histamine responsible for most of the symptoms experienced during allergy) found in the blood samples of patients.

More recent studies have identified individual proteins that are recognized by IgE from a patient's blood serum. One group of wheat proteins, the α-amylase inhibitors, has been identified as containing the most important allergens. A number of other factors found in wheat, however, have been reported to be recognized by IgE (meaning that they can trigger the allergic reaction mediated by IgE) from patients with baker's asthma.

In a development that bears additional research, several of these factors have also been reported to be active in the dietary allergy to wheat as well as in the respiratory response seen in baker's asthma.

WHAT'S FDEIA?

In very rare instances, people who eat a certain food and then exercise vigorously can experience Food-Dependent Exercise-Induced Anaphylaxis (FDEIA). A recent study published in the *Journal of Investigational Allergology and Clinical Immunology* found that of all of the cases of anaphylaxis reported in an emergency department, FDEIA was identified in 2.4 percent of cases. Anaphylaxis to a food allergen occurred in 29 percent of the cases. Since many individuals might not realize that their symptoms are related to FDEIA, the actual incidence rates could be higher.

FDEIA is caused by the combination of the offending food and subsequent physical exercise. Although a number of different foods have been linked to FDEIA, wheat is the most widely reported food associated with this condition.

DIETARY PROBLEMS WITH WHEAT

Allergic responses to eating wheat can be divided into two types. Wheat-Dependent Exercise-Induced Anaphylaxis (WDEIA) is a clearly defined syndrome associated with the major subgroup of proteins called gliadins. Patients with WDEIA display a range of clinical symptoms from skin rashes and hives to severe allergic reactions including severe and possibly fatal breathing difficulties.

The other type of response is more general and also includes atopic dermatitis (skin rash), urticaria (hives), and anaphylaxis, which can result in respiratory arrest (see above). These responses appear to be related to a range of wheat proteins; they may vary between populations and may be related to age and symptoms.

The responses and mechanisms of wheat allergy have been studied less than other phenomena related to gluten. Consequently, wheat allergy is the most likely underdiagnosed form of reaction to gluten exposure. Like many other forms of food allergies, wheat allergies may also be on the rise, but more systematic studies are needed to appreciate the real clinical impact of this form of gluten reaction.

WHEN FOOD BECOMES DANGEROUS: SIGNS OF ANAPHYLAXIS

Along with reactions typical of wheat allergy, watch for these signs of anaphylactic shock, which can be fatal if not treated promptly:

- Chest pain
- Swelling of throat
- Rapid heartbeat
- Severe difficulty breathing
- Pale blue skin color
- Dizziness or fainting

If these symptoms occur, call 911 and seek emergency help immediately. Wear a medical bracelet that identifies your allergy to emergency medical personnel and others.

WHEAT ALLERGY: SYMPTOMS AND DIAGNOSIS

Symptoms in both children and adults can occur within a few minutes or a few hours after ingesting or inhaling wheat. They include nasal congestion and swelling of the nasal passages; itching or irritation and swelling of the mouth and/or throat; itchy and watery eyes; stomach cramps, diarrhea, nausea or vomiting; difficulty breathing; and hives with an itchy rash or swelling of the skin.

HOW IS WHEAT ALLERGY DIAGNOSED?

As with any food allergy, diagnosis of wheat allergy can be tricky. It becomes even harder because some form of wheat is present in so many foods. Along with symptoms, your doctor will review family and medical history and perform a physical exam.

Helpful tests include skin prick tests that measure allergic reactions to a variety of substances, blood tests for specific antibodies, and behavior-based tests. These include keeping a food diary and undertaking an elimination diet and/or a food challenge to reintroduce the food being tested.

ARE THERE TREATMENTS FOR WHEAT ALLERGY?

If you suffer from wheat allergy, you must avoid all foods containing wheat and wheat derivatives. Here's where a dietitian's help is invaluable, especially with children, to ensure that proper nutritional needs are being met on a wheat-free diet.

You can take antihistamine medications to help reduce discomfort from the swelling of sinus passages and itching. Check with your doctor about what type to take.

People with potentially life-threatening allergies to wheat and other food products should carry an emergency kit that contains epinephrine to inject as needed.

CHAPTER FOUR

Making Sense of Gluten, Leaky Gut, and Autoimmunity

"An oven whose door does not shut does not bake its loaves."
—**MALTESE PROVERB**

LOWERING THE DRAWBRIDGE

The human intestine is a deceptively complex organ. Lined by a single layer of cells, it's exquisitely responsive to stimuli of innumerable variety. The gut is populated by a complex community of microbial partners that are far more numerous than the cells of the intestine itself.

We can think of the multitude of microorganisms living in our gut as a parallel civilization with its own rules and organization. This miniature society includes a communication network with its host—that is, our body—through the intestinal mucosa.

Under normal circumstances, the intestinal cells form a tight but selective barrier; they have to distinguish between friends and foes from the external environment. Think of your body as a medieval city surrounded by a wall. Microbes and most environmental substances are held at bay outside the wall of the city. Nutrients from the essential to the trivial are allowed in because they are recognized as useful. They are absorbed efficiently.

Moreover, as in a medieval city, the drawbridge can be lowered to allow the passage of substances from the environment into our bodies through the space between neighboring cells. These bridges, technically called "tight junctions," regulate the passage of substances in and out of the intestine in a dynamic but still poorly understood manner.

Scientists at the Center for Celiac Research have been studying the regulation of gut permeability for years. In 2000 our group discovered zonulin. The only physiologic modulator of gut permeability identified by scientists to date, it holds many unexplored mysteries.

There is one thing, however, that is becoming increasingly clear about a "leaky gut." In this condition in which the drawbridge is defective and cannot be completely closed, the indiscriminate passage of molecules from the environment (for example gluten), is associated with a large number of local and systemic disorders, including many autoimmune diseases.

OPENING THE GATES OF THE GUT

I'm very encouraged about the eventual reality of a "celiac pill" as a safety net to protect against cross-contamination (see Chapter Sixteen). Research from our Center has been instrumental in the early development of Larazotide acetate, a compound now being tested by Alba Therapeutics. As so often happens in science, the development of this anti-zonulin drug resulted from a serendipitous outcome.

It's my personal experience that scientific discoveries are made by a constellation of failures alternated by rare successes. What we read in the literature is the sci-fi story that leads to significant results. This doesn't necessarily reflect the role that serendipity quite often plays in important discoveries.

Serendipity is unquestionably my favorite English word. It's a word that expresses the wisdom, the unforeseen, the unpredictable, and the design of nature that overcomes our plans. Here's the real story with the role that serendipity played in discoveries made at the Center that led us to formulate a new paradigm of celiac disease pathogenesis. In turn, those discoveries have led us to create a new frontier of treatment alternatives to the gluten-free diet.

SERENDIPITY AND CELIAC DISEASE: A STORY IN FIVE ACTS

Act One: From Vaccine Failure to New Discoveries

As a gastroenterologist, I've always been interested in understanding the mechanisms leading to diarrheal diseases in children. In the late 1980s, I joined the Center for Vaccine Development at the University of Maryland School of Medicine in Baltimore, Maryland, to develop a vaccine against cholera. We then believed that cholera caused the devastating diarrhea that affects children in so many developing countries through a very powerful weapon called cholera toxin.

I was asked to design a cholera vaccine by deleting the gene encoding this powerful toxin. On paper, this approach looked like it would definitely work and protect children around the world against cholera. What an achievement this would be for a young and idealistic scientist!

But when we administered the vaccine to volunteers, it caused enough residual diarrhea to make it clinically unacceptable. Years of hard work literally went down the toilet. When this happens you give up and move on, or you sit down with your data and attempt to understand what nature is trying to tell you with these unanticipated results.

I teach my students that this is the time when scientific advancement requires perseverance in the face of experimental failure. And it was an act of perseverance that led us to discover a new toxin, elaborated by vibrio cholera, which would eventually open a new pipeline of research.

Act Two: New Paradigms of Bacterial Pathogenesis

In the late 1980s, the general wisdom was that diarrhea was induced by bacterial toxins in the gut that directed intestinal cells to pour water and salt into the intestine. Therefore, the discovery of a toxin that caused diarrhea by affecting intestinal permeability by opening the gates in between cells (tight junctions) was definitely out of the ordinary. These spaces were thought to be so completely sealed that the myriad of enemies threatening the intestinal lumen couldn't get easy access into the human body.

In the early 1990s a series of seminal discoveries clarified that these gates are highly dynamic and can be opened and closed under certain circumstances. What was still missing was exactly how these dynamic structures were modulated. In other words, what made them open and close?

At that point we knew that there must be a system to command the lowering and lifting of the drawbridge, but we had no idea what it was. That would come later. But for now, our discovery of this new toxin that we called "zot" for zonula occludens toxin provided a valuable tool that shed some light on how tight junctions are modulated.

Act Three: Learning from the Bacterial Civilization

While studying how zot was able to open these gates in between cells, we realized that the system was too complicated to have evolved simply to cause biological harm to humans. Rather, it became clear to me that the toxin vibrio was clever enough to learn how we regulate the permeability of our gut and develop its own tool, that is, zot, to take advantage of it. Following the trail of zot and its mechanisms for permeating the intestinal barrier led me to hypothesize that the toxin was mimicking the mechanism of an unknown molecule that we use for the same purpose, namely as a key that can open the gates at will.

Five years after I formulated this hypothesis, we discovered zonulin, the human counterpart of zot. Zot is a cholera protein that can regulate tight junctions; zonulin is the human protein that is in charge of modulating gut permeability. In other words, zot mimics zonulin in its process of opening and closing the tight junctions. Zonulin is what we use in our intestine to regulate the opening and closing of the intestinal epithelial barrier. It plays the leading role in the development of leaky gut.

Act Four: Celiac Disease: A New Paradigm of Autoimmunity

While counting the number of people with celiac disease in the United States in the early 2000s, I realized that a large percentage of celiac patients had increased intestinal permeability. From there, it was simply an act of faith, coupled with logical connect-the-dots strategy, that made us realize that the increased gut permeability in celiac patients was because of an exaggerated production of zonulin.

From these results, we expanded our horizon to search the scientific literature for clinical conditions in which intestinal permeability was increased. To my major surprise, we realized that many autoimmune diseases, including type 1 diabetes, multiple sclerosis, rheumatoid arthritis, and inflammatory bowel disease (IBD), all had leaky gut as a common denominator. So we expanded our zonulin research to these other conditions and realized that zonulin is indeed involved in many other autoimmune diseases.

Act Five: The "Holy Trinity" that Causes Celiac Disease

So what's the outcome of this serendipitous story of the discovery of zonulin? Contrary to our previous beliefs, we learned that to develop an autoimmune disorder like celiac disease, not only do you need to be genetically predisposed and exposed to the environmental trigger (gluten), but you also need impaired intestinal barrier function to allow the offending protein to gain access into your body.

This new theory implies that each one of the three elements of this "holy trinity" (genes, environmental triggers, and leaky gut) is needed to develop autoimmunity. I realized that removing any of the three elements needed to develop autoimmunity would be a valid therapeutic option.

We surely can't eliminate genes, because they are too numerous and too important to simply get rid of them. Removing the environmental trigger is only feasible for celiac disease, since we don't know the triggers that cause other autoimmune diseases. And as we discuss in other parts of this book, the complete avoidance of gluten presents its own challenges.

But maybe by removing the third element, the intestinal barrier defect, we could create a possible therapeutic alternative for autoimmunity. In Chapter Sixteen, I'll talk about this exact scenario in the current clinical trials using the zonulin inhibitor called Larazotide acetate. But before we learn more about Larazotide acetate, let's delve a little deeper into the fantastic and complicated world of our immune response.

ABCs OF IMMUNE RESPONSE

As a crucial and complex component in the development of gluten-related disorders, the immune system is designed to protect us from disease. The evolution of the immune system, which fights an array of invaders from viruses to parasites, tells a fascinating story. As described in Chapter Two, cells develop into specific tissues, organs, or systems including the immune system.

Imagine the scenario of these immune cells moving around during the nine-month period when the fetus matures into a little baby. The immune cells are studying the composition of the baby's body to understand how it is made and storing this information in the baby's immune system "database." From the time that we're born until the time we pass on to a better life, our immune system is constantly on alert. It's checking to see if the molecules it encounters "belong" to our body or not. In other words: are they part of the database?

If indeed these molecules or agents are part of our body, the immune system is instructed to stay put, which is what we technically call tolerance. If, on the other hand, they aren't in the database, they are considered to be enemies that could potentially harm our body. In this case, the immune system is instructed to deploy "special unit" soldiers as first responders to an enemy attack, what we technically call an immune response.

IS IT RAPID OR SOPHISTICATED?

The most ancient branch of our immune system, the innate immune system, orchestrates this response. It enacts a rapid chain of events: First: I see a molecule. Second: I check my database, and it's not there. Third: By default, it must be an enemy. Fourth: I immediately deploy my soldiers, that is, immune cells to get rid of it.

The innate immune system has the advantage of being a fast responder. But its great limitation is in not being able to engage in war for a long period of time. If the enemy is resilient and survives this first intervention, the innate immune system needs to call on reinforcements. Those reinforcements come from the more-recently evolved and more sophisticated branch of the immune system called the adaptive immune system.

The adaptive immune system is much more efficient in fighting enemies because it can customize weapons against a specific enemy. We call these weapons antibodies. To deploy these weapons, the adaptive immune system needs time to study the characteristics of the enemy. It then creates antibodies designed specifically to fight the invader.

Although the adaptive immune system isn't effective for an immediate response, it's ideal for a prolonged fight. The adaptive immune system develops a memory of the enemy, and if the invader returns, the antibodies can be produced faster and more easily. Incidentally, this is the mechanism behind the development of vaccines.

In autoimmune diseases, including celiac disease, both the adaptive and innate branches are involved. More specifically, it's a miscommunication between the two branches that leads to the auto-attack of the immune system against its own body. Conversely, in gluten sensitivity, it seems that only the innate immune system is involved. That explains why there is no intestinal destruction typical of celiac disease.

REDEFINING CELIAC DISEASE

When Samuel Gee described celiac disease more than a century ago, there was a general perception that it represented an allergic reaction to gluten. This concept slowly faded and was replaced by the concept of it as an intolerance, with no clear understanding of what mechanisms were involved in its onset.

The scene changed in the 1960s with new diagnostic procedures like Watson's capsule and improved endoscopy techniques (see Chapter Five). Researchers were able to view clearly the damage to the small intestine, which became the defining hallmark of the celiac disease diagnosis.

It soon became clear that this condition was much more than an allergic reaction. We learned that the destruction of the machinery that allows us to digest and absorb food was mediated by an attack from the immune system. Celiac disease then became defined as an immune-mediated enteropathy, or disease of the intestinal tract.

Because the intestine became damaged after exposure to gluten, some researchers, myself included, concluded that we were dealing with an autoimmune disease in which the immune system attacks and destroys its own tissue. By initiating and following a strict gluten-free diet, most of the time this tissue damage could be reversed.

Nevertheless, even the most open-minded and expert colleagues and immunologists were reluctant to support the view of celiac disease as an autoimmune disorder. Indeed, even now, autoimmune diseases are considered irreversible conditions. Once the immune system starts to fight against its own body, there's no way to stop it. Many physicians and scientists still believe this is a defining precept of autoimmunity.

TAKING ANOTHER LOOK AT AUTOIMMUNITY

Two main theories have been formulated to explain autoimmunity. The first theory claims that components of invading microorganisms, mainly infectious agents or viruses, are very similar to our own components. An immune system not finely tuned in this war against environmental enemies may mount a response that targets the body component that is structurally similar. This theory is called "antigen mimicry."

A second theory states that insults to our body, including infections, may cause cell destruction. As the cells deteriorate, components from inside begin to leak outside the cell. The immune system perceives these leaks as extraneous material and mounts a defense to get rid of them. This theory is called "bistandard effect."

Both theories imply that once this reaction is triggered, the immune system goes into automatic, meaning the chain of events cannot be stopped or reversed. But what if that's not necessarily the case? Let's take a closer look at celiac disease, the only autoimmune disorder for which we know the trigger, and see what else we might find.

TAXING THE IMMUNE SYSTEM

As humans evolved, the immune system developed to fight one enemy: dangerous microorganisms. We either died from accidents or natural calamities like the eruption of Mt. Vesuvius, or we died from infectious agents. The immune system evolved to fight these infectious agents.

Until recently, these were the only targets of the immune system. No manmade chemicals, no artificial substances, no unusual stuff that isn't really food; such things didn't exist. Now our immune system faces enemies far more complex than its evolutionary system might be able to handle.

Surprisingly, it does quite well most of the time. Not so surprisingly, sometimes it makes mistakes. The immune system has to adapt its weaponry against these different enemies. In the case of a mistake, as in the targeting of gluten as an enemy, tissues like the intestinal mucosa become a casualty in the battle of the immune system to guard against invaders. The resulting collateral damage is called celiac disease.

Three key elements, a genetic predisposition, an environmental trigger, and a "leaky gut," are needed to trigger an autoimmune response. The third element, the leaky gut, allows the environmental trigger (gluten) to interact with the immune system that is genetically skewed to attack its own body rather than getting rid of the enemy gluten. This process leads to the autoimmune destruction of the gut. If these three elements are needed for autoimmunity, you could reverse or prevent autoimmunity by taking away any one of the three, at least in theory.

A PARADIGM SHIFT IN TREATMENT OF AUTOIMMUNITY?

With celiac disease, we know the trigger is gluten. When you remove the trigger by implementing a gluten-free diet–surprise!– the intestine repairs itself and the autoimmune disorder is reversed. Someone who has celiac disease and is successfully treated with the gluten-free diet is indistinguishable from someone without the disorder. If the third element in the equation, the leaky gut, is removed, we should be able to reverse the autoimmune response in other conditions.

Progress in any discipline, whether it is biology, music, sociology, or economics, comes from incremental shifts in our outlook about what has long been accepted as undeniable fact. In wheat allergy, we know the body's response is an allergic reaction. With celiac disease, our Center contributed to the revolutionary concept that celiac disease is a true autoimmune disorder.

It became the first autoimmune disorder to be treated by removing its cause. The more we learn about the molecular makeup of celiac disease, the more promising becomes the possibility of treating other autoimmune disorders.

A CLINICAL CHAMELEON

Scientists now generally accept that celiac disease represents the autoimmune response to gluten that leads to the self-destruction of the intestine. As described earlier, celiac disease was long perceived by clinicians as a gastrointestinal disorder of childhood characterized by a malabsorption syndrome with chronic diarrhea and weight loss.

Indeed, classical features of children with celiac disease closely resemble malnourished children from the third world. With big bellies and the complete disappearance of subcutaneous fat, these are indeed the features of extreme malnutrition. But the child suffering from malnutrition in Africa looks emaciated because the child doesn't have enough to eat.

Some children with celiac disease have a similar appearance even though they are eating. Their bodies are simply not able to make use of the food they eat, as it moves through the intestine without proper absorption of the nutrients.

For reasons that are still partially unknown, the clinical characteristics of celiac disease changed in recent years in the Western world. Its onset occurred in older children. The symptoms became milder and rarely characterized by the "celiac crisis" that was responsible for the high mortality associated with celiac disease in cases like the Saharawi people of Western Sahara.

The advent of more specific and sensitive diagnostic tools in the late 1980s revealed that celiac disease was much more than malnutrition in childhood. Indeed, we learned that rather than being a gastrointestinal disorder, celiac disease may affect every organ or tissue in our body. In an editorial in the *New England Journal of Medicine* published in 2007, I describe celiac disease as a clinical chameleon that "can range from chronic diarrhea, weight loss, and abdominal distention to symptoms and conditions that can affect any organ system."

Besides the classical gastrointestinal symptoms described above, we started diagnosing celiac disease in patients with other gastrointestinal complaints including nausea, vomiting, stomachache, bloating, and even constipation. The last symptom is quite a counterintuitive concept, since celiac disease was originally defined as a malabsorption syndrome and usually associated with diarrhea.

Even more intriguing was the manifestation of celiac disease as "extraintestinal" or outside of the intestine. What was originally defined as atypical celiac disease became the most frequent way that the disease presents itself. Anemia, osteoporosis, joint pain, the skin rash called dermatitis herpetiformis, neurological symptoms, behavioral changes, miscarriage, and infertility are some of the examples of the multifaceted expression of celiac disease.

A NEW CLASSIFICATION OF CELIAC DISEASE

With these developments, the new classification of celiac disease in its clinical form moved from the old form that defined celiac disease as typical, atypical, and silent. Now we define it as 1) symptomatic: people who experience symptoms; 2) asymptomatic: people who have positive autoantibodies and intestinal damage but no clinical symptoms; and 3) potential: subjects with positive autoantibodies but no intestinal damage.

The multiform way that this disease presents itself is partially responsible for the original misconception of celiac disease as rare in the United States. The early epidemiologists were looking in the wrong direction. They were searching for young children with big bellies, something clinicians had encountered in the 1930s with the "banana babies" (see Chapter Fourteen). This manifestation is no longer the clinical hallmark of pediatric celiac disease.

This clinical vulnerability is also responsible for a phenomenon that is unique among all autoimmune diseases. Most patients affected by other autoimmune diseases such as rheumatoid arthritis, multiple sclerosis, and type 1 diabetes are diagnosed, but only a small percentage of people with celiac disease have been correctly identified and treated.

Another consequence of this complex presentation is the enormous delay in the diagnosis of celiac cases in the United States. Many studies suggest that the lag period between the onset of symptoms and the time of diagnosis is measured in years (sometimes more than ten years) in the United States, with obvious consequences in public health including health-care costs and the quality of life of the affected individuals.

Why does an autoimmune disease that destroys the intestine present itself with symptoms that have nothing to do with the gastrointestinal tract? The answer is partly related to the physiology of the gut. But we have to look beyond the gut to the bigger picture.

THE GUT IS NOT LIKE LAS VEGAS: WHAT HAPPENS IN THE GUT DOESN'T STAY IN THE GUT

Take the example of iron-deficiency anemia, the most common symptom currently seen in celiac disease patients. Iron is absorbed exclusively within a few inches of the small intestine, in an area located downstream from the stomach.

If this region of the intestine is destroyed by the gluten-induced autoimmune attack, we have no backup to absorb iron. We develop anemia, a blood disorder. The remaining spared intestine may subsidize the lack of digestion and absorption of foodstuff and prevent the onset of gastrointestinal symptoms. For the same reason, destruction of a neighboring region of the intestine that specializes in the absorption of calcium and vitamin D can lead to osteopenia or osteoporosis (degenerative bone disorders), without causing any gastrointestinal symptoms.

Other extraintestinal symptoms include infertility and miscarriage (reproductive system), joint or muscular pains (orthopedic and musculoskeletal systems), and neurological or behavioral symptoms. Neurological symptoms run the gamut from gluten ataxia, which is loss of coordination and balance, to migraine headaches, and tingling in the extremities.

Behavioral symptoms can include anxiety and depression. Immune cells armed by the exposure to gluten can leave the intestine and target specific organs or areas, such as the brain or the joints, which leads to local inflammation. This mechanism can create conditions that explain the almost bewildering array of clinical symptoms caused by gluten in genetically predisposed people.

MAKING THE CELIAC DISEASE DIAGNOSIS

We know that celiac disease is an autoimmune disorder triggered by the ingestion of gluten that does not spare any age, race, or gender. When a physician has the clinical acumen to suspect celiac disease, he or she has some of the best diagnostic screening tools available in clinical care. Usually the clinician looks for high levels of autoantibodies in the blood of patients suspected to have celiac disease before confirming the diagnosis with an intestinal biopsy.

The time of diagnosis represents one of the most challenging parts of my professional responsibilities. The typical response of a patient newly diagnosed with celiac disease is anger, frustration, anxiety, depression, and denial, which sometimes come all at once.

As a physician, I'm very sympathetic with this complex combination of emotions. I never minimize the feelings of someone who has just realized that his or her life has been changed forever by this restriction on one of the most enjoyable activities of humankind, that is, eating. More than 10,000 years ago, the gluten-free diet was a way of life. Now gluten-containing grains are so intertwined with our cuisines that removing these grains seems a daunting proposition.

But once I've given my patients time to fully express their feelings, I begin my cheerleading speech. Actually, it's more of a fable or fairy tale. I tell them that they have wisely chosen the kind of chronic condition that will affect their life. And although they might see the glass as half empty, I want them to imagine that I have a special power.

My power is to take their celiac disease away. But of course, there is a condition, as there always is in fairy tales. They must trade their celiac disease with another chronic condition. They can chose from a list that includes diabetes, Crohn's disease, rheumatoid arthritis, multiple sclerosis, or any type of cancer.

When I put their situation in these terms, most of my patients appreciate the fact that although celiac disease is a lifelong chronic condition, its current treatment is, after all, a diet. It's painful at the beginning. It's complicated to implement, but still, it's a diet with no side effects and no complications. They will have no changes in their physical appearance like hair loss or puffy faces.

Most important, once they are on a gluten-free diet, their life expectancy becomes comparable to that of a person without celiac disease. The destiny of people affected by the other autoimmune diseases and conditions I've offered to them is very different, with a future that, at least for now, cannot be controlled as we can with celiac disease through the gluten-free diet. Now let's look at how someone receives a celiac disease diagnosis.

CHAPTER FIVE

Getting the Right Diagnosis

"My bowels boiled and rested not;
the days of affliction came upon me."
—JOB 30:27

WATSON'S CAPSULE

In the early years of my training, diagnosing celiac disease was a cumbersome journey for both patient and physician. With no specific screening tests and the recognition that it's a lifetime diagnosis, we used a three-step approach recommended by the European Society for Pediatric Gastroenterology and Nutrition.

The first step included identifying typical childhood symptoms including diarrhea and failure to thrive. As previously discussed, at that time it was considered strictly a disease that originated in childhood. Other signs of malabsorption were fat in stools and the lack of absorption of a sugar marker called xylose.

If these criteria were met, the child would then undergo the first biopsy, or removal of intestinal tissue for examination. At that time endoscopy, the use of a long, lighted tube inserted through the mouth, was not routinely performed. The biopsy was obtained with a special device called Watson's capsule, which only allowed for one tissue sample.

It was an unpleasant procedure, since the child was only mildly sedated and had to swallow a capsule the size of an olive pit. The capsule was attached to a long tube that the operator had to maneuver to bring the capsule first into the stomach and then to the proximity of the pylorus, the valve that divides the stomach from the intestine.

I've done hundreds of these procedures. Every time it was very painful to see the restrained child fight the introduction of the tube that always caused gagging and extreme discomfort. After getting the tube inserted, the operator used an X-ray monitor called a fluoroscope to position the capsule in the proper spot. This could take hours.

Once the capsule reached the duodenum (the first part of the intestine), air from the tube was aspirated by a syringe to close a little guillotine in which a small piece of intestine was trapped. The operator then recovered the capsule with the tissue sample intact. If the biopsy showed the typical intestinal damage of celiac disease, then the next step was put in place.

TAKING REPEATED BIOPSIES

The second step was placing the child on a gluten-free diet and monitoring the child's condition to see if the symptoms disappeared. After one year, the child underwent a second biopsy through the same cumbersome process using Watson's capsule to see if the damage had been healed. But that wasn't necessarily the end of the story—or the end of Watson's capsule.

The child would be reexposed to gluten and monitored for a reappearance of symptoms. If this occurred, the child would undergo a third biopsy to confirm the findings of intestinal damage.

Of course the entire process was extremely stressful for the child, the family, and the physician performing the procedure. So it's not surprising that tremendous effort was placed in developing good screening tests to simplify this complicated and painful diagnostic journey.

The advent of the nonspecific anti-gliadin antibodies (AGA) followed by the very specific antiendomysium antibodies (EMA) in the mid-1980s changed the diagnostic landscape. We had new recommendations for diagnosis.

If the child had signs or symptoms compatible with celiac disease, if the child tested positive in the blood screening of antibodies, if an intestinal biopsy showed typical intestinal damage, and symptoms resolved on a gluten-free diet, then the diagnosis of celiac disease was confirmed.

YOU CAN'T FIND IT UNLESS YOU LOOK FOR IT

Over the years the diagnosis of celiac disease has become even more challenging since we've learned that the disease can affect people at any age and present with a myriad of symptoms. And despite a growing awareness of its many clinical faces, celiac disease remains largely underdiagnosed. In developed countries, for each diagnosed case an average of five to ten cases remains undiagnosed (the submerged part of the celiac iceberg), usually because of atypical, minimal, or even absent complaints.

Screening studies in the United Kingdom indicate that more than 90 percent of celiac disease in schoolchildren is missed. In the United States the projected number of patients with celiac disease is approximately three million, yet fewer than 200,000 have been diagnosed to date. Dr. Peter Green, director of the Celiac Disease Center from Columbia University, reported that in New York City between 1981 and 2004 the delay between the onset of symptoms and diagnosis decreased from eleven years before 1981 to a still unacceptable four years after the year 2000.

Physicians who see patients with diarrhea, the classic hallmark of celiac disease, often don't initially consider the disorder, as examples of long lag times from first symptoms to diagnosis demonstrates. The Canadian Celiac Health Survey of 2,681 patients with biopsy-proven celiac disease diagnosed between 1998 and 2002 showed a delay in diagnosis after an onset of symptoms of 11.7 years.

In 2004 a survey performed in Southern California revealed that only about one-third of primary care physicians had ever diagnosed a patient with celiac disease. It also showed that only 44 percent of the physicians were aware that specific autoantibody testing could be used for diagnosis.

A CRUMBY WORLD

By Sharone Jelden

At age nineteen I realized that something wasn't right with me. To feel healthier, I became "earthy crunchy granola." That meant I frequented my college health-food store and bought whole-wheat vegan sprout sandwiches that tasted like Timothy hay. I turned vegetarian and became more tired, allergic, itchy, and sick. Poor dairy—I blamed it for a lot of problems and cut it out of my diet periodically. Goodbye, sweet butter.

While other kids pounded beers and scarfed down late-night pizza, I boiled a concoction of stinky Chinese herbal healing tea made out of twigs, roots, and stems that had been wrapped in brown paper and twine. I did this on a single electric burner in my dorm room. My poor roommate had to adjust to the delightful scent of decayed rodent layered with subtle undertones of manure. For a person who tried to eat a healthy diet, exercise regularly, drink water, and avoid a lot of bad stuff (aka fun stuff), I didn't feel the way I thought I should feel—or the way it appeared others felt.

Over a twenty-three-year period from college until several years ago, I cycled through the following, some on a daily basis: sinus pain, sinus infections, congestion, allergies, headaches, migraines, joint pain, stomach and digestive problems galore, exhaustion, difficulty with pregnancies, pleurisy, dehydration, anemia, eye pain, episcleritis, conjunctivitis, and bronchitis and pneumonia, as well as issues with skin, hair, and gums.

Looking back, I can say that my "normal" was feeling as if hundreds of balloons had been filled with air and placed inside my body and inside my stomach, my internal organs, my head, and everywhere else. And the leftover space in there was infused with lead; everything felt heavy and sore. This is what it felt like to be in a state of constant inflammation.

My primary care physician either offered me lame halfhearted solutions with no overall plan or directed me to a specialist. Headaches? Neurologist. Sinus infections? Eye, Ear, Nose, and Throat doctor. Low iron? Eat liver. That is just mean.

I suggested that it might be lupus and all these symptoms could be connected. (Probably too much time spent online trying to diagnose myself.) My lupus test came back negative; my doctor now had confirmation of my hypochondria.

I persisted and went back to her complaining of extreme exhaustion. Driving toddlers around with your eyes at half-mast, brain lost in a fog of apathy and confusion, is not only frightening, but it's also very sci-fi. The doctor suggested I create a reward sticker chart for my youngest daughter, who wasn't sleeping well at the time, as this would help us all get more sleep. Then I wouldn't feel tired. Never mind my low iron, low cholesterol, and low vitamin D. Excuse me? A *sticker chart?!*

My doctor didn't realize that I had celiac disease. When I developed pneumonia, my sister convinced me to try a more holistic doctor. The new doctor spent an hour just talking with me as she carefully reviewed my health and history. She had a sign in her office with the words "Don't Ever Give Up."

In the first five minutes, she noticed that I wasn't absorbing food well (apparently a total cholesterol of 108 is not only extremely low, it's downright unhealthy). She immediately asked me if I'd been tested for celiac disease and since I hadn't, told me she planned to do the blood test that very day. Then she urged me to go home and eat a stick of butter. Now that was a high point.

I got the call right before I sat down to a dinner of steaks, grilled vegetables, and pasta. My new doctor told me that my celiac panel test came back positive. My numbers were so off the charts that they were unreadable. She urged me to stop eating all gluten immediately and go to a gastroenterologist who specialized in celiac disease.

I had an endoscopy, the gold standard, to confirm the diagnosis. The gastroenterologist who performed the procedure told me he believed that I'd had the disease since childhood due to the mucosal scalloping and flattening of my intestinal villi.

After a week of gluten-free eating, I felt as if every single one of those balloons in my body had popped. No more pain, pressure, and bloating. That heavy sensation of being infused with lead disappeared. My head stopped pounding. Everything improved in a major way. Even environmental allergies and cat allergies, which had plagued me since childhood, disappeared. I remember sitting outside at a table covered in pollen, shocked at the lack of affect it had on me. Suddenly I was able to press my face into the body of any feline and feel fine! (Don't do this, by the way; cats do not like it.) It was an exhilarating physical change.

The big downside is that the diet is extremely restrictive. The FDA concluded that for some people with celiac disease, intestinal damage can begin after consuming just 1/200th of a teaspoon of wheat flour. That is so damn little. And when you have to avoid even a crumb, wheat or gluten seems to be everywhere.

Mentally, I felt locked in "food jail" at the beginning. That feeling dissolved and only resurfaces at the tasty memories of, say, Pizzeria Regina or Kit Kat bars. Time helps. Decent cooking also helps. I committed myself to learn all I could about gluten-free living, cooking, and baking.

That happened several years ago. Since then I've discovered that my youngest daughter has celiac disease as well. For a six-year-old child to maneuver herself safely through all those crumbs is a daily challenge. Luckily, improved health was her rapid reward.

My daughter adjusted to the new diet a lot better than I did. The only hiccups we've had involve gatherings elsewhere with lots of glutinous baked goods. We've learned to bring our own desserts. Sometimes her cupcake looks and tastes better than everyone else's; that's how far gluten-free products have come. Trader Joe's Gluten-Free Chocolate Cupcakes with Buttercream Frosting are stiff competition for anything out there.

I recently met Dr. Alessio Fasano at the Center for Celiac Research Visiting Day at Boston's MassGeneral Hospital for Children. He has gathered a top-tier team of scientists, connected with other research centers, and is rapidly uncovering what's happening inside the gut of a celiac. Dr. Fasano explained that once one autoimmune disease "puzzle" is deciphered, it may help to understand others, such as type 1 diabetes and rheumatoid arthritis.

As Dr. Fasano walked us through a tour of his bright, open laboratory overlooking the harbor in Charlestown, Massachusetts, a palpable feeling of hope seemed to fill that space and all those who work there. The words "Don't Ever Give Up" reflected off every test tube and beaker.

From the viewpoint of a patient it was overwhelmingly uplifting and inspiring. Of all the issues to deal with, one that creates a more thoughtful and selective approach to eating is not the worst thing a person can have. I feel grateful that we're dealing with celiac disease; it's manageable and it seems like the future holds a solution. And I can still have my butter.

IS IT SPECIFICITY OR SENSITIVITY?

Many people find the process of being tested for celiac disease confusing. Let's talk some science first to see if we can make it easier to understand.

Two terms—specificity and sensitivity—will help you when it comes to understanding how accurate the blood tests for celiac disease can be. Sensitivity is related to positive results: If everyone with the disease returns a positive result, then that test has 100 percent sensitivity.

Specificity is related to negative results: If everyone without the condition returns a negative result, it means that the test is 100 percent specific. So if a test has very high sensitivity, it will diagnose celiac disease accurately most of the time. If it has a very high specificity, it will correctly rule out the condition most of the time. None of the blood tests have 100 percent sensitivity or specificity, but some tests are extremely accurate.

DISCOVERY OF TISSUE TRANSGLUTAMINASE

One of the landmarks on the journey of celiac disease diagnostics was the discovery by a brilliant German scientist, Dr. Detlef Schuppan, of tissue transglutaminase (an enzyme that is present within human cells that turned out to be instrumental for the pathogenesis of celiac disease), as the target of the EMA.

We knew this meant that we might be able to abandon the very cumbersome EMA test and develop an enzyme-linked immunosorbent assay (ELISA) to detect antibodies against the tissue transglutaminase. At that time, the only commercially available tissue transglutaminase was from guinea pigs. We were among the first research labs to develop a test using the guinea pig substrate.

But the results were discouraging. We lost both the superb specificity and the sensitivity that had characterized the earlier EMA test. When we went back to the drawing board to find out why it didn't work, we realized that human tissue transglutaminase would be the best target to use in the ELISA.

In a fortunate coincidence, as so often happens in science, at that time there was a visiting researcher in our lab from Trieste in northeastern Italy, Daniele Sblattero, who was able to clone and produce human tissue transglutaminase. We became the first lab in the world to develop and report on the human-based anti-tissue transglutaminase (tTG) ELISA. It's the same test now used worldwide to diagnose celiac disease.

To validate the test, we went back to the blood donor samples and repeated the screenings. They showed that the prevalence in this cohort was not one to 250 as we previously reported, but rather one to 125, which was very similar to what we found with our large epidemiological study published in 2003 (see Chapter One). These results demonstrated that our old screening approach, namely the AGA test followed by the EMA test, might have missed half of the patients!

The development of the anti-tTG antibodies ELISA was a special moment for our Center. Another pivotal moment was when we became the first research team to publish material about the important development of the anti-tTG antibody test. It's now recognized as a critical milestone in the modern history of celiac disease.

THE ROLE OF GENES IN DIAGNOSIS

As research progressed, celiac disease became defined as an auto-immune disorder, which implies that there is a genetic component involved in its development. Scientists began to look more closely at the role of HLA-DQ2 or -DQ8, two genetic markers associated with celiac disease.

Several studies from Europe proved that the presence of either one or both genes was almost universal among celiac disease patients, while present in only one-third of the general population. The bottom line is that these genes seem to be absolutely necessary for the genetic predisposition of celiac disease. But along with the genetic component, there has to be some environmental trigger along with the gluten that kicks off the autoimmune process (see Chapter Four).

Based on this observation, we were extremely interested in using this approach as a diagnostic tool. But in the late 1990s, there were some major obstacles to the general application of this technique. The search for HLA-DQ2 and -DQ8 required cumbersome and extremely expensive techniques along with large amounts of blood to be drawn from each patient.

Once again it was the acumen of two fellows in our lab, Sandro Drago and Maria Rosaria di Pierro, which led to a revolutionary new technique that allowed us to perform HLA research using only a few drops of blood from each patient. This new protocol is now used around the world to determine the genetic component of someone's celiac disease diagnostic portrait.

NEW DIAGNOSTIC CRITERIA FOR CELIAC DISEASE

Now that all the pieces of the diagnostic puzzle are joined together, it should be obvious to patients and physicians that there is no single tool, whether it is blood tests, HLA typing, or intestinal biopsy, which can lead to celiac disease diagnosis with absolute certainty.

Instead, it's the combined analysis of symptoms, positive serological and HLA testing, an intestinal biopsy showing mucosal damage typical of celiac disease, and a clinical and serological response to the implementation of a gluten-free diet that guides us to a conclusive diagnosis.

SEARCHING FOR LOST CELIAC PATIENTS

By the beginning of the new millennium, we finally had all the proper tools to make an accurate diagnosis using a state-of-the-art algorithm to look for celiac patients. Therefore, we were finally in a position to tackle the iceberg of celiac underdiagnosis. How to approach this task remains a matter of debate in the scientific community.

Initially, there were valid arguments in favor of mass screening:

1. Celiac disease is a common disorder causing significant morbidity in the general population.
2. Early detection is often difficult on a clinical basis.
3. If not recognized, celiac disease can manifest itself with severe complications that are difficult to manage, including infertility, osteoporosis, and, in rare cases, lymphoma.
4. There is an effective treatment: the gluten-free diet.
5. Sensitive and simple screening tests are available, such as the anti-tTG antibody test.

The economic benefits of mass screening for celiac disease using serological tests followed by intestinal biopsies for positive cases show that it yields $44,491 per each year of life saved for screening compared to no screening. This price tag is an estimation of how much it costs to society in terms of lab tests performed, procedures, use of the health-care system, loss of productivity, decrease in quality of life, and increased morbidity and mortality in each case of undiagnosed celiac disease each year.

TARGETING POPULATIONS FOR TESTING

Nevertheless, we need to look more closely at the cost-effectiveness performance of celiac disease screening. Although we know that patients with untreated celiac disease may develop complications, the natural history of undiagnosed and untreated celiac disease, particularly the so-called "silent" form, remains unclear.

Treatment with a gluten-free diet is likely to interfere greatly with a person's quality of life, especially in adults, and its implementation should be carefully conducted. Despite the high sensitivity of current blood tests, the ability to predict a confirmed celiac diagnosis by intestinal biopsy decreases when the blood tests are applied to the general population in whom the risk of celiac disease is low (approximately 1 percent).

Conversely, in patients at risk for celiac disease (people with symptoms or family members of a celiac patient) in whom the risk is higher (5 to 15 percent), the positive predictive value of serological celiac disease markers is much higher.

Furthermore, the appropriate age for celiac disease mass screening is still undetermined, since we now know that celiac disease can develop at any age, even among the elderly. For all these reasons, the best approach to the iceberg of undiagnosed celiac disease seems to be the serological testing of at-risk groups, a procedure defined as "case-finding" that minimizes costs and is ethically appropriate.

A primary care practice provides the best opportunity to first identify individuals who are at risk for celiac disease and need referral for definitive diagnosis. Our Center undertook a multicenter, prospective, case-finding study using serological testing (IgA class anti-tTG antibody determination) of adults seeking medical attention from their primary care physician in both the United States and Canada. We were looking for cases of celiac disease in populations at a higher risk for the disorder than the general population.

By applying simple and well-established criteria for finding celiac disease in a sample of adults, we achieved a thirty-two- to forty-three–fold increase in the diagnostic rate of this condition. Many people who were newly diagnosed reported a long-standing history of symptoms, which should have raised the suspicion of celiac disease long before the screenings.

Our study published in 2007 was the first demonstration that an active case-finding strategy in the primary care setting is an effective means to improve the diagnostic rate of celiac disease in North

America. Subsequently, other studies confirmed the validity of the approach, which we recommended in lieu of mass screening of the general population.

WHEN CELIAC DISEASE IS OVERDIAGNOSED

Although both the number and the accuracy of diagnostic tests have increased since 1996, celiac disease overdiagnosis can also be a problem. A mistaken positive diagnosis often occurs through confusion about the definition of celiac disease, since health-care professionals sometimes interpret a positive AGA as a clear and sufficient sign of the disease.

Shifting from the recommended three-biopsies approach to a single biopsy diagnostic process that rarely includes a gluten challenge also increases the possibility that the patient is placed on a gluten-free diet for life without conclusive evidence of the diagnosis. But the most common reason for celiac disease overdiagnosis is misinterpretation of diagnostic tests.

HOW GOOD ARE CURRENT SCREENING TESTS?

The specificity of serological celiac disease markers is not 100 percent. As you recall, specificity is the likelihood that the test will be negative among people who don't have the condition. Although IgA anti-tTG antibodies and EMA antibodies are both close to 100 percent in specificity, other celiac disease serological markers exhibit a lower diagnostic accuracy. This may be the source of some diagnostic errors.

The specificity of IgG class AGA is only 40 to 80 percent in adults and between 60 to 90 percent in children, which suggests that AGA testing for celiac disease has a limited role. For reasons that are only partially understood, a false positivity of both IgG and IgA-AGA can be found in patients with other gluten-related disorders or in inflammatory or infectious diseases.

It's possible, however, that an increased absorption of gluten and its peptide fragments can be followed by a humoral immune response (production of antibodies) to the nonself antigen (gluten). In the most recent test developed for the diagnosis of celiac disease, the diagnostic accuracy of serum antibodies directed against deamidated gliadin (anti-DGP), seems to be higher. The determination of IgG-based antibodies, the IgG anti-tTG antibody and, more recently, the IgG anti-deamidated anti-gliadin antibody (DGP) is useful in patients with selective IgA deficiency.

Preliminary studies of children who are at genetic risk of celiac disease have shown that even the best serological marker of the condition that is currently available, the IgA anti-tTG antibody, may fluctuate over time from a borderline positive to a normal value and vice versa. The quantitative assessment of the IgA anti-tTG antibody level is useful to help determine who should receive an intestinal biopsy during the screening process.

CAN GENES PREDICT WHO GETS CELIAC DISEASE?

The role of HLA-DQ2 and HLA-DQ8 is well known, as almost all celiac patients carry the genetic markers encoding these genes. Most individuals with celiac disease (approximately 95 percent) produce HLA-DQ2 and the remaining individuals are usually HLA-DQ8 positive.

HLA-DQ2 is common in the general population, however, and is carried by approximately 30 percent of Caucasians. Even so, only about 3 percent of people with this gene will develop celiac disease. Thus, HLA-DQ2 or HLA-DQ8 is necessary for disease development but not sufficient, as its estimated risk effect is only 36 to 53 percent.

Thanks to the Center's contribution, testing for HLA-DQ is now much more affordable and is increasingly being used for diagnostic purposes. One such application is in doubtful cases or in at-risk groups. The ability to rule out celiac disease by HLA-DQ is impressive and the proportion of false negatives (celiac disease patients who do not carry these genes) is extremely small. Therefore, HLA testing is useful to rule out celiac disease but not to confirm the diagnosis.

Recent data from our Center, however, suggest that, while the absence of HLA-DQ2 and -DQ8 pretty much rules out celiac disease, the presence of two copies (one inherited from our mother and the other from our father) of the HLA-DQ2 greatly increases the risk of developing celiac disease in people with a positive family history.

The genetic tests also are particularly effective for people who have implemented a gluten-free diet without having the proper antibody screening tests and intestinal biopsy beforehand. Indeed, a negative result may help them avoid a gluten challenge, since these patients are almost surely not affected by celiac disease. It's more likely that they're suffering from gluten sensitivity.

By contrast, the positive predictive value of HLA testing is poor. The reason that HLA testing is almost worthless to predict celiac disease is the high frequencies of the DQ risk alleles among unaffected individuals.

Villi: From Healthy to Damaged

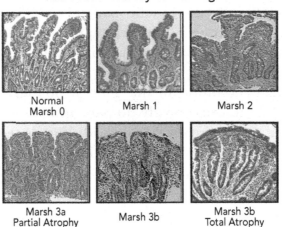

Normal
Marsh 0

Marsh 1

Marsh 2

Marsh 3a
Partial Atrophy

Marsh 3b

Marsh 3b
Total Atrophy

IS THE INTESTINAL BIOPSY STILL THE GOLD STANDARD?

Although the important role of small intestinal biopsy in the diagnosis of celiac disease is indisputable, there are a number of interpretative issues that can lead to diagnostic errors. Changes in the lining of intestinal tissues that occur in celiac disease follow a sequential course classified by the system developed by Dr. Michael Marsh and modified by Dr. Georg Oberhuber into five stages (type 1, 2, and 3a, 3b, and 3c). As the disease progresses, the villi eventually become completely eroded, leaving a flat surface.

In cases of the most severe damage to intestinal villi, which is defined as Marsh-Oberhuber 3 lesion, we see several classic characteristics. There is a deepening of the valleys in between the villi, more intraepithelial lymphocytes (immune cell soldiers), and a range of damage from mildly blunted to completely eroded villi. These tissue changes are not specific to celiac disease, however, and can be caused by several other diseases of the intestinal tract, such as infectious diarrhea, autoimmune enteropathy, radiation insults, and food allergy.

As you can see from the preceding illustration, the amount of tissue damage can go from extremely minimal to total destruction of the villi. For example, a type 1 lesion (the least damage possible) is characterized by normal villi structure and the presence of immune cells (so-called intraepithelial lymphocytes) on the "gut battlefield."

Going back to the parallel of the walled city, it is as if the presence of the enemy (gluten) is detected and soldiers (immune cells) are deployed on the wall of the city ready to fight. The battlefield is set, the two camps are ready to engage in battle, but no shots have yet been fired and, therefore, no damage is detectable at this early stage.

This should be accepted as possibly indicative of celiac disease only when other diagnostic evidences are very strong as in the clear-cut and persistent positivity of IgA anti-tTG antibodies and the presence of HLA-DQ2 and/or -DQ8. The poor specificity of a milder enteropathy is an even bigger problem in less-industrialized countries where the prevalence of so-called "environmental enteropathy," which can arise from infections and malnutrition, is high.

In addition, the evaluation of small intestinal biopsy specimens is influenced by a number of technical aspects. The first one is the site the sample comes from. In one study, celiac disease–associated villous atrophy was occasionally detected only in the duodenal bulb, which is the very first part of the small intestine. This site was generally avoided by gastroenterologists in the past because of possible difficulties in interpreting the tissue because of the presence of a type of cell not typically seen in the small intestine.

A second difficulty can be patchiness of the mucosal lesion, which is not often uniformly distributed. For diagnostic purposes we need to take a minimum of three tissue samples in one endoscopic procedure, incorporating a duodenal bulb biopsy, to make sure we can detect villous atrophy. A five-biopsy regimen, however, is recommended for recognition of even the most minimal of patchy lesions.

A third consideration is that the correct handling and processing of biopsy specimens is required for a proper evaluation of changes in the intestinal tissue, especially when the degree of damage is less severe. If the villi are not sectioned along their longitudinal axis, cuts made at a different angle can result in samples that simulate shortness of the villi, leading to an incorrect diagnosis of celiac disease.

Evaluating any damage to the intestinal tissue relies heavily on the observer's judgment and experience, the fourth technical aspect. While there is no doubt that the Marsh-Oberhuber scoring of intestinal damage is an efficient diagnostic tool, this system has been criticized because of too many diagnostic categories, which may lead to reduced consensus among observers, and eventually to misdiagnosis.

THE FIVE PILLARS OF DIAGNOSIS

We've come a long way since I performed my first procedure using the cumbersome Watson's capsule. In 1989 the European Society for Gastroenterology, Hepatology and Nutrition issued guidelines centered on five criteria that needed to be met in order to diagnose celiac disease. They are:

1. Signs or symptoms compatible with celiac disease
2. Positive serological screening tests (at that time only EMA tests were available)
3. Presence of genetic markers HLA-DQ2 or -DQ8

4. Intestinal damage typical of celiac disease detected
   by endoscopy
5. Symptom resolution following the implementation
   of a gluten-free diet

With these criteria met, the diagnosis is final; no repeated endoscopies are needed.

Over the years, we've adhered strictly to these guidelines. Nevertheless, we've experienced several exceptions to these rules, to the point that recently Dr. Carlo Catassi and I questioned the appropriateness of these rigid diagnostic algorithms.

As usual, it was our clinical experience that indeed suggested that this rigid algorithm might cover the vast majority, but not all, cases of celiac disease. Reviewing the five criteria shows us what kind of exceptions we've experienced for each one.

THE "SILENT CASES" OF CELIAC DISEASE

The first criterion is signs and symptoms compatible with celiac disease. We've discussed at length what kind of signs and symptoms people affected by celiac disease might experience. There are also possible cases without symptoms that we classified as the "silent form" of celiac disease.

So how did we initially find out about these silent cases? When we learned that celiac disease is an autoimmune disorder and, as such, it has a genetic component, we actively looked for cases of celiac disease among first- and sometimes second-degree relatives. Our 2003 epidemiological study in the United States is a typical example of this approach.

Sure enough, we found out that relatives of celiac disease patients have between a two- and ten-fold higher chance of being affected with the condition. We also learned that many of these relatives who had the disease had no symptoms whatsoever, fulfilling the definition of silent cases.

Many other studies performed worldwide confirmed that there is a subgroup of celiac disease patients who exhibit no symptoms of any kind. We still uncover these cases at the Center when we screen family members of recently diagnosed celiac disease patients as recommended by the current protocols.

How is it possible that someone with an autoimmune disease that is destroying his or her intestines can have no symptoms? To answer this question, keep in mind that the small intestine is a long tube that's approximately 18 to 23 feet long.

Therefore, if the damage occurs in a region that is not specialized in any specific task, that is, absorption of iron, calcium, and vitamin D, the rest of the intestine subsidizes the lost ability in the local region to digest and absorb nutrients. In this case, no clinical symptoms appear. But eventually, the damage can progress until the critical mass of intestine is affected leading to the appearance of symptoms. So it's not surprising that the first diagnostic pillar—signs and symptoms—is not always present.

WHEN THE BLOOD TEST AND BIOPSY DON'T MATCH

The second criterion is positive serological screening tests. If we follow the diagnostic algorithm recommended for celiac disease, first we screen the subject in search of the antibodies specific for celiac disease. If the results are positive, we perform an endoscopy in search of the typical damage. This is also the approach we've taken to establish the sensitivity of the tTG test. Sensitivity, you'll recall, is the ability of the test to identify all cases of celiac disease.

This is a self-fulfilling prophecy, however, since endoscopies are done only if the antibodies are positive. Once again, our clinical practice has taught us otherwise. Specifically, we've seen cases in which gastroenterologists decide to perform an endoscopy just based on symptoms, and they find intestinal damage typical of celiac disease.

To validate the finding, they order the antibody test, and the results may come back negative. Another scenario that occurs is when the physician considers celiac disease as a possible diagnosis and correctly performs the blood test but gets negative results. Despite the negative results, they may decide to perform an endoscopy in search of other causes of the patient's symptoms and detect the intestinal damage typical of celiac disease.

Based on our clinical experience and recent data just published, we estimate that roughly 10 to 20 percent of celiac disease patients test negative to the serology screening test. Therefore, pillar number two of the diagnosis is challenged on clinical and research grounds.

The third diagnostic criterion is the genetic markers of HLA-DQ2 or -DQ8. Even if it's almost impossible to develop celiac disease without having the proper HLA-DQ and/or -DQ8, there are still 2 to 3 percent of people with celiac disease who don't have these genes. It happens rarely, but sometimes diagnostic pillar number three is also not absolute.

The fourth criterion is measurable damage to the small intestine. We have always considered the presence of the intestinal damage as the "gold standard" for celiac disease diagnosis. All clinicians familiar with celiac disease know all too well, however, that the damage may be patchy and can sometimes be missed when biopsies are taken.

There also is the possibility that the damage occurs farther down the gastrointestinal tract in an area that can't be reached by the endoscope and can be missed. Therefore, even clinical pillar number four, our gold standard, has lost its shiny characteristic. It might be only silver or even bronze in nature.

The fifth clinical pillar is that symptoms must resolve after the implementation of a gluten-free diet. There are several possible reasons why someone may not respond to a strict gluten-free diet for long time, despite good adherence and compliance. This complicated scenario can confuse both patients and health-care professionals.

ELIMINATING THE INTESTINAL BIOPSY

While the vast majority of people with celiac disease will fulfill all five diagnostic criteria listed above, there are still exceptions for each of the five clinical pillars to justify what Dr. Catassi and I suggested as the most rational approach to diagnose celiac disease. If indeed, our suggestions are followed, four of the five criteria satisfied should be sufficient to cover all people affected by celiac disease.

For example, if you have clear signs and symptoms of celiac disease; if your screening test is clearly positive (antibody levels are at least 10 times more than normal); if you have the proper HLA-DQ2 and or -DQ8, and your symptoms go away following the implementation of the gluten-free diet, an intestinal biopsy can be avoided, particularly in the pediatric population.

Our recommendation has been adopted by the European Society for Pediatric Gastroenterology, Hepatology and Nutrition, which has recently revised its guidelines to reflect this recommendation. Do you remember Aladdin's lamp from my Introduction? Here we satisfy wish number three: to eliminate the need for repeated intestinal biopsies, especially in children.

NON-RESPONSIVE CELIAC DISEASE

Sometimes we see patients who continue experiencing symptoms and have high levels of anti-tTG antibodies at their six-month follow-up visit, despite their adherence to a gluten-free diet. In these cases our dietitian, Pam Cureton, goes on a detective mission to discover any possible cross-contamination or poor compliance to the diet.

Sometimes she comes up with some interesting discoveries. Take the case of Betsy, who repeatedly and vigorously claimed absolute adherence to the gluten-free diet. One day she clarified that she maintained her stringent diet Monday through Saturday, while on Sunday she enjoyed her bowl of pasta! Most of the time, however, Pam can't identify a clear reason why the patient isn't improving, even though he or she is following the correct gluten-free diet.

Non-responsive celiac disease, which occurs in 10 to 15 percent of patients, is one of the most challenging areas I face as a physician treating gluten-related disorders. Normally, when you follow a gluten-free diet, your body and immune system relax because they finally feel "safe" from the gluten invaders. Your body begins the healing process as the immune system stops attacking body tissue. But with non-responsive celiac disease, your immune system remains on high alert.

If you follow a strict gluten-free diet for one year, and yet your blood tests show elevated levels of anti-tTG antibodies, or your endoscopy shows continued damage to the villi of your small intestine, you have non-responsive celiac disease. For most people with non-responsive celiac disease, inadvertent gluten ingestion is the most common cause. Nevertheless, other factors can come into play, which sometimes make it a serious and difficult-to-treat condition. Even for patients who follow the diet rigorously, there is a high percentage who show persistent villi damage.

GLUTEN GUARDS GO ON HIGH ALERT

Let's go back to our picture of your body as a fortress against foreign invaders, with your immune system as the soldiers or guards at the gate. Most people with celiac disease can safely ingest up to 10 milligrams (mg) of gluten a day before the "gluten guards" go on alert and start wreaking havoc on your immune system. (Ten mg of gluten is equal to about one-eighth of a teaspoon of flour.)

In other words, the immune system of most patients with celiac disease won't go into high alert over a few crumbs. But if you have non-responsive celiac disease, you have hyper-reactive gluten guards. And for someone recently diagnosed with celiac disease, sometimes it takes a while for those gluten guards to relax a little and give up their defensive positions.

In this scenario, all gluten is considered a threat, including the 10 mg that is usually easily handled by a well-functioning immune system. In the case of non-responsive celiac disease, absolutely all traces of gluten must be removed for the immune system to return to normal. If tests show that gluten is getting through in spite of strict adherence to the gluten-free diet, this is the most likely reason you're still suffering from symptoms.

WHEN IT'S REALLY *NOT* JUST CELIAC DISEASE

For patients with non-responsive celiac disease, the first step is to examine your diet carefully (see "Eliminate Those Gluten Invaders" on page 88). Inadvertent gluten ingestion is the most common reason for non-responsive celiac disease.

But just as celiac disease often masquerades as another condition, fooling the best diagnosticians, the reverse can be true and celiac disease can be misdiagnosed. Or celiac disease can coexist with other conditions. Some conditions that mimic celiac disease symptoms include pancreatic insufficiency, IBS, small intestinal bacterial overgrowth, lymphatic colitis, collagenous colitis, ulcerative jejunitis, T-cell lymphoma, pancreatic cancer, fructose intolerance, protein-losing enteropathy, cavitating lymphodemopathy, and tropical sprue.

THE FASANO DIET

When our patients don't respond to the gluten-free diet, our first step is to review their dietary habits and symptoms. If the symptoms don't improve after several months of strict adherence to the diet, we suspect a case of non-responsive celiac disease. We often then put the patient on the "Fasano Diet." A dietitian with expertise in celiac disease can help you decide if the Fasano Diet is right for you and get those gluten guards properly trained.

We developed the Fasano Diet to ensure the full removal of all gluten from a patient's diet and promote calming of the immune system. The three-month diet allows your body time to adjust, time to heal, and time to retrain the gluten guards. Staying on the Fasano Diet for three months allows your body to settle into its new non-inflamed, recovery state.

With the elimination of processed foods, the Fasano Diet focuses on fresh fruits and vegetables, highly tolerated grains such as rice, and meats such as turkey and chicken. While similar to an elimination diet, the Fasano Diet is designed to eliminate even trace amounts of gluten from your diet while emphasizing healthful choices.

A word of caution here: Before starting on this or any elimination diet, you must have your diet carefully reviewed by a knowledgeable dietitian to find and eliminate any possible sources of gluten sneaking into your diet. Never begin any diet or other nutritional therapy without the assistance of your health-care team.

REFRACTORY CELIAC DISEASE

Based on data collected at the Center during the past seven years, almost 80 percent of patients with non-responsive celiac disease improve on the Fasano Diet. The remaining 20 percent are affected by refractory celiac disease, also known as refractory sprue.

Approximately 1 to 5 percent of patients diagnosed with celiac disease develop refractory celiac disease. It's a very rare but sometimes life-threatening condition in which there is an absence of long-term improvement on the gluten-free diet. This is when our patients with celiac disease, almost exclusively adults, face the most challenging scenario.

Patients continue to lose weight, and symptoms tend to worsen rather than improve. It is defined as persistence of severely damaged villi in patients on a strict gluten-free diet for at least one year in which other specific causes have been ruled out. Refractory celiac disease usually presents with symptoms of severe malabsorption.

There are two types of refractive celiac disease. Type 1 accounts for 25 percent of cases with the remaining 75 percent classified as Type 2. With a normal intraepithelial lymphocyte population (remember our immune soldiers on the battlefield?), Type 1 carries a good prognosis and a five-year survival rate of more than 95 percent. Conversely, Type 2 has an aberrant intraepithelial lymphocyte population, and 50 to 60 percent of patients with Type 2 refractory celiac disease develop a lymphoma within five years.

ELIMINATE THOSE GLUTEN INVADERS

- Recheck the food labels of your favorite, everyday foods as ingredients can change without notice.
- Contact manufacturers of products you use that contain the statement "manufactured in a plant that also produces or is used on a machine that also processes wheat" to ask about the manufacturer's cross-contamination avoidance procedures. This is a voluntary allergen statement, and it may or may not be reflective of contamination. Likewise, products that do not contain this statement and do not declare "gluten-free, made in a dedicated kitchen," may be manufactured in a plant that also produces or is used on a machine that also processes wheat. When in doubt, call the manufacturer.
- Recheck all over-the-counter and prescription medications with the manufacturers to be sure they are gluten free. Visit www.glutenfreedrugs.com for help with your medications. Caution: do not stop any medications without first consulting your physician.
- Recheck all products that go in your mouth including toothpaste. While it is highly unlikely that mouth products would contain gluten, it is important to recheck everything.
- Use a gluten-free communion host or the low-gluten wafers offered by the Benedictine Sisters. These wafers, described as low-gluten, are labeled as 0.01 percent gluten and are considered safe. Visit http://altarbreads-bspa.com/lowgluten.php.
- Evaluate the frequency and strategies you use for eating out. For more tips on dining in restaurants, refer to Chapter Eight.
- Look for sources of cross-contamination at home. Be sure you use a dedicated gluten-free toaster. Thoroughly clean kitchen counters. Use separate cooking and serving utensils. Use separate pans for baking pans with crevices such as muffin tins. Always use a clean knife and a "one-dip policy" for common condiment jars.

CHAPTER SIX

Gluten and Your Brain

*"A crust eaten in peace is better than a
banquet partaken in anxiety."*
—AESOP

GLUTEN AFFECTS MORE THAN THE GUT

After I graduated from the University of Naples in 1986 as a pediatric gastroenterologist, I was eager to begin treating patients. In Italy, I began to see many patients with celiac disease. Many of the children had the typical symptoms of celiac disease: gastrointestinal distress, diarrhea, bloated belly, and poor growth.

It was almost as though we viewed celiac disease through a black-and-white lens. In those days, if you didn't have those symptoms, then it wasn't celiac disease. And almost always, it was diagnosed only in children. Many physicians believed that children could outgrow celiac disease, much as a child might outgrow an allergy.

Now we know the story is very different. We know that celiac disease can strike anyone at any time of life. We also know that it's not something that you will ever outgrow, but a condition that must be managed permanently by strict adherence to a gluten-free diet. In the intervening years, I've also learned to appreciate the many different ways that celiac disease presents itself clinically.

Health-care practitioners on the inside track of the celiac disease story have seen a shift in its clinical presentation. We've watched the monochrome snapshot of gastrointestinal symptoms become transformed into a cinematic, systemic disease that can touch every single organ or tissue.

In retrospect, I can see that the brain was somehow systematically involved in the clinical presentation of celiac disease all along. Now that we also know that gluten reactions go way beyond celiac disease, the preferential targeting of the brain has become even more apparent to me.

In our clinic, it's extremely rare to come across a patient with a possible gluten-related disorder who doesn't have some symptoms that involve the brain or the nervous system in general. Headaches, migraines, anxiety, depression, tingling of the fingertips, and foggy mind are among the most frequent symptoms reported by our patients. Gluten ataxia, the loss of coordination, is a less-common manifestation of the effect of gluten on the brain.

Many mysteries about gluten and the brain still remain, but there is one thing I know for sure. When patients with behavioral and/or neurological symptoms secondary to gluten-related disorders are placed on a gluten-free diet, most of them experience an almost magical relief from symptoms that have plagued their lives for years. This is one of the most rewarding experiences I've enjoyed in the care of these patients, as the scenario below illustrates.

A DIFFICULT DIAGNOSIS

Eleanor was a fifty-two-year-old associate college professor at a state university. She began experiencing mild gastrointestinal symptoms and then began suffering from cognitive decline, including memory loss and disorientation. Because of the gastrointestinal issues, she was tested for celiac disease. Although the anti-tissue transglutaminase (tTG) antibody test was positive (indicating celiac disease), she did not have a follow-up endoscopy nor was she placed on a gluten-free diet. It seems her mental state was deteriorating so rapidly that all the focus was placed on diagnosing her mental condition. The positive anti-tTG antibody test was overlooked.

In the meantime, her mental health declined so much that she had to be admitted to an inpatient psychiatric ward. The team of clinicians couldn't come up with a definitive diagnosis, although Alzheimer's disease was the suspected cause of her condition.

By this time, her family and friends were frantic with the puzzling and rapid decline of their mother and colleague. The son recalled the positive blood test that pointed toward celiac disease and started searching for any possible connection to his mother's mental deterioration.

That's when we got involved. Eleanor's son and a supportive family friend brought her to our clinic. We repeated the blood screening and confirmed a positive result for anti-tTG antibodies. We performed an endoscopy, which showed intestinal damage, and the diagnosis of celiac disease was confirmed. Eleanor was placed on a gluten-free diet and began to respond positively. Within several months, her mental condition had improved, and she was discharged from the psychiatric institution. Several years later, she returned to work at her former job at the same state university.

Eleanor's story is a dramatic and highly unusual case of how untreated celiac disease can have tragic consequences. Nonetheless, the whole topic of gluten and its effects on the brain remains highly debated. Conflicting research results and skepticism on the part of many health-care professionals about gluten's role in neurological diseases contributes to the controversy.

Why does gluten have a detrimental effect on the mental health of only some people and not others? There are several explanations out there, and I've boiled them down to two basic schools of thought.

THE ENDORPHIN EFFECT VERSUS INFLAMMATION

As I have mentioned in other parts of the book, there are fragments of gluten that cannot be completely digested. Some investigators believe that a few of these fragments bear a structural resemblance to chemicals called endorphins, which are produced in our brain. Endorphins share a similar chemical structure to morphine, and they naturally relieve pain and reduce stress.

Supporters of this theory call the gluten fragments "gliadorphins." They hypothesize that the gliadorphins somehow cross the intestinal barrier, enter the bloodstream, and cross the blood-brain barrier. Once across the blood-brain barrier, the gliadorphins interact with the endorphin receptors and cause the behavioral changes described above.

This theory can explain the behavioral changes experienced by patients with celiac disease and gluten sensitivity. It doesn't adequately explain, however, symptoms like neuropathy, an abnormal and usually painful state of the nervous system, or the tingling of the hands and feet that I often detect in these patients.

This apparent contradiction can be explained by the second theory, which suggests that brain involvement in gluten-related disorders is secondary to an inflammatory process. This inflammation is a continuum of immune responses starting in the gut.

The first few steps in the process overlap with the first theory: specific gliadin peptides are generated from gluten, and they cross the intestinal barrier. But the picture changes after that. The breakdown of the gliadin peptides generates a chain of events that leads to an inflammatory response.

When these fragments "breach the walls of the city" by crossing the intestinal barrier into places they don't belong, the immune soldiers mount a response to get rid of the enemy. The immediate immune response (or the innate immune response) in the intestine is the first step leading to what could become symptoms of gluten-related disorders (see Chapter Four).

If only the innate immune system (I think of them as the special response units deployed after an attack from the enemy) is involved, the outcome is likely to be gluten sensitivity. If the more sophisticated adaptive immune system is involved (I think of these guys as infantry settling in for a long siege), then the autoimmune response of celiac disease will most likely emerge.

But remember, my philosophy is that the gut is not like Las Vegas: What happens in the gut doesn't stay in the gut. These immune cells may leave the intestine and travel to other districts, including the peripheral nerves or the brain. There they can cause inflammation leading to the behavioral and/or neurological symptoms I described earlier. Clinical trials and research studies supporting this second theory have increased in recent years.

WHY DOES GLUTEN ATTACK THE BRAIN?

Of the two theories, the second one makes more sense to me. It correlates with what we already know in terms of the development of inflammation in the pathogenesis of gluten-related disorders.

But why do clinicians see more and more patients suffering from these symptoms? And why is the brain one of the most preferred targets of this inflammatory attack triggered by gluten? As more research is focused in the area of gluten's effects on the brain, I'm confident that in the next few years we'll know a lot more about this fascinating and yet disturbing aspect of gluten-related disorders.

As you might imagine, two areas that have been among the most controversial in regard to gluten and the brain are Autism Spectrum Disorder (ASD) and schizophrenia. Let's look at the facts and fantasies surrounding these two devastating conditions.

DIAGNOSING THE PROBLEM

Early in my career as a pediatric gastroenterologist at the University of Maryland Medical Center, I witnessed another dramatic turnaround. I had just arrived in Baltimore and was experiencing a new city, a new country, a new language, and new customs. Nevertheless, my basic instincts as a doctor kicked in when I heard a child's screams coming from a room in the pediatric clinic in 1993.

I thought, "Oh, the nurses must be having trouble getting an intravenous line in." I walked into the room to see if I could help. I was surprised to see only a mother and a child of about five years of age. He was just screaming for no apparent reason. I asked his mother what was wrong, and she answered, "He does this most of the time, and I don't know what the problem is. We haven't been able to find out what's wrong with him."

The boy was scheduled for a test to rule out cystic fibrosis because of a recent bout of severe diarrhea. He was not even scheduled to see a physician that day. He had already lost some of his developmental milestones, including specifically his speech and communication skills. After talking to his mother about his symptoms, I realized that the combination of diarrhea and behavioral changes could indeed be due to celiac disease. I decided to screen him for the condition.

Sure enough, his blood samples came back positive for celiac disease. We scheduled an endoscopy of his upper intestine, never an easy procedure on a five-year-old. The results showed extensive inflammation and the villous blunting of his small intestine typical of celiac disease.

We immediately started him on a gluten-free diet. A few months later I received an interesting letter. It was from the boy's speech therapist. She was amazed by the progress the child had made in such a short period of time. She wanted to know what we had done to cause such an amazing transformation in him.

In less than six months, he went from knowing a handful of words to speaking in full sentences. Instead of acting like a two- or three-year-old, the point at which his development became delayed and his behavior deteriorated, he began acting like an age-appropriate five-year-old.

I also was astonished when I saw him a few months later. Not only could he communicate properly for his age, but he also had changed from a child living in his own world to a very spirited little boy with a sparkle in his eyes that I had never seen before. One of my most gratifying moments as a physician came that day when his mother said, "Thank you for giving me my son back."

ONE IN EIGHTY-EIGHT CHILDREN

ASDs are mixed neurodevelopmental disorders that affect approximately 1 percent of the general population. Children and adults on the autism spectrum show impaired communication, poor or nonexistent social skills, repetitive behaviors, and a narrow range of interests. When autism was first recognized as a distinct clinical entity in the mid-1940s, it was thought to be caused by a combination of inborn biological errors and psychological factors.

In the mid-1960s, Bruno Bettelheim published the book *The Empty Fortress: Infantile Autism and the Birth of the Self.* In this treatise,

Bettelheim identified emotionally distant "refrigerator mothers" as the primary cause of autism.

His influential treatise was initially well received, but later came under more critical scrutiny as other factors in the development of autism emerged. In 1977 British researchers Susan Folstein and Martin Rutter published the first twin study that indisputably proved the existence of a genetic component in the genesis of autism. Regardless of the causes, today approximately one in 88 children is diagnosed with an ASD, according to the Centers for Disease Control and Prevention.

The disorder affects an estimated 1.5 million individuals in the United States and tens of millions of children and adults around the world. Boys receive the diagnosis three to four times more frequently than girls. Estimates show that one out of 54 boys in the United States are on the autistic disorders spectrum.

MULTIPLE CAUSES OF ASD

Researchers generally agree that there are multiple causes for the outcome of ASD, with both genetic and environmental components placing children and adults somewhere on the autistic spectrum. Indeed, some evidence suggests that environmental factors play an important role in the pathogenesis of ASD.

These factors include increased concerns about environmental exposure and neurodevelopment in general. More specific aspects include some provocative data on how environmental exposure might cause autism; epidemiological data on environmental exposure and autism; and, most important, regional differences in autism prevalence and descriptive data on the recent rise in autism.

But which environmental factors are involved in this ASD epidemic? Several theories exist, but there are few certainties concerning the culprits that trigger ASD in genetically susceptible children. Among these theories genetic mutations, oxidative stress, metabolic disorders, intestinal dysbiosis (an imbalance of healthy microorganisms in the gut), exposure to heavy metals, and food sensitivities have all been named as causing ASD. With few facts or evidence-based research, many therapeutic approaches have arisen to treat autism and related disorders.

Many children and adolescents with ASD suffer from gastrointestinal problems. Their symptoms include constipation, gastroesophageal reflux, gastritis, intestinal inflammation (autistic enterocolitis), maldigestion, malabsorption, flatulence, abdominal pain or discomfort, lactose intolerance, enteric infections, and other symptoms.

It's hard for us to measure the impact of these gastrointestinal symptoms, since nonverbal or minimally verbal children can't tell us about some of their symptoms. Estimates of ASD children suffering from gastrointestinal symptoms as reported in medical literature range from 9 to 90 percent. Researchers are now starting to more closely examine the relationship between gastrointestinal disorders and ASD.

ALTERNATIVE VERSUS TRADITIONAL TREATMENTS

Of the almost fifty treatments proposed for ASD, seven (antifungal therapy; chelation, the removal of heavy metals from the bloodstream; enzymes; gastrointestinal treatments; intestinal parasite therapy; nutritional supplements; and dietary options) specifically target the gastrointestinal tract. Although subjects with ASD frequently experience gastrointestinal symptoms, the prevalence and nature of the symptoms remain elusive along with the most effective treatments.

The different, and not necessarily mutually exclusive, theories on what causes ASD and the subsequent myriad of proposed treatments have generated tremendous confusion and skepticism. Experts are engaged in a heated debate that has divided them into two major camps.

The alternative medicine camp claims that each and every one of the nearly fifty proposed treatments is a valid approach to treat ASD. The traditional medicine camp regards most (if not all) of the proposed treatments as not evidence-based and illegitimate. When these extreme positions arise, it's my opinion that the most appropriate approach is a compromise between the two camps.

THE GLUTEN-FREE DIET AS TREATMENT

To present my case, I'll focus on one of the fifty proposed treatments and the one that is most pertinent to the focus of this book: the gluten-free diet, alone or in combination with the casein-free diet. In a recent survey involving more than 27,000 parents of autistic kids, avoidance of gluten (approximately 9,000 cases) and/or casein (approximately 7,000 cases) were the most frequent treatments they implemented with their children.

The survey results from the Autism Research Institute showed a better to worse ratio of thirty to one and thirty-two to one, respectively, for these dietary interventions. This means that for every one child whose behavior deteriorated on the gluten-free diet, thirty children had improved behavior (from a total of 4,340 children), and for every one child whose behavior deteriorated on the casein-free diet, thirty-two children improved (from a total of 6,950 children).

Therefore, from the point of view of caretakers who experience firsthand the burden of ASD, the gluten-free diet is judged to be one of the most effective interventions to treat the condition. To challenge these conclusions, scientists have performed several double-blind studies. In these studies, both the family of the ASD child and the investigator are unaware if the child is in the treatment group (gluten-free diet) or the placebo group.

A recent systematic review reported in the literature by researchers for the Cochrane Collaboration identified six double-blind randomized trials. Three studies showed that a gluten-free diet was beneficial. The remaining three studies detected no improvement in the behavior of ASD children after implementation of the diet. The authors concluded:

> *Research has shown of high rates of use of complementary and alternative therapies for children with autism including gluten and/or casein exclusion diets. Current evidence for efficacy of these diets is poor. Large-scale, good-quality randomized controlled trials are needed.*

These are interesting conclusions that, in my humble opinion, will bring more inconclusive results if more trials are conducted as suggested. What I find most intriguing is that even though researchers agree that the path to the final destination of ASD can differ from child to child, some researchers are still looking for the "holy grail" single treatment approach to fix all ASD cases. Let's try something else.

TAKING A MORE TARGETED APPROACH TO RESEARCH

To continue presenting my case, let's hypothetically assume that I have enrolled one hundred children with ASD in a double-blind study to verify the efficacy of the gluten-free diet. Let's further assume that twenty children out of the one hundred followed the "gluten path" to arrive at the ASD final destination.

In other words, gluten was the environmental trigger that somehow led these twenty children down the path to an autistic outcome. But in this trial, we don't know which of the one hundred children might be sensitive to gluten.

At the end of this trial of the gluten-free diet, I detect an improvement of ASD only in the twenty children with sensitivity to gluten. The remaining eighty show no difference in their behavior.

This tells me that the diet has only 20 percent efficacy (the gluten-free diet improved ASD in only twenty children out of one hundred). Therefore, I conclude that the gluten-free diet failed to have a meaningful effect on ASD.

Now let's repeat the trial with the same one hundred children but with a different approach. Let's assume that I have biomarkers (biological red flags) to identify the twenty children among my original one hundred who followed the gluten path to get to the final destination of ASD. Let's target them for my clinical trial (this approach is called population stratification).

Now I perform my double-blind, gluten-free diet trial on these twenty children and twenty matched children who are not sensitive to gluten as our control group. My final result will be astonishingly different: all twenty children who are sensitive to gluten will respond to the diet, while the children with no sensitivity to gluten will show no difference in their behavior. In this study, the gluten-free diet has 100 percent efficacy.

Of course, to make my case, I have oversimplified a story that most likely is much more complicated. It's possible that the several paths leading to ASD are interconnected and influence each other. One unifying theory to connect the dots would link gluten ingestion, gut microorganism composition, and leaky gut.

LOOKING FOR ANSWERS TO ASD

As stated earlier, gut dysbiosis is an imbalance in microoganisms in the gut. Expose this intestinal environment to some gliadin fragments, and this might cause the release of zonulin that leads to a leakiness of the gut. This is just like a breach in the wall of our medieval city. It allows enemies, including components of foodstuffs such as gluten and casein, to cross the intestinal barrier and gain access behind the city walls. Our immune cells, the soldiers that protect us against the enemies, can then cause inflammation both in the intestine (autistic enterocolitis) and in the brain (ASD).

An alternative to the inflammatory hypothesis in ASD patients is the proposition that the defect in the intestinal barrier allows the passage of neuroactive peptides of food, the gliadorphin peptide from gluten, into the bloodstream. The toxic peptide could then travel to the cerebrospinal fluid to interfere directly with the function of the central nervous system.

Whichever theory might be correct, a gluten-free diet can change the intestinal microbiome: the community of microbes in the gut. This change could result in the elimination of the instigating enemy that arms our immune cells causing inflammation. It could correct the leaky gut and thus prevent the inflammation and the resulting symptoms and damage. It's possible that at least a subgroup of ASD children could benefit from this therapeutic approach.

This is the working hypothesis that scientists at the Center, in collaboration with colleagues from the California Institute of Technology and the University of California, Davis, are currently testing. With the support of a grant from Autism Speaks (a leading advocacy organization for ASD awareness and research), we are committed to working as hard as we can to test our hypothesis, and we hope to contribute to solutions for this devastating condition.

AUTISM SPECTRUM DISORDER AND THE ROLE OF THE GUT

What are some common symptoms that ASD children and adolescents might exhibit if they are having gastrointestinal issues?

Obvious signs and symptoms include chronic constipation; stomachaches, with or without diarrhea; and underwear soiling. Behaviors that could point to gastrointestinal problems include vocal behaviors such as screaming, frequent clearing of throat, tics, swallowing, sighing, whining, moaning, and more; motor behaviors such as unusual posture, putting pressure on the belly, wincing, constant eating, gritting teeth, and more; and/or changes in the overall state such as sleep disturbances, noncompliance with requests that typically elicit proper response, increased irritability and more.

What should families do if they think their autistic child has gastrointestinal issues?

Families should be referred to a pediatric gastrointestinal specialist familiar with ASD-related gastrointestinal disorders. One thing to avoid is undertaking any remedy, either alternative or traditional, to resolve gastrointestinal issues before seeking medical advice. This can complicate the diagnosis and proper management needed to help the child.

Should they insist that their child be tested for celiac disease or gluten sensitivity?

If a child with ASD is also experiencing gastrointestinal symptoms, it's valid to raise the possibility of celiac disease or gluten sensitivity as the cause of the behavioral and intestinal symptoms.

For more information on autism research, visit www.autismspeaks.org.

GLUTEN AND SCHIZOPHRENIA

An inability to distinguish between reality and delusion, so beautifully portrayed in the semiautobiographical film, *A Beautiful Mind*, about Nobel Prize–winning scientist John Nash, is the hallmark symptom of schizophrenia. Someone suffering from this severe brain disorder may suffer from hallucinations (visual or more often auditory), delusions, and disordered thinking and behavior.

Statistics show that about 1.5 million people in the United States, or one-half of 1 percent, are diagnosed with schizophrenia. The condition begins in young adulthood and can be chronic and disabling for the rest of the person's life. The lifespan of a person with schizophrenia is approximately twenty-five years less than the general population, and typical treatment, which includes psychotropic medication, is only marginally successful.

According to the World Health Organization, "The chronic course and debilitating effects of schizophrenia combine to create a disease which imposes very considerable clinical, social and economic consequences on societies throughout the world, resulting in it being a leading contributor to global and regional levels of disability and the overall disease burden."

MIXED RESEARCH RESULTS

The role of gluten in schizophrenia has long been debated, going back to the 1940s, contemporary to Dr. Dicke's observation that linked gluten to celiac disease. A clinical link was made during World War II, when clinicians saw a decrease in schizophrenia in Europe paralleled by an increase of the disease in the United States.

Among all the environmental factors considered, gluten was suspected as one of the major instigators. Because of wheat shortages during World War II, its consumption had declined in Europe but had increased in the United States, where wheat was becoming increasingly important in the diet.

This circumstantial observation was followed by several small studies with patients with schizophrenia who underwent gluten withdrawal in clinical trials. Researchers, some of whom used methods that have since been discredited, obtained mixed results. Some studies suggested a correlation, while others disputed the role of gluten in the pathogenesis of schizophrenia.

Just as in the studies on gluten and ASD, the two camps (believers and nonbelievers) became more and more divided on the topic. The reasoning of the two schools of thought was based on a false presumption that, in my opinion, deviated from what would have been the proper focus: explaining how gluten can have an impact on the condition of schizophrenia or ASD.

Some proponents support the notion that gluten consumption can explain all cases of schizophrenia, a thesis that is difficult to support with the facts. Nonbelievers make the argument that since celiac disease is not extremely frequent among patients with schizophrenia, then, by default, gluten cannot be a player except in rare cases of celiac disease and schizophrenia.

Given these biased presumptions, I think that both camps are incorrect. We now know that gluten is associated with other disorders, not only celiac disease. We need to investigate the role of gluten sensitivity as well as celiac disease in people with schizophrenia. We also know that multisystemic disorders, such as schizophrenia and ASD, are final destinations that can be reached by following different routes, including the "gluten route."

LOOKING FOR GLUTEN REACTIONS

My clinical and research attention never included a focus on gluten and schizophrenia until a few years ago. Two colleagues from Baltimore, Dr. William Eaton from Johns Hopkins Bloomberg School of Public Health, and Dr. Nicola Cascella, from Johns Hopkins School of Medicine, contacted me to talk about doing a collaborative study on gluten and schizophrenia.

Dr. Eaton collaborates with researchers from Denmark. Their work, which suggests a link between schizophrenia and autoimmunity, resulted in findings that show that among all the environmental triggers considered in the pathogenesis of schizophrenia, gluten surfaces as a strong candidate.

Dr. Eaton and Dr. Cascella have access to a large collection of blood samples of people diagnosed with schizophrenia. It was a no-brainer for me to join them in what seemed to be a very simple scientific exercise. We'd look for signs of gluten reaction in the blood samples of these patients.

As expected, we found only a handful of people with celiac disease. The prevalence rate was approximately 2 percent, or two times the rate in the general population. These results support the group of nonbelievers, since ostensibly 98 percent of patients with schizophrenia wouldn't benefit from the implementation of the gluten-free diet.

Not as expected, however, we also found that approximately one-fifth of the patients mounted an immune response against gluten, suggesting a possible inflammatory mechanism triggered by gluten. These results could support the other school of thought about gluten and schizophrenia. But to me, it clearly suggests that only a portion of people diagnosed with schizophrenia have developed the disorder through an adverse reaction to gluten.

Following our research, other groups published similar results reinforcing our overall hypothesis that gluten may play a role in a subgroup of people diagnosed with schizophrenia. The question remained, were these just coincidental findings or does this immune response to gluten indeed play a role in the pathogenesis of schizophrenia?

PUZZLING BLOOD TESTS

These results prompted us to conduct the next series of experiments that I believe led to more direct evidence of this link. One thing that really bothered me about our original studies was an apparent discrepancy that I had never experienced before.

Because we used historical samples, we couldn't confirm a diagnosis of celiac disease by the usual method of intestinal biopsy (we only had blood samples). So, as we'd done before, we decided to restrict our criteria for celiac disease to a positive test for anti-tTG antibodies followed by a positive test for antiendomysium antibodies (EMA) (see Chapter Five).

In general these two antibodies work in parallel, meaning that with few exceptions, a strong positive anti-tTG antibody is almost always associated with a positive EMA. When we can't complete an endoscopy on a patient for whatever reasons in our clinic, we almost always use this approach to diagnose celiac disease.

For the first time, however, I observed a disconnect between these two autoantibodies. Nearly 15 percent of the patients with schizophrenia tested strongly positive for the presence of anti-tTG antibodies but negative for EMA.

We published this data in our original report. Subsequent research both confirmed and criticized our findings, but we remained puzzled by this high percentage of people diagnosed with schizophrenia who tested negative for celiac disease but positive for tTG.

TRACKING DOWN DIFFERENCES IN tTG

I started brainstorming to find a possible logical explanation for this apparent dichotomy. It then occurred to me that this tTG comes in different types, known as isoforms.

One isoform, the tTG2 type, is very specific to the intestine. Another, the tTG3 isoform, is found only in the skin. This isoform results in dermatitis herpetiformis, the skin manifestation of celiac disease. There is a third isoform, tTG6, which is found only in the brain. EMA strictly correlates only with the antibodies against the tTG2 form.

I asked our lab technician if the kit we used to screen the samples was specific to detect tTG2. In other words, did it measure only antibodies against the tTG2 form?

The lab technician asked the kit's vendor who confirmed that the test was specific for tTG2 since the test is for the diagnosis of celiac disease. Not satisfied with the answer, I visited the company's website. I wanted to find out if their methods would specifically pinpoint only the tTG2 isoform.

I found out that they assume the tTG form is tTG2, since more than 95 percent of the tTG found in the gut is in the tTG2 isoform. Nevertheless, at least on paper, their test could also pick up the other isoforms, including the brain-related tTG6 isoform.

I decided to employ the kit that specifically identified antibodies against tTG6 and run the samples again. And sure enough, the vast majority of the patients who were negative for EMA but who tested positive for tTG antibodies showed elevated anti-tTG6 antibodies. And that, for me, confirmed what I suspected about gluten and people diagnosed with schizophrenia.

TAKING A CLOSER LOOK AT THE ROLE OF tTG

Now we have more than just circumstantial evidence that gluten may cause neuroinflammation in people with schizophrenia. The way I see the story is summarized in the following chain of events:

1. The person eats gluten.
2. Small fragments of gluten remain undigested.
3. Some of these fragments cross the intestinal barrier because of increased permeability caused by the release of zonulin triggered by gluten.
4. These fragments are perceived as enemies and induce an inflammatory immune response, which is originally confined to the gut.
5. Some of these armed immune cells leave the gut and migrate to the brain where they cause a local inflammation that leads to the destruction of brain cells with a subsequent leak of the tTG6 enzyme outside the cell.
6. For the first time, the immune system sees this enzyme as nonself and mounts an immune response, leading to the production of tTG6 antibodies.

PATIENTS RESPOND TO TREATMENT

Our latest research includes looking at the brains of schizophrenic patients preserved after death. We're hoping to confirm what seems to be more than just circumstantial evidence of the link between gluten and schizophrenia.

At the same time, we're collaborating with colleagues from the Maryland Psychiatric Research Center (MPRC) at the University of Maryland School of Medicine on pilot studies of the implementation of the gluten-free diet with selected patients with schizophrenia. Under the leadership of Dr. Deanna Kelly from MPRC, we've completed a proof-of-concept study on two patients diagnosed with schizophrenia. One tested positive for anti-tTG6 antibodies and the other tested positive for anti-gliadin antibodies (AGA).

In both cases, the implementation of the gluten-free diet caused improvements in their schizophrenic symptoms. It also caused robust improvements in some of the side effects caused by almost all drugs currently used to treat schizophrenia. Arising from the region of the brain that controls movement and coordination, these "extrapyramidal side effects" involve both nerves and muscles.

These side effects include abnormal muscle spasms, tremors, involuntary and repetitive movement, including tics and other Parkinsonian-type movement disorders, slurred speech, and agitation. Because both subjects in the study saw improvement in these areas, a larger and more long-term study is needed. Even though these are very preliminary results, they are remarkably promising. Dr. Kelly has now obtained enough funding to allow us to perform these clinical trials on a larger scale.

Although the gluten-free diet is not a panacea for all patients with developmental or brain disorders, it does appear to hold promise for a subgroup of these patients. When I founded the Center in 1996, I never imagined that one day our research on celiac disease, a condition that was supposed to be strictly gastrointestinal with no relation to mental health, might have a profound impact on the quality of life for people with schizophrenia.

PART TWO

Learning to Live Without Gluten

CHAPTER SEVEN

Living Well on the Gluten-Free Diet

"One should eat to live, not live to eat."
—BENJAMIN FRANKLIN

"EXCUSE ME, DR. FASANO, BUT WHAT DO WE EAT?"

In the early years before celiac disease was recognized as a common disease, patients really had a hard time leading normal lives. An individual might finally receive the correct diagnosis after many years of struggle, but beyond that, there was very little support from the health-care community for follow-up care and nutritional counseling.

Patients started their own support groups to share information about the gluten-free diet, the availability of gluten-free food, health-care professionals, and other things to make their lives more livable. Those early support groups were focused on recipe exchanges, and people often brought their own food samples to share with one another.

My expertise was in clinical symptoms and the medical and molecular science behind celiac disease; it was not in cooking gluten-free meals. Along with other experts from the Center I began to give talks at support group meetings, where I spoke about celiac disease. Along with raising awareness, we also solicited volunteers for the blood screenings for the prevalence study through the support groups.

My eyes were opened to the plight of these patients at one of my earliest visits to a support group in Washington, D.C. I stood at the front of the room and began my lecture about celiac disease, its symptoms, its diagnosis, and other clinical issues. I showed my accompanying slides of mucosal damage to the intestinal villi (remember, this was pre–PowerPoint).

We were all looking at how the fingerlike tentacles lining the wall of the small intestine become blunted through malabsorption, which is the diagnostic hallmark of celiac disease. Suddenly a hand shot up from the back of the room and an older lady stood up. She said, "Wait a minute, Dr. Fasano, we thought you were here to give us recipes. We don't know what to eat!"

I was shocked that in the most medically advanced country in the world, people were struggling with the most basic of human needs: how to eat a healthy diet. Receiving little or no guidance from doctors, people diagnosed with celiac disease relied on each other for information on gluten-free food sources, recipes, and referrals for knowledgeable health-care professionals, including dietitians.

I think this is why the celiac community evolved into such a strong and tight-knit group that has accomplished so much for public advocacy and reform. Many people with celiac disease have learned to eat safely through the support of a celiac group. National and local organizations have extensive information on the gluten-free diet, the topic of our next discussion.

I've diagnosed thousands of children and adults with gluten-related disorders. I've seen the panic that sometimes ensues when they first hear the words "gluten-free diet." Now that celiac disease and gluten sensitivity are becoming more widely known, it's not nearly as scary as it was back in the early days of the Center when there were so few resources—and no Internet or smartphones!

In this section, you will learn about how to eat safely on the gluten-free diet, which is something that took years of advocacy from the celiac community and the Center to achieve.

HOW MUCH GLUTEN IS TOO MUCH?
(The Real Story on the Food Labeling Journey in the U.S.)

The brief story of the meeting in Washington, D.C., that I just shared with you now seems light-years from our current reality. About ten years after that story, I found myself again in Washington, D.C. This time I was providing testimony to the U.S. Congress about celiac disease to aid in the passage of the Food Allergen Labeling and Consumer Protection Act (FALCPA) of 2004.

FALCPA states that if any ingredient used in food contained any of the top eight allergens (milk, egg, fish, shellfish, nuts, tree nuts, soy, and wheat), it must be labeled in plain English. It took until August 2013 for all the components of FALCPA to become fully implemented, including a definition of gluten-free food as containing less than 20 parts per million (ppm).

The Center for Celiac Research had a great deal of influence on this piece of legislation. The story begins more than a decade ago, when Andrea Levario, who was working as a lobbyist in Washington, D.C., gave me a call. Andrea, whom you will meet again in Chapter Eleven, had a husband and son with celiac disease. She told me that the bipartisan U.S. House of Representatives Committee on Energy and Commerce was holding discussions on a piece of legislation, which was introduced by Rep. Nita Lowey, about food allergens and appropriate food labeling.

Although the Republican Party had already chosen its scientific expert to provide advice on the drafting of the law, the Democratic members were still making up their minds. The U.S. Senate Committee on Health, Education, Labor, and Pensions, which was also instrumental in the bill's success, reached out to me through Andrea's intervention. I remember when I got the call from an assistant on behalf of one of the Senate sponsors of the bill, Senator Ted Kennedy, to testify in front of the congressional committee. I was thrilled, but, at the same time, somewhat intimidated.

When I read legal documents, they always look to me as though they are written in a foreign language. Nevertheless, the first thing I noticed was that the word "celiac" was nowhere to be found in that lengthy document of the proposed legislation. So the first order of business was to try to get celiac disease included in the bill.

I vividly remember my first experience giving witness as an expert to the Senate Committee in 2002. That was during a period when the two major political parties were still able to work together and reach a compromise. Even if the opinions were quite different, we had a very constructive discussion.

The expert chemist engaged by the Republican Party made the very appropriate point that, in principle, the food manufacturing industry was not opposed to a piece of legislation that would regulate thresholds of specific foodstuffs, including gluten. They were very skeptical, however, that without indisputable scientific evidence, choosing an arbitrary threshold would expose manufacturers to frivolous legal suits that ultimately would have a negative impact on consumers.

While I accepted the argument put forward by my colleague, I, on the other hand, stressed the point that it would not be prudent to ignore the need for a threshold, and that the law should be expanded to include celiac disease. Otherwise, the same mistakes would be made that had been made with tobacco and asbestos, which became the targets of major lawsuits that cost those industries dearly in both money and public reputation.

Ultimately, the committee agreed that scientific evidence was needed to set an appropriate threshold for levels of gluten. For that reason, the Center embarked on the landmark study that determined 20 ppm as the safe threshold for people with celiac disease.

Ted Kennedy's committee was instrumental in encouraging us to move forward with this study. Without his visionary commitment, celiac disease today would still be without proper recognition in the legislation regulating appropriate thresholds of gluten intake.

We had a false sense of accomplishment when the bipartisan Congressional efforts succeeded in passing FALCPA in 2004. Celiac disease, described as a chronic digestive disease that damages the small intestine and interferes with absorption of nutrients from food, was listed among the conditions that would benefit from this piece of legislation. The findings from our prevalence study, which determined that one in 133 people in the United States has celiac disease, were also included.

What we didn't realize at the time was that this was just the beginning, rather than the end of the process. For the next ten years, the FDA was involved in the lengthy process of translating the legislation into real results for consumers. FALCPA went into effect in January 2006, without a gluten-free labeling threshold established.

The legislation required the FDA to "issue a proposed rule that will define and permit the voluntary use of the term 'gluten free' on the labeling of foods by August 2006 and a final rule no later than August 2008." Finally in August 2013, the gluten-free labeling ruling was enacted with the 20 parts per million threshold. Compliance with the gluten-free food labeling regulation by manufacturers is voluntary.

During this decade, we continued to play a key role in providing expert input to the FDA and keeping the gluten-free labeling agenda in the public eye. Since the implementation of FALCPA, people who follow the gluten-free diet have a much wider variety of safer, more palatable, and less costly products. In this chapter, you will learn about the many options available to people first implementing the gluten-free diet.

THREE LITTLE WORDS: WHEAT, RYE, AND BARLEY

There is a general misconception that Italians eat only pasta and pizza. When I was young, we enjoyed our pasta and bread, but many of the ingredients and recipes from my childhood were naturally gluten-free. I didn't know it at the time, but our cuisine included the basic ingredients of a healthy gluten-free diet (see Chapter Nine). As you embark on this new way of eating, keep in mind that international cuisines are a great place to look for many healthy and delicious gluten-free alternatives to the gluten-filled way of eating often seen in the United States.

In some ways, the gluten-free diet is very simple—if you start with the basics. Think about when you were an infant. You started life with either breast milk or formula, and foods were added as you grew. Go back to that basic idea of your diet as a blank slate, and think about all the healthy foods that you can eat that don't contain gluten.

On the gluten-free diet, there are basically three items to avoid: wheat (contains gluten), barley (contains secalin), and rye (contains hordein). As discussed earlier, these three grains contain peptides from these proteins that can trigger a gluten-related reaction in susceptible individuals. For convenience and easier communication, when we refer to the gluten-free diet, we include all three grains, wheat, barley, and rye, in the word gluten-free.

The gluten-free diet sounds simple. It becomes complicated when you consider all the forms that these three grains, especially wheat, can take in someone's individual diet. Not only do we have bread, pasta, cookies, and cakes to consider, there's also candy, soy sauce, processed meats, salad dressings, and energy bars.

As for barley, that's a main ingredient in barley soup and beer, not to mention breakfast cereals in the form of malt. And just think of all the tantalizing varieties of rye bread: pumpernickel, light and dark rye, and caraway.

As you can already see, implementing the gluten-free diet might not be as easy as eating well in Southern Italy a few decades ago. So in Part Two of *Gluten Freedom,* I've engaged the help of some experts to help us navigate safely through this gluten-filled landscape.

> **VERY IMPORTANT:** Before starting a gluten-free diet, make sure that you've been fully tested for celiac disease. Once you stop eating gluten, your body no longer produces the antibodies in your blood that are the diagnostic markers for celiac disease. A blood test for celiac disease could return a false negative result. Celiac disease can't be properly diagnosed while you're on a gluten-free diet.

DON'T GO IT ALONE

Currently, the only treatment for gluten-related disorders is a gluten-free diet. People with celiac disease must eliminate gluten for life. Depending on their symptoms, individuals with either gluten sensitivity or wheat allergy might not have to adhere as strictly or as permanently to a gluten-free diet.

This chapter will describe a strict gluten-free diet for celiac disease and can be individualized for persons with other gluten-related disorders. To make sure that your nutritional needs are being met, always work with a knowledgeable dietitian. The Academy of Nutrition and Dietetics (formerly the American Dietetic Association) offers comprehensive information on following the gluten-free diet (see Resources section at back of book).

I happen to have one of the best in the field working with me. Pam Cureton is an integral part of the history of the Center for Celiac Research. I've relied on her savvy expertise for accurate information on following the gluten-free diet.

Research shows that people who have individual instruction and social support are more likely to stick to the gluten-free diet. After your diagnosis, look for a celiac support group in your area or join an online support group. You'll have more success as you adjust to the challenges of the gluten-free lifestyle (see Part Three for tips on adjusting to the gluten-free lifestyle).

Your dietitian can assess your current food and nutrition intake. She can also reevaluate your nutritional profile to create a balanced nutrient intake of important vitamins and minerals such as calcium, iron, vitamin B complex, and vitamin D and make sure you are getting enough fiber.

Other areas a skilled dietitian can assess include:
- Knowledge, beliefs, or attitudes that demonstrate a readiness or reluctance to implement a gluten-free diet
- Social and religious beliefs impacted by a gluten-free diet
- Factors affecting access to both food and nutrition-related supplies, such as availability and cost of gluten-free foods
- Medication and herbal or other supplement use

WHERE'S GLUTEN FOUND?

Gluten is found in common foods such as breads, cereals, baked goods, and pasta. Because it's used in processed foods as an additive or preservative, gluten is also found in a wide variety of foods and nonfood items from prescription medication to Play-Doh®. If you're the food shopper in your family, you must learn to read labels very carefully to comply with a gluten-free diet.

THINGS TO AVOID ON THE GLUTEN-FREE DIET

Grains That Contain Gluten (or similar proteins)
- Wheat, including all types such as spelt, seitan, couscous, einkorn, emmer, kamut, and durum
- Barley, barley malt, extract or flavoring
- Rye
- Triticale (a hybrid grain made from wheat and rye)

THINGS TO EXAMINE CAREFULLY ON THE GLUTEN-FREE DIET

Questionable Foods
- Imitation bacon
- Imitation seafood
- Marinades
- Broth/bouillon/soup
- Candy
- Seasonings
- Salad dressings
- Sauces and gravies
- Low-fat foods
- Packaged flavored rice and potato mixes

Questionable Nonfood Items
- Herbal supplements
- Vitamins
- Prescription or over-the-counter medications (check with your health-care provider or pharmacist)

THINGS YOU CAN EAT ON THE GLUTEN-FREE DIET

You can eat fresh and dried fruits and vegetables, eggs, meat, fish, poultry, seafood, dairy products (or products made with soy, rice, or almond if lactose intolerant), nuts, beans, and legumes, which are the main components of the gluten-free diet. But watch out for marinades, sauces, broths, and gravies used with any of these fresh and unprocessed foods. These items often contain some form of flour or gluten as a thickener. In your own kitchen, cornstarch and arrowroot are safe alternatives for thickening sauces and stews.

Gluten-Free Grains, Flours, Seeds, and Starches
- Amaranth
- Arrowroot
- Buckwheat
- Cassava
- Corn
- Flaxseed
- Nut flours
- Millet
- Montina™
- Gluten-free oats (see following section)
- Quinoa
- Rice
- Sago
- Sorghum
- Tapioca
- Teff
- Wild rice

HOW DO OATS FIT IN?

Including gluten-free oats (approximately one-half cup of dry oats per day) is generally safe, improves compliance, and increases the nutritional profile of the gluten-free diet. Studies indicate that the vast majority (approximately 95 percent) of people with celiac disease can tolerate oats that haven't been cross-contaminated through exposure to gluten. Oats can become contaminated both through farming practices and by processing in a facility that processes wheat.

For oats to be considered gluten-free from the field (free of contamination from byproducts of wheat harvesting), they must be grown in a field that has been free of wheat, barley, or rye for five years. This is not an FDA requirement; the only requirement for oats is that they test to less than 20 ppm of gluten.

Oats can be highly contaminated with gluten-containing grains, so only oats labeled gluten-free should be used. There are a small number of people with celiac disease, however, who cannot tolerate the protein in oats. Make sure you check with your physician or dietitian to see if oats are safe for you. The introduction of oats should be delayed until all symptoms have resolved and all testing is back to normal before adding oats.

SAFE INGREDIENTS LIST

Prior to changes in the labeling law in 2004, consumers were confused about what ingredients might contain gluten. Now we know that the ingredients below are indeed safe to include in a gluten-free diet:

- Vinegar (except malt vinegar)
- Distilled alcohol
- Caramel color
- Citric acid
- Spices
- Monosodium glutamate
- Maltodextrin
- Mono- and diglycerides
- Artificial flavor and color
- Natural flavor and color

SO WHAT CAN I EAT?

Before FALCPA was passed in 2004 and partially implemented in 2006, label reading was a daunting task that left the consumer with more questions than food to eat. Wheat could be mysteriously disguised as a component of ingredients that required phone calls to manufacturers to solve the mystery. As we learned more from manufacturers, scientists, and the FDA, ingredients previously thought to contain gluten were discovered to be safe.

Vinegar was a questionable ingredient before FALCPA, and it still raises concern from time to time. It was once listed as an ingredient to avoid unless the manufacturer was contacted to verify ingredients. Then food chemist Don Kasarda, one of the leading experts in wheat biochemistry, reported that if the vinegar originated from wheat, the distillation process would remove the harmful gluten protein.

In addition, the FDA defines the lone term "vinegar" as being "apple cider" only. This opened up a welcome world of ketchup, mustard, and salad dressing to the celiac community! The bottom line with vinegar: you can consume all vinegars except malt vinegars.

Although FALCPA isn't perfect, it did greatly improve the consumer's chances of getting gluten-free foods. As noted above, according to FALCPA, any ingredient used in food that contains any of the top eight allergens (milk, egg, fish, shellfish, nuts, tree nuts, soy, and wheat) must be listed on the label in plain English. This can be done by putting the allergen in parentheses next to the ingredient, i.e. Durham flour (wheat) or under a "Contains" statement, i.e., Contains: milk, egg, wheat.

With FALCPA, wheat is no longer a hidden ingredient. If a product contains modified food starch, it is safe to use unless the word (wheat) is listed next to it or if a "Contains" statement lists: Wheat.

LEARNING TO READ LABELS

Thanks to FALCPA there are only six words to look for and avoid in an ingredients list of a food product not labeled "gluten-free":

- Wheat (listed in ingredients list or "Contains" statement)
- Barley
- Rye
- Malt (unless a gluten-free grain is named as the source, such as "corn malt")
- Oats (unless labeled gluten-free oats)
- Brewer's Yeast

EXCEPTIONS TO FALCPA

As useful as FALCPA is, it's far from foolproof in terms of the gluten-free diet. The law does not apply to:

- Barley (malt), rye, or oats
- Meat, poultry, and egg products (see USDA below)
- Over-the-counter or prescription medications
- Alcoholic beverages
- Ingredients added unintentionally that can cause cross-contamination

---

THE BEER, THE WINE, AND THE GLUTEN

The good news is that people with celiac disease can consume most alcoholic beverages. The distillation process eliminates the gluten peptides so distilled products are generally safe (watch for added flavorings in cocktail mixes, wine coolers, and flavored alcoholic beverages, etc.).

The bad news is that beer, ales, and lagers are made from barley and hops and are not distilled. Nevertheless, the gluten-free beer market is rapidly expanding with some adventurous flavors.

The other good news is that wines are also gluten-free. According to WineAmerica, the National Association of American Wineries, no wheat, rye, or barley is used in the processing, finishing, or "finings" of wine production in the United States.

Labels on Alcoholic Beverages
The labeling of major allergens in alcoholic drinks remains optional. In 2006 the Alcohol and Tobacco Tax and Trade Bureau (TTB) issued a proposed rule for the mandatory labeling of wines, distilled spirits, and malt beverages (TTB 2006). At the time of this writing, this rule has not yet been finalized.

BARLEY (MALT), RYE, OR OATS

Once you have scanned the label for the word wheat and it does not appear, the next step is to read carefully the list of ingredients for the words: barley, malt, rye, and oats. These ingredients will appear if they are used in a product and are not hidden as a component of other ingredients. (Manufacturers do not use barley to make modified food starch nor do they use rye to make dextrin.)

Although technically malt could be hidden under the term "natural flavoring," manufacturing practice is to list this ingredient separately. If the product contains malt, malt flavoring, malt syrup, or malt extract, it is not gluten free. If it contains maltodextrin, isomalt, maltose, or any other form that sounds like a chemical, it is a highly processed sugar/alcohol and is gluten free.

WHAT'S THE USDA GOT TO DO WITH GLUTEN?

The United States Department of Agriculture (USDA) regulates meat, poultry, egg products (meaning any dried, frozen, or liquid eggs, with or without added ingredients), and mixed food products that generally contain more than 3 percent raw meat or 2 percent or more cooked meat or poultry meat. Foods under the regulation of the USDA are not subject to FALCPA.

Nevertheless, 90 percent of manufacturers do comply with FALCPA voluntarily (to determine if a product is regulated by the USDA, look for the USDA seal). To help determine if a USDA product is following FALCPA, look for a "Contains" statement or other FALCPA-type allergen labeling on the label of a food product regulated by the USDA. This indicates voluntary compliance with FALCPA.

A QUICK CHILI DINNER
Turkey Chili with a Tropical Twist
From Susie Flaherty

Ingredients:
- 2 tablespoons olive oil
- 2 cups cooked shredded turkey or 1 pound ground turkey
- 1 clove garlic
- 1 medium onion, chopped
- 1 can (15 oz.) white pinto beans
- 1 can (15 oz.) red pinto beans
- 1 can (28 oz.) yellow tomatoes
- 1/2 cup diced mango (very ripe)
- 1 teaspoon cumin
- 1/2 teaspoon cayenne pepper
- 1 tablespoon chili powder
- dash of Tabasco sauce (or more if desired)
- 1 tablespoon brown sugar
- 1/2 teaspoon salt
- 1/2 teaspoon ground black pepper
- parsley or cilantro sprigs

If using ground turkey, heat 1 tablespoon of olive oil in large skillet or pot and cook turkey over medium heat until brown, remove from skillet, place in bowl and set aside. Heat 1 tablespoon of olive oil in skillet and add garlic and onion. Cook over medium heat until soft.

Return ground turkey to skillet or add shredded turkey to the onion and garlic. Add beans, yellow tomatoes, mango, spices, Tabasco sauce, sugar, salt, and pepper. Cook on low heat for at least 30 minutes. The longer it cooks, the better the flavor. Garnish with fresh sprigs or parsley or cilantro. Makes 4 to 6 servings.

MINI CORN MUFFINS
From Susie Flaherty

Ingredients:
- 1 cup yellow cornmeal
- 1/2 cup corn flour (masa harina)
- 1/2 cup gluten-free flour
- 1/4 cup brown sugar
- 1/2 teaspoon salt
- 1/2 teaspoon chili powder
- 2 teaspoons baking powder
- 1/2 teaspoon baking soda
- 2 eggs, beaten
- 2 tablespoons butter or margarine or other shortening
- 1 cup plain yogurt

Combine dry ingredients in large bowl and set aside. In smaller bowl, beat eggs, then add melted shortening and yogurt and mix together. Pour this mixture into bowl with flour and mix together until just blended. Fill mini-muffin tins two-thirds full with batter. Bake at 375 degrees until golden brown (about 15 to 20 minutes). Insert toothpick into muffin to test for doneness. If it comes out clean they are ready to eat! (Don't overcook or they will be dry.) They are best served hot from the oven. Makes 24 mini-muffins or twelve large muffins.

Serve your chili with the corn muffins and a garden salad for a delicious dinner anytime. But make sure your salad dressing is gluten-free and don't use croutons unless they are also gluten free.

GOOD NUTRITION ON THE GLUTEN-FREE DIET

Although there are many attractive gluten-free commercial products, place your emphasis on eating fresh and unprocessed food for the best results from your gluten-free diet. Planning ahead and making a menu for the week with a list of needed ingredients will help you stay on track when you're shopping.

Shopping in the perimeter of the store will help you hit the gluten-free areas (think produce, dairy, meats, eggs, fish, and seafood) and avoid processed and highly refined products. Watch out for lunchmeat and other processed meats as they may contain gluten as fillers. Other gluten-free items to shop for include plain rice, corn tortillas, dried beans and legumes, peanut butter and other nut butters, cooking oils (olive oil is a healthy option), and spices and herbs.

Many supermarkets now offer gluten-free breads, bagels, and pizza crusts in the frozen section. Purchase commercial gluten-free treats such as cookies, crackers, cakes, and pastries only occasionally as special treats. These products can be much higher in fat and caloric content than their gluten-free counterparts.

Remember: even though you're on a gluten-free diet, there are some special nutritional considerations. Work with your registered dietitian to have your iron, vitamin D, and vitamin B levels monitored. The gluten-free diet, without the enriched wheat products typically found in baked goods, means you must pay special attention to your nutrition.

Make sure you select a gluten-free vitamin supplement that meets 100 percent of the recommended daily allowances, including calcium. Generally, with exceptions just mentioned, if you eat a well-balanced diet, you'll get an adequate amount of most nutrients.

HOW CAN I TELL ABOUT MEDICATIONS?

FALCPA regulations that apply to foods do not apply to either over-the-counter or prescription medications. They do, however, apply to supplements such as vitamins and herbal supplements. Drug manufacturers are not required to disclose whether excipients (inactive ingredients) are obtained from one of the top eight allergens.

Check with a knowledgeable pharmacist to determine if the excipient is gluten free. You can also visit glutenfreedrugs.com, a website authored and maintained by a clinical pharmacist.

YES, YOU CAN LICK THAT ENVELOPE!

Gluten does pop up in some unlikely places—like soy sauce, licorice, and cream of crab soup. But one place that you won't find gluten is in envelope or stamp glue. According to the Envelope Manufacturers Association based in Alexandria, Virginia, there is no gluten used in the glue that is used on lickable envelopes.

The glue has a cornstarch base, with no wheat, rye, or barley used in the process. And according to the U.S. Postal Service, stamp glue (less than 2 percent of stamps sold are not self-sticking stamps) is gluten-free.

Some unlikely places where gluten might show up, however, include lipstick and other cosmetics. A recent survey by *Gluten-Free Living* analyzed lipstick ingredients. The magazine found that the most gluten you could ingest through lipstick daily would be approximately 1.4 ppm of gluten—well below the standard of 20 ppm established by the FDA in 2013.

Play-Doh® is another nonfood source that contains gluten. Young children can ingest Play-Doh or lick their fingers while using the modeling compound. There are gluten-free options in modeling compounds, as well as cosmetics and other nonfood items with gluten. If you have doubts about a product, contact the manufacturer or supplier directly, talk to your local celiac support group, and don't believe everything you read on the Internet!

WHAT'S CROSS-CONTAMINATION?

FALCPA applies to the ingredients in foods. It does not cover the possibility of contamination of products by contact from the milling, manufacturing, or transporting process. Allergen advisory statements or "may contain" statements are voluntary statements. The voluntary statements (i.e., manufactured in a plant that contains wheat) used in labeling products could indicate the potential or unintended presence of a food allergen.

Such statements may benefit and adequately inform food-allergic consumers, as there is no safe threshold of contamination for severe allergic reaction. This is not the case, however, for celiac disease patients, as the recent ruling passed by the FDA for labeling products gluten free allows a safe threshold level of less than 20 ppm. Ten milligrams of gluten is equivalent to less than one-eighth teaspoon of flour (see table below).

You don't have to avoid all products that carry voluntary advisory statements. Products with these types of statements are not necessarily contaminated. Consumers must also realize that products without voluntary advisory statements are not necessarily free of contamination.

FALCPA PART II

FALCPA required the FDA to develop and implement regulations for the voluntary labeling of gluten-free foods. Under the FDA regulations, the term "gluten free" refers to a food that includes the following guidelines:

- The food does not contain a prohibited grain, such as wheat, barley, rye, and triticale.
- The food does not contain an ingredient derived from a prohibited grain that has not been processed to remove gluten, such as farina, hydrolyzed wheat protein, and barley malt flavoring.
- If the food contains an ingredient derived from a prohibited grain that has been processed to remove gluten, such as wheat starch or modified food starch, use of that ingredient in the food product may not result in the food product containing 20 ppm or more of gluten.
- The food product contains less than 20 ppm of gluten.

WHY 20 PARTS PER MILLION?

Research shows that consuming products containing up to 10 mg (approximately one-eighth teaspoon of flour) of gluten per day is safe for most people with celiac disease. Our double-blind studies measured intestinal changes of three groups of celiac patients in remission (meaning good compliance with the diet, no symptoms, and no increased serum autoantibodies) who consumed 0, 10, or 50 mg of gluten daily. The group that ingested 0 and 10 mg showed no changes while the 50 mg group did exhibit intestinal injury typical of celiac disease.

The study evaluated the usual daily intake of gluten-free foods of the participants, which was 300 grams (a little more than 10 ounces). The following chart shows the amount of gluten an individual would be exposed to based on the gluten contamination levels in parts per million and the total amount of gluten-free foods consumed daily.

The contamination level is uniform throughout the food product. A person could eat a product contaminated up to 200 ppm and be safe if they only eat 50 grams (less than 2 ounces) of gluten-free products daily. A person could consume up to 300 grams of a gluten-free product containing 20 ppm, however, and remain safely below the level of 10 mg.

Gluten-Free Products Consumed

	50 g Gluten-Free Products	100 g Gluten-Free Products	200 g Gluten-Free Products	300 g Gluten-Free Products
200 ppm	10 mg	20 mg	40 mg	60 mg
100 ppm	5 mg	10 mg	20 mg	30 mg
50 ppm	2.5 mg	5 mg	10 mg	15 mg
20 ppm	1 mg	2 mg	4 mg	6 mg

WHAT'S WHEAT STARCH?

When protein, which is the source of the peptides that can trigger celiac disease, is removed from wheat, wheat starch (the highly refined carbohydrate food source) is what is left. There is some variation on the use of wheat starch in gluten-free products in Europe versus the United States. The bottom line, according to the FDA, is that products labeled gluten-free (containing less than 20 parts per million) that contain wheat starch are safe to consume on the gluten-free diet.

Now that you've got the basics of the gluten-free diet, it's time to set up your gluten-free kitchen and go shopping with Jules.

CHAPTER EIGHT

Gluten-Free Cooking and Dining

"Acorns were good until bread was found."
—Francis Bacon

IT'S JUST A DIET, RIGHT?

You've been diagnosed with celiac disease or gluten sensitivity. So it's no more gluten for you. Maybe you've tried some kind of diet before—either to lose weight or to feel healthier. You think: How hard can it be to give up gluten? Then you start to dig a little deeper into the details of the gluten-free diet. And you realize that this is not going to be a typical diet with easy-to-follow rules. There's a lot more to going gluten free than just cutting out bread, beer, and pizza. Your nutritional health is at stake.

Even though I have many years of expertise in treating patients with gluten-related disorders, I never dare to instruct my patients on the particulars of the gluten-free diet without assistance. Indeed, it's fair to say that the most powerful tool in the hand of any physician, the ability to heal, does not apply here. That capability rests in the hands of a knowledgeable dietitian. This health-care professional is the key figure for the proper treatment of celiac disease and other gluten-related disorders.

As I discussed in the previous chapter, following a gluten-free diet can result in certain mineral and vitamin deficiencies. Consult with your doctor or health-care practitioner to find a registered dietitian who can help you properly implement the gluten-free diet to maintain the best health possible.

But always remember that the most important person involved in your healing is you. After learning the basics of the gluten-free diet, you must learn to apply the diet in a wide variety of situations to keep yourself eating safely. These begin in your kitchen and travel with you to work and social situations that include dining out and traveling. If you're the parent of a child who has difficulty with gluten, you'll encounter a whole new set of challenges in the school setting.

I've consulted experts and friends of the Center for Celiac Research to help guide you safely through the maze of gluten-free eating at home or on the road. In this chapter, we'll teach you how to set up a gluten-free kitchen and find substitutes for your old gluten-filled favorites.

We'll also walk you through what it takes to eat safely in the restaurant of your choice, whether it's down the block or on another continent. With the right attitude and information, eating gluten-free can become an exciting adventure into a healthier life for you and your family.

ADJUSTING TO YOUR DIAGNOSIS

I've seen how overwhelming the diagnosis of celiac disease or gluten sensitivity can be. There's a strong sense of loss that accompanies the inability to enjoy your favorite foods. Food and the act of eating pervades all aspects of our lives as social human beings—whether it's going out on a date, meeting for a business lunch or hosting a family dinner, which is why limiting our food choices can feel so devastating.

While everyone experiences some form of initial disbelief, grief, or even depression, each person's unique concerns are different. I remember one young patient who couldn't believe she wouldn't be able to eat Girl Scout cookies any more. At the other end of the spectrum, people diagnosed late in life often find it quite difficult to change the basic eating habits of a lifetime.

That's why it's so important to feel truly satisfied with your personal version of gluten freedom. Eating nutritious and satisfying gluten-free food is the key to first regaining, and then maintaining, your health and positive attitude. Be patient with yourself as you begin this new lifestyle and keep in mind your long-term goal of renewed health and vitality. Each day will get easier . . . and tastier!

CREATING YOUR GLUTEN-FREE HAVEN

You've grasped the basics of the gluten-free diet from Chapter Seven. The next step in your gluten-free revolution is setting up your gluten-free kitchen and learning how to make simple gluten-free dishes and baked goods. Once you can prepare your own food safely and deliciously at home, the challenges of living with celiac disease or other gluten-related disorders will be far more manageable.

Think of your home, and especially your kitchen, as your safe, gluten-free haven. No matter what else is happening in your busy life, always keep delicious gluten-free food and snacks available in a clean, uncontaminated environment. It's easier than you think. Knowing that you can always find a safe meal in your own home will help ease the inevitable feelings of insecurity and loss that come along with your diagnosis.

There are some excellent books and websites by experts on learning to live without gluten (see Resources section at end of book). I asked one of these experts, Jules Dowler Shepard, to tell us how to set up this gluten-free haven.

I first met Jules when she visited the Center for Celiac Research after she moved to Maryland. She came to the Center for help in managing her celiac disease. I met Jules first as a patient, and then as a gluten-free author and baker. Trust me, her chocolate chip cookies taste just like the real "gluten-filled" thing!

I recommend her books and recipes to all my patients who are just starting the gluten-free diet. She brings a unique perspective as a patient with celiac disease, a gluten-free cooking expert, and a former lawyer who uses her advocacy skills to lobby for transparency in gluten-free labeling laws. Using Jules's suggestions, let's get started on setting up your new kitchen.

THE BAG, THE BOXES, AND THE NOTEBOOK

It's time to clean out, reorganize, and fully stock your new gluten-free kitchen. The tools that Jules recommends for the first step of clearing and cleaning out are a large trash bag, two cardboard boxes, and a notebook. Old food goes into the trash bag, food with gluten and questionable items go into separate boxes, and your list of food favorites and suggestions goes in the notebook. Grab a friend and head to the pantry with your bag, boxes, and notebook.

Have your friend go through the items and read the expiration dates. Toss anything that's older than two years into the trash bag. Consuming expired food items is never worth the risk. And that goes for that food in the side door of your refrigerator as well, but we'll get to that later.

After you toss the expired food, read the labels again to see which of the remaining items contain gluten (see list in Chapter Seven for names of possible gluten-containing ingredients and explanation of labeling laws). Products with gluten go into the box, and items without gluten go back into the pantry. Write down your favorite gluten-containing products in the notebook. Set aside products that you're unsure about after you list them in your notebook.

Before returning the gluten-free items to the cupboard, wipe down the shelves and doors, making sure that all traces of crumbs and flour are gone. Jules recommends that you wipe down the countertops, stove, sink, and other kitchen surfaces at the same time.

CLEANING OUT THE CRUMBS

While you're spring-cleaning your kitchen, look around for items that might need to be replaced to avoid cross-contamination. One item that will have to go is the old toaster; you'll need a new one for your gluten-free kitchen. It's impossible to clean out all those crumbs in all those tiny crevices.

Indeed, when I clean out my toaster, no matter how many times I shake it down those toasted crumbs keep coming out like magic. It reminds me of Mary Poppins's magic carpetbag with endless objects emerging from it! Donate or segregate your old toaster for gluten-filled items only, and buy a new one for your gluten-free baked goods.

As you create your gluten-free haven, keep in mind that mixing bowls, skillets, and pots and pans are not a source of cross-contamination if you follow good basic hygiene rules: wash in between uses by hand with hot soapy water or in the dishwasher. Pay special attention to the rims of pots, skillets and lids to catch all those gluten crumbs if you're cooking products containing gluten.

If your pots and pans are particularly scratched, or if the non-stick coating is compromised, it's time to replace them anyway. Gluten contamination from those deep scratches is just another reason not to use them anymore.

Here's another great tip I got from Jules: Whenever you can, use condiments that come from squeeze bottles and keep a few empty squeeze bottles on hand. Make your house a "one-dip" house with the rule that silverware and spatulas only go into a jar once. Once that knife with peanut butter meets bread or crackers containing gluten, those crumbs can end up back in the jar on the second dip. Don't take the risk!

As you go through the favorite food items on your list, make sure that you know the latest on gluten-free food labeling laws (see Chapter Six). If you're still unsure about an item, whether it's food, medicines, or vitamins, contact the manufacturer for accurate information.

GIVING UP THE GLUTEN BOX

Now that you have your remaining items sorted into gluten-free (in the pantry), gluten-full (in a box), and questionable (listed in your notebook), what comes next? This depends on the makeup of your household and whether other family members intend to continue consuming gluten-containing products or not. Everyone in your home can eat the gluten-free foods you'll be bringing home or making, but not everyone can eat the gluten-full foods.

With Jules's suggestions, you can create a separate section in the pantry—or you can use clearly labeled plastic boxes—for gluten-containing foods. Even a person with celiac disease living alone could use a separate area to keep foods with gluten for family and friends who are not on a gluten-free diet. How about an old-fashioned breadbox?

If no one in your household will be eating those gluten-filled foods, donate what you can of the unopened items to a local food bank or shelter. This way you'll feel doubly good about beginning this gluten-free journey!

For those favorite gluten-filled items you can't eat anymore, don't worry. In time, you'll find suitable replacements for almost all of your favorites. In nearly twenty years of practicing medicine in the United States, I've seen the portfolio of gluten-free goodies grow from a few in the mid-1990s to the thousands of products now available.

Now gluten-free items are found not just in specialty food stores, but also in mainstream supermarkets and big-box stores, too. But remember, our dietitian cautions against eating too many highly processed gluten-free food substitutes, which often contain high levels of fat and sugar to compensate for improved flavor and texture. Eating fewer processed foods is a great nutritional goal, so let this goal guide your food purchases on the gluten-free diet.

GLUTEN IN THE ICEBOX?

An ingredient in many processed foods, gluten shows up in the most unlikely places. Now that you've thrown out your old food and segregated your gluten-free items from your gluten-full items in your pantry, it's time to tackle that icy last frontier: the family refrigerator.

Review the list from Chapter Six with foods that might contain gluten and also watch out for processed meats of any kind, including pork products (sausage, hot dogs, and spare ribs in barbecue sauce); imitation seafood or fish products; all sauces or gravies, including soy sauce and steak sauce; and other marinades or sauces; and certain condiments (ketchup and mustard are okay).

That side door is a place that can hide a lot of not-so-obvious gluten-filled favorites, so read the labels carefully and act accordingly. List in your notebook any favorites that you had to toss, along with questionable items.

Freezer items can also contain gluten. The obvious ones are frozen dough or bread and baked goods, pizza, pies, and cakes. Also watch out for certain kinds of ice cream, such as chocolate chip cookie dough or ice cream with candy and other processed foods. In many cases when it comes to gluten and processed foods, when in doubt, throw it out.

REPLACING YOUR OLD FAVORITES

Now you're ready to look at your list of favorite and questionable foods. Items from that favorite food list could include foods with ingredients you don't recognize as well as items with gluten. Let's tackle the questionable foods first.

If you can't figure it out from the label, a quick call to customer service is often the easiest way to get answers. Many company websites also have e-mail addresses listed for customer inquiries. The customer service representatives will either clarify the gluten-free status of their products to your satisfaction, or they will not.

If they don't answer your gluten-free, cross-contamination, or ingredient questions, or if they are unclear, then, as Jules says, "that's your answer." You'd better toss it in the trash bag.

If, on the other hand, they clarify their labels for you, explain their cross-contamination–avoidance procedures, and make an effort to address your concerns, there's your answer. There are too many good, safe gluten-free foods out there to take risks or give your food dollars to companies that haven't taken the time to make safe gluten-free foods their priority.

The next step Jules advises is to look over the favorite items you've listed in your notebook that contain gluten. What would you really miss? It's time to find that gluten-free substitute. Better yet, says Jules, find a recipe and make it yourself! Cooking at home can be easier than you think, it's safer, and it's nearly always cheaper.

Celiac disease community or Internet support groups, gluten-free Facebook pages and blogs, and the knowledgeable staff at your local market all have favorite product suggestions. With the gluten-free items you already have, reorganize your pantry and make space for the new items to replace your old gluten-filled favorites.

RESTOCKING YOUR KITCHEN

The next step is shopping! Take the lists you made in your notebook, as well as the product recommendations you've collected, and head to the stores and online for the many gluten-free options available.

Find a knowledgeable clerk to tour the aisles with you at the local supermarket. You'll be amazed at the array of gluten-free choices, especially all the baked goods and cookies and snacks for occasional treats. Make sure to visit several health-food and specialty grocery stores, which feature a wide variety of items along with helpful advice.

Whatever venue you visit, ask for a guide who specializes in the store's gluten-free product line. Nowadays, most large chain supermarkets have gluten-free sections clearly labeled to make it easier to find gluten-free products.

The local farmer's market or community co-op is often a great source, not only for fresh fruits and vegetables, but also for meats, fish and seafood, dairy products, and specialty items like honey and jams. At the local supermarket, it will probably take several trips for you to become familiar with the gluten-free items in your local supermarket. But don't get discouraged. Remember that much of what you might already buy for basic meal preparation and snacks is naturally gluten-free.

Depending on your needs, there are several ways to approach meal planning and shopping as you stock your gluten-free haven. To replace your favorite foods, with your list in hand, check off all the snacks, treats, staples, and other items that need gluten-free replacements. Pick the ones you want to include in your gluten-free cupboard and add them to your shopping list.

PREPLANNING YOUR MEAL PREPARATION

I like to cook and enjoy reading cookbooks and planning meals (see Chapter Nine). Much of the cuisine of Southern Italy, where I am from, is naturally gluten-free with fish, meat, fresh produce, great dairy products, and the world's finest olive oil. So cooking gluten-free meals is something I learned early in life.

To develop your skills, buy some good gluten-free cookbooks or develop menus and meal plans from the many good Internet sources. If you belong to a support group, talk to members about their favorite menus and food sources. If you don't, now's a great time to join. A little preplanning into your family's mealtime will make it an easier and more enjoyable time for all. If you develop meal plans, add these items to your shopping list.

Whether you are a carnivore, vegan, or somewhere in between, stock your refrigerator, freezer, and pantry with the basic protein sources: meats, fish, seafood, eggs, tofu, legumes, and beans. Next add fruits and vegetables along with dairy and soy products.

Check with a registered dietitian about the best procedure to follow with dairy and soy products when you first begin a gluten-free diet. Celiac disease can sometimes trigger secondary lactose intolerance, which will usually disappear after the intestine heals. Some people suffer from primary lactose intolerance, which is a genetically determined lack of lactase, the enzyme that breaks down the carbohydrate called lactose in dairy products. If you have this condition, you can take lactase pills or eat and drink lactose-free dairy products.

Nonperishable snacks to keep on hand include nuts and nut butters, dried fruit, popcorn, gluten-free granola or protein bars, and gluten-free pretzels and potato chips (for occasional treats). Keep dinner staples in your pantry, including rice, gluten-free pasta, quinoa, corn tortillas, and other gluten-free basics such as gluten-free bread or wraps (or a gluten-free flour or mix to make your own) for sandwiches.

The all-purpose flour that Jules has developed is my top choice for every recipe that calls for flour. With it, you can make any gluten-free food from sandwich bread to tortillas, or birthday cake to fish and chips.

Developing a relationship with the gluten-free expert at your local supermarket and health-food or organic store will make a world of difference in your gluten-free shopping experiences. If you know a product is good, ask your supermarket or health-food store to put it on the shelves.

BAKING WITH JULES: THE ICING ON THE GLUTEN-FREE CAKE
By Jules Dowler Shepard

To round out your new gluten-free kitchen, you need gluten-free baking supplies. You might be thinking, "What? I can't bake! I've never baked anything in my life!" Don't panic. It's easy enough to get started with the right tools, and the results will be far more rewarding than anything you'll buy on the store shelves. Baking your own fresh, hot cookies, cakes, and breads is one of the greatest rewards of eating gluten free.

Baking gluten free once meant reinventing the wheel in each person's kitchen. Luckily, that's not the case anymore. You don't have to purchase 15 different gluten-free flours, a binding agent with a crazy name like xanthan or guar gum, and any number of new cookbooks. Time and the patient experimentation of others before you have made gluten-free baking easier than ever before.

Many people find themselves contending with other food restrictions like dairy, egg, nuts, or other ingredients. Baking at home allows you to tailor those ingredients, increase the nutritional value, and make fresh food to suit your family's tastes.

With that in mind, add these basic supplies to your first shopping list:

- Gluten-free all-purpose flour (one that already includes a binder like xanthan or guar gum)
- Baking powder
- Baking soda
- Sugar (white and brown) or unrefined sugar alternative like coconut palm sugar

- Molasses, maple syrup, agave nectar, and applesauce for sweetening
- Butter or nondairy alternative suitable for baking and/or shortening
- Spray baking oil (without flour—check label)
- Baking pans: muffin tins, loaf pans, 8x8 and 9x13 baking pans, two cookie sheets, pie plates, cake tins, and parchment paper
- Rubber spatulas and wire whisk
- Large mixing bowl
- Mixer (countertop mixers can be more versatile than hand mixers)

If you already have a recipe you love—maybe grandma's famous casserole or the cookies your kids devour—use all-purpose gluten-free flour to substitute for wheat flour. Follow the manufacturers' directions for substitutions, as some brands require more moisture in a recipe.

If you use all-purpose flour that doesn't already contain a binder like xanthan or guar gum, you will need to add this as well. Some all-purpose gluten-free flours act very much like regular all-purpose wheat flour and require little, if any, recipe tweaking to make your old favorite recipes gluten-free.

The first flour you buy may not be the perfect one for you, so keep experimenting. There are now so many choices. If you notice an odd aftertaste in your recipes, steer clear of bean flours or other ingredients in the mix that might affect the taste. If your recipes are crumbly or gritty, use a mix made with more refined starches that have had more of the bran, hull, and fiber removed during processing. With an all-purpose flour you like, you'll be amazed at how easy it is to bake your own great tasting gluten-free goodies.

Visit www.julesglutenfree.com for additional recipes and gluten-free baking tips.

If you don't like a product, tell the store buyers so they can make better buying choices for their customers. If it really tastes terrible, take it back to the store and ask for a refund.

EMBRACING GLUTEN FREEDOM

With your gluten-free haven fully stocked with equipment, food, and baking supplies, it's time to heed the words of Gusteau from the movie *Ratatouille.* He reminds us that anyone can cook, but only "the fearless can become great chefs." So it's time to summon up your courage and go back to your notebook. Review the recipes, dishes, or treats that you thought you had to give up when you went gluten free.

Armed with your meal plans and recipes from cookbooks and the Internet, get creative in the kitchen, and don't be afraid to experiment. You're bound to have failures, but the culinary world (just like the scientific world) is replete with stories of discovery from failed recipes and experiments.

Many people worry about preparing safe food on the gluten-free diet. But soon the same people are saying that going gluten-free has been such a gift for them and their families: a gift of good health, of renewed energy and vitality, and of family unity.

Jules and I have both seen families grow closer through their new gluten-free lifestyle. They bake holiday cookies together and share favorite family foods with friends and neighbors. Family pizza night can become a time when everyone gets their hands in the dough and makes the pizza from start to finish, instead of simply calling the delivery guy.

As Jules can confirm, living gluten free can be a really remarkable transformation to good health and happiness in so many ways—if you let it. So after you follow the steps above, put on your new gluten-free chef's hat and apron, relax, and enjoy the haven of your new gluten-free zone with your family and friends.

Two Recipes From Our Favorite Gluten-Free Baker
GLUTEN-FREE CHOCOLATE CHIP COOKIES
From Jules Dowler Shepard

Ingredients:
- 8 tablespoons (1/2 cup) butter or nondairy alternative (Earth Balance® Buttery Sticks)
- 8 tablespoons (1/2 cup) shortening (or Earth Balance® Shortening Sticks)
- 1 cup firmly packed light brown sugar
- 1/2 cup granulated cane sugar
- 3/4 teaspoon sea salt
- 2 teaspoons gluten-free vanilla extract (Neilson-Massey® Madagascar Bourbon Vanilla)
- 2 large eggs (or reconstituted Ener-G egg replacer or applesauce)
- 1 teaspoon baking soda
- 1/2 teaspoon baking powder
- 2 1/2 cups Jules Gluten-Free™ All Purpose Flour or other brand
- 12 ounces semisweet chocolate chips or dairy-free chocolate chips, peanut butter chips, white chocolate chips (available dairy-free!), M&Ms, or a mixture

Bring the butter and shortening to room temperature and then beat together with sugars until light and fluffy (several minutes). Mix in the vanilla extract and eggs until combined. In another bowl, whisk together dry ingredients. Gradually stir these dry ingredients into the sugar mixture. Stir in chips and nuts, if so desired.

Scoop dough into a container (metal, if possible) and cover tightly. Refrigerate or freeze until very cold (overnight is ideal). Preheat oven to 350 degrees (static) or 325 degrees (convection). Drop by measured tablespoonfuls onto a cookie sheet lined with parchment paper, at least 1 inch apart. Bake for 8–9 minutes, or until the tops are lightly browned. Let them stand 5 minutes before removing them to cooling racks.

Makes approximately 60 cookies.

GLUTEN-FREE SCONES WITH "WHATEVER YOU LIKE!"
From Jules Dowler Shepard

What you add to this delicious scone recipe is up to you (or what you have on hand).

Some folks have asked for chocolate chip scones, others for berry scones, still others for cinnamon-raisin. The thing I like about my scone recipe is that it is perfectly suited to any of these twists, and its light, moist, semisweet crumb makes it the ideal recipe for breakfast, tea, or dessert.

As with many of my baking recipes, yogurt is a key ingredient for sustainable moisture, but it shouldn't be overlooked for flavor as well. There is just no reason to use plain yogurt in a baking recipe! Take advantage of the opportunity to liven up your creations by experimenting with yogurt flavors (piña colada yogurt, anyone?), and try some of the great new coconut or soy yogurts out there if you are avoiding dairy.

Whatever your twist, be sure to try this amazing recipe, and you'll wish you'd discovered it years ago. It has become my favorite go-to-breakfast-in-a-hurry recipe, as it takes only 5 minutes to whip it up and 12 minutes to bake. It almost takes all the fun out of our crazed morning routine of scrambling to get the kids to the bus stop on time. OK, even though breakfast is ready, my kids still somehow wind up racing to the corner with untied shoes and unzipped book bags!

Ingredients:
- 2 cups Jules Gluten-Free™ All Purpose Flour or other brand
- 1/4 cup granulated cane sugar
- 2 teaspoons baking powder
- 1/2 teaspoon baking soda
- 1 teaspoon cinnamon
- 4 tablespoons butter or nondairy alternative (Earth Balance® Shortening Sticks)
- 2 large eggs (or egg substitute like 2 tablespoons flaxseed meal steeped in 6 tablespoons warm water)

- 3/4 cup yogurt, dairy, or nondairy (So Delicious® Vanilla, flavored, or plain coconut yogurt)
- 1/2 cup peeled and diced fresh peaches*, fresh or frozen berries, raisins, chopped nuts, chocolate chips, or whatever else you have on hand
- cinnamon sugar to sprinkle on the tops before baking

Preheat oven to 400 degrees. Whisk together all dry ingredients in a large-bottom bowl. Cut butter or shortening into the dry ingredients using a pastry cutter or two knives. Stir in the eggs and yogurt. Gently fold in fruit, nuts, chocolate chips, etc.

Turn dough out onto a clean counter or pastry mat dusted with gluten-free flour. Pat into a rectangle to a thickness of about 3/4 inch. Cut into triangles with a bench scraper or butter knife. Place onto a parchment-lined baking sheet and brush the tops with butter or nondairy substitute (optional) and sprinkle with a premade cinnamon and sugar mixture. Bake for 8–10 minutes, just until the tops are lightly browned. Do not overcook!

(*Note: If you're using fresh cut fruit like peaches, the dough will be much wetter and more difficult to pat out and cut. If the dough is very wet, simply dollop large spoonfuls of dough onto the parchment-lined baking sheet for "drop biscuit" scones. Bake as directed above.)

Makes approximately 12 scones.

GLUTEN-FREE EATING AWAY FROM HOME

There's nothing like having a great meal with family and friends in the comfort of your own home. But in my opinion, dining out in a great restaurant comes in a pretty close second. For many people diagnosed with gluten-related disorders, especially celiac disease, dining out safely becomes a challenging experience many people want to avoid.

Statistics show that after receiving a diagnosis of celiac disease, many patients restrict their dining out activities because they're afraid of eating gluten inadvertently. A 2007 survey of Canadians with celiac disease showed that 81 percent of the respondents avoided restaurants all or most of the time. The danger lies not only in consuming foods that contain gluten, but also when eating gluten-free foods prepared on surfaces or in dishes that have been used for foods containing gluten (called cross-contact or cross-contamination).

So how do you overcome these obstacles and eat safely no matter what the setting? You've probably figured out by now that proper planning ahead of time is one answer. Another key is to find good recommendations and reliable information, which is getting easier all the time. With the Internet revolution and mobile phone applications, you have information on gluten-free menus and restaurants at your fingertips (see Chapter Thirteen). And remember to check with celiac disease support group members for their favorite dining spots.

For many chain restaurants and private establishments, the words celiac disease and gluten-free are no longer mysterious medical terms. The National Restaurant Association listed gluten-free cuisine number five in its annual culinary forecast of "What's Hot in 2014."

More than 1,300 chefs across the United States named locally sourced meats and seafood and locally grown produce (all naturally gluten-free) as the top two items on their "hot" list for 2014. Number one in top trends for "Starches/Side Items" was nonwheat noodles and pasta, followed by quinoa and black and red rice. Gluten-free cuisine was listed second in the culinary themes, and gluten-free beer made the "Alcoholic Beverages" category at number four.

Gluten-free dining is here to stay, but the responsibility for safe eating still rests primarily in your hands. The most important thing to remember when dining out is to be assertive and ask questions of the waitperson, the chef, or the manager (see box on opposite page).

Your food safety is of paramount importance, and most restaurants are eager to make sure you have a great dining experience. If the restaurant personnel are unable to answer your questions to your satisfaction, vote with your feet and find another place to eat.

"WANT FRIES WITH THAT GLUTEN-FREE BURGER?"

Pam Cureton, our registered dietitian whom you met in Part One, stresses how important it is to ask the right questions to ensure you're getting a gluten-free meal. Things to ask include:

- What are the ingredients used to prepare my dish? (This is the most important question!)
- Will my food be prepared on a "clean" cooking surface and in "clean" containers using "clean" utensils? (In other words, is it free of flour contamination or contact from foods with gluten?)
- Will my French fries be cooked in the same fryer, pan, or oil that is used for cooking foods with gluten, such as flour-coated chicken, fish, or vegetable pieces? (Ask for fries to be cooked in dedicated fryer or clean pot.)
- Are the hamburgers and hamburger buns cooked together on the same surface? (Ask for hamburger or other grilled meats to be cooked in clean pan or aluminum foil on top of grill.)
- Does the marinade or sauce used on my meat or fish contain soy or teriyaki sauce, which usually contains gluten? (You can bring your own gluten-free soy sauce, or ask for a different sauce that does not contain gluten.)
- Will my gluten-free pasta be cooked in fresh water with clean utensils?
- Has my chicken or fish been dusted with flour before pan-frying?

Many restaurants train personnel in serving people with food allergies. The Food Allergy and Anaphylaxis Network provides material about food allergies (including material on celiac disease) for restaurant workers. http://www.foodallergy.org/files/WelcomingGuests2010.pdf).

DO YOUR HOMEWORK

Before you step into a restaurant, make sure you know the basics of your gluten-free diet. A knowledgeable dietitian can teach you what foods to avoid, the less obvious sources of gluten, and where contamination might occur. Read labels on prepared foods (cream soups and mashed potato mixes are two examples of gluten in prepared foods), watch cooking shows, and talk to experienced cooks who really know about the gluten-free diet.

Many restaurants with gluten-free menus list their dishes and ingredients on their websites, which makes a good first step to an enjoyable gluten-free dining experience. Once you've picked out a place, calling the restaurant ahead of time is a good second step. Try to call at off-hours, which are usually 2 to 4 P.M. (it's a good idea to eat at off-hours too if possible) and ask to speak to the chef directly. Let the chef know what your dietary restrictions are and ask if the restaurant can handle your needs. The chef might have a creative way to celebrate your special occasion or evening out.

When you arrive at the restaurant, make sure the staff knows that you have a medical condition with certain dietary restrictions. It might help to practice the explanation of your dietary needs before you arrive, especially if you are anxious about speaking up, or you're in a big group. Your dietitian can help with this. "I am on a medically required diet," and "I have a severe reaction to wheat," are two useful phrases.

We advise our patients to use the term "wheat" instead of gluten or celiac disease. Although it's changing rapidly, many food servers still aren't familiar with the word "gluten." Use the term "wheat" and walk them through the steps in the food preparation where wheat might be used. Some examples are adding croutons or bread sticks to your salad, grilling your gluten-free hamburger bun on same grill as wheat buns, or frying your gluten-free food in the same fryer used for breaded or floured foods.

In addition to asking about any wheat or flour included in any food preparations, also ask if malt vinegar, barley, or rye is used. Most knowledgeable consumers might know where rye and barley would show up in food preparation, but gluten is a less-obvious ingredient in restaurant food preparation. Wheat flour can show up in some pretty surprising and unexpected places!

Whether you have celiac disease, gluten sensitivity, or a wheat allergy, another great phrase is "food allergy." Even if the term is strictly speaking incorrect (you should know by now that celiac disease and gluten sensitivity are not food allergies), it's a buzzword that gets the food server's attention, making him or her take special care with your meal.

SAY IT WITH A DINING CARD

Some of our patients use "dining out cards," also called "cook cards," which list dietary restrictions that can be given to the chef (see Appendix 1 for Dining Card website). You can download dining cards in various languages from the Internet, or do what one of our globetrotting patients did: She put her dining restrictions on the back of her business card. She just hands that to the waitperson and asks that it be given to the chef.

Many restaurant workers are trained in preparing meals for people with dietary restrictions or food allergies and are more than willing to help. If you get the sense that the waitperson doesn't understand your needs, ask to talk to the manager, or better yet, speak directly to the chef.

Even if a restaurant has a published "Gluten-Free Menu," you still must cover the bases with your server or the manager. You must make sure that they know how to prevent cross-contamination by making your meal only with gluten-free ingredients and delivering it to the table gluten-free as well.

Of course, if it's a very busy meal service and a chaotic kitchen, it might be harder to communicate your needs. If you have any doubt about whether you will receive a safe meal, trust your instincts, and always talk to the chef. If you feel like the chef or manager is not responsive or doesn't understand your needs, don't take the risk and go elsewhere to eat. (This is why it's always good to have backup food with you such as gluten-free granola bars, fruit, or nuts.)

When you have a specific dish or meal in mind, first ask about the ingredients and then about the method of preparation. Ordering simple dishes, or dishes with sauces on the side or omitted altogether, will improve your chances of getting a safe gluten-free meal. Anne Lee, registered dietitian with the Schär company (an international manufacturer of gluten-free products), calls it "naked food." (For tips on more adventurous eating, see "Working with the Chef" by Bob Levy of Bob and Ruth's Gluten-Free Dining and Travel Club in this chapter.)

In a busy restaurant, dishes can get mixed up or delivered by different servers. When you get your meal, ask the waitperson or server, "Is this my gluten-free meal?" to make sure you've got the right dish. If something is obviously wrong (for example, croutons on the salad or burger served with a bun), call the waitperson back and ask for a replacement. Keep the dish at your table while your replacement meal is being prepared. That way, the restaurant staff will not be tempted to just remove the items containing gluten, but will replace the entire dish.

After you've enjoyed your delicious gluten-free meal, make sure you show your appreciation to the chef and the wait staff. Making people happy with food is the goal of most chefs and restaurant workers, but it's always nice to be acknowledged. And spread the word among the celiac and gluten-free community when you have a great dining experience. As you eat out safely and successfully, you'll gain confidence in your ability to eat safely and deliciously no matter where you are.

LEARN TO SPEAK THE LANGUAGE TO EAT SAFELY

Knowing the ingredients in any dish is the key to eating out safely in any situation. This is a partial list of cooking terms that might mean wheat is an ingredient in the preparation of your dish.

Watch Out for This Menu Term: Wheat Alert!

Au Gratin	Browned topping of breadcrumbs and grated cheese
Béchamel	White sauce made by thickening milk with roux
Beef Wellington	Filet steak coated with paté and duxelles (mixture of cooked mushrooms, onions, shallots, and herbs) wrapped in puff pastry and baked
Beurre Manie	Butter and flour mixture used to thicken sauces
Cordon Bleu	Dish with meat (chicken, veal, or ham) and cheese dipped in bread crumbs and sautéed
Dusted	Lightly sprinkled with a dry ingredient, such as flour
Encrusted	Flour or breadcrumbs used to bind ingredients to food item
Farfel	A soup garnish made of minced noodle dough
Fricassee	A stew of meat or poultry in gravy, usually thickened with flour
Fritter	Food dipped into batter (flour and liquid ingredient) and fried
Gnocchi	Dumplings made from a paste of flour, potatoes, and egg
Pan Gravy	Sauce made from meat juices and often thickened with flour
Marinade	May contain soy sauce
Meuniere	Dusted with flour and sautéed in butter
Raspings	Very finely grated stale bread
Roux	Butter and flour mixtures used to thicken sauces and soups
Scallopini	Thinly sliced meat dredged in wheat flour, cooked in small amount of oil until tender, and covered with tomato or piccata sauce
Soy Sauce	Sauce made from fermented soy beans and sometimes roasted wheat or barley
Teriyaki Sauce	Contains soy sauce
Tempura	Shrimp, seafood, chicken, and vegetables coated in flour-based batter and fried
Veloute	Sauce thickened with roux, often used as base for soups, stews, fricassee
Welsh Rarebit	Cheese sauce made with ale or beer served over toast or crackers

TAKING IT ON THE ROAD

Bob and Ruth Levy of Bob and Ruth's Gluten-Free Dining and Travel Club escort people all over the world to experience top-notch travel and dining experiences. Kenya, Dubai, China, Scotland, South Africa, and Australia are just a few of their destinations. Diagnosed with celiac disease in 1995, Bob views his condition not as a hindrance, but as an opportunity to explore a whole new world of spices, herbs, ingredients, and cooking methods from countries such as Mexico, Thailand, Korea, Brazil, China, India, and Italy.

I first met Bob in the late 1990s. Since then, I've had the pleasure of sharing in his gluten-free travel adventures. He's always generous in sharing his tips for getting great gluten-free food, along with his great travel tales. I thought it was impossible to make good bread with just rice flour, but Bob proves me wrong in this account from a trip to China.

IS THAT BREAD REALLY MADE FROM RICE?
By Bob Levy

In most regions of China, bread made isn't a mainstay of the diet. We certainly didn't expect to have it on the menu during our first riverboat cruise on the Yangtze River. But one afternoon, as we were relaxing on the ship's deck, a slight, elderly man stepped out of a small Chinese junk from alongside our boat. He disappeared into the ship's hold.

Several hours later, he emerged from the galley carrying his specialty: bread made from black and white rice flour. With a wide grin on his face, he broke open the bread to show us the purple bread inside. It was fantastic—moist, spongy, and delicious!

Visit bobandruths.com for more information on gluten-free travel adventures.

WORKING WITH THE CHEF

Whether he's in China or Catonsville, Maryland, Bob is passionate about great food. He does his utmost to ensure that his customers get a great dining experience no matter where they go. His greatest enemy is what he calls "conference food," the bland fare often served to people with food allergies epitomized by a plate with boiled chicken, a baked potato, and steamed broccoli.

I've known Bob for many years. I appreciate how this kind of food offends his highly developed culinary sensibilities. He is convinced, and rightly so, that people with celiac disease and other gluten-related disorders have the right to enjoy high-quality cuisine. Bob is also convinced, that with a little patient persuasion, people with celiac disease and gluten-related disorders can get a great meal by working directly with the person who prepares it.

GETTING AROUND THE WORLD GLUTEN-FREE
By Bob Levy

When you're traveling around the world, it can be a lot more challenging to eat safely with a gluten-related disorder. That's the bad news. The good news is that many countries, especially European ones, are more familiar with the gluten-free diet; they provide delicious gluten-free substitutes in grocery stores and restaurants. Going gluten-free around the world can be a joyful event with lots of new taste sensations. So pack your common sense, throw in some gluten-free snacks, and let's go!

The Airport
Packing food for your trip is a very personal choice, but there are several guidelines that will make it easier as you move from home to your final destination. Remember that you can't take liquids of any more than 3 ounces through any U.S. airport, so even your bottle of water will be confiscated at the security gate.

You can buy water and usually some kind of gluten-free snack in the airport kiosks. Some people like to take cereal in crush-proof containers for a quick breakfast or snack. Fruit and vegetables can be tricky to take internationally because of custom regulations, but within the continental United States, you can bring food onto your flight. One gluten-free expert takes her leftover homemade Pad Thai on long flights to carry her through meals with no problem.

If we're going to be on a long flight, and most of our flights are long, Ruth makes sure that we have some favorite snacks on hand. Whenever possible, visit a grocery store or local market to pick up some fruits and veggies to supplement your diet while you're on the road.

The Plane Trip

When you're flying to an international destination, always order a gluten-free meal well in advance to eat during your flight (most domestic airlines don't offer free meals in the continental United States). When you check in, verify that you'll be getting a gluten-free meal. And then make sure you have your backup food accessible in your carry-on bag. For those of you who are parents, traveling anywhere when you have a gluten-related disorder is kind of like traveling with small children—you always have to be prepared with food on hand.

Be prepared to be disappointed or pleasantly surprised with the gluten-free meal you get on the plane. I often find the entrees to be questionable and sometimes downright unpalatable. The fruit, salad, or side dish, however, might be just fine.

The Hotel

Before we book the hotel for our groups, we have extensive discussions with the manager and executive chef to make sure that our diners will be eating safely. Be your best advocate for a good gluten-free experience in your hotel restaurant.

If possible, talk to the manager or chef beforehand about your dietary restrictions so the restaurant staff will be prepared when you come down for breakfast. Book a room with a refrigerator (and a kitchen, too, if you can) and buy produce and dairy products at the local market.

The Cruise Ship

If you're using a travel agent to make reservations for tours, cruises, or resorts, be skeptical when they tell you not to worry about your gluten-free diet. I've heard too many horror stories of people telling me that they were assured their dietary restrictions were listed on their reservations only to find that the dining options were not gluten-free.

Whether it's a cruise or destination resort, don't worry, you won't starve. Salad fixings, grilled meats, seafood, vegetables, and fresh fruit are always on the table. Some cruise lines offer minimal gluten-free options, but in most cases, minimal is the key word. Remember that those tasty soups (think flour as thick-ener) and sauces, breaded foods, cakes, pies, and desserts won't be available to you. But relax, we know this will only get better. It's just a matter of time.

Before you step onboard, contact "Special Services" of the cruise line. Tell them you are on a gluten-free diet and request a meeting with the executive chef to be scheduled as soon as pos-sible after you board the ship to depart. Have them confirm your meeting by phone or e-mail.

Before you sign on the dotted line for a resort, make sure you have a chat with the executive chef or food and beverage director to ensure a safe dining experience while on vacation. I don't consider my gluten-free diet as a life sentence to bland and boring food. I view it as an adventure every day, and it can be a very rewarding adventure indeed. Bon voyage and bon apétit!

Gluten-Free Summertime Favorites
MOUTHWATERING CRAB CAKES FROM THE CHESAPEAKE BAY
From Maureen Murphy, Sudlersville, Maryland

Ingredients:
- 1 pound Chesapeake Bay crab meat (backfin or lump)
- 3/8 cup plain gluten-free breadcrumbs
- 1/2 cup mayonnaise
- 1 tablespoon wet mustard
- 1 tablespoon "Old Bay" seasoning
- 1 egg
- 1 tablespoon sugar
- 2 tablespoons olive oil

Combine all ingredients except crabmeat and olive oil and mix thoroughly. Gently mix in crab, which has already been cooked and "picked" from the shell. Form into patties, wrap each patty in waxed paper, and refrigerate for one hour. Heat olive oil over medium heat and fry crab cakes for several minutes, until lightly browned on both sides. Makes approximately six crab cakes.

THREE SIMPLE SUMMER SALADS
From Mary Frances McFadden, Jackson Township, New Jersey

Using the same dressing for a base, you can create three different salads with a bit of mixing and matching. Feel free to get creative once you get the basics!

BASIC SALAD DRESSING
Ingredients:
- 1/2 cup water
- 1/4 cup apple cider or white vinegar
- 1 teaspoon white sugar
- 1/4 teaspoon salt
- Pinch of black pepper
- 1 teaspoon celery seed
- Fresh herbs of your choice (parsley, rosemary, thyme, dill, or other)

CUCUMBER SALAD

Peel one or two cucumbers and slice into rounds. Use English cucumbers or peel if skin is tough. Place in bowl. Thoroughly mix or shake ingredients for dressing and pour over cucumbers. Chill well in refrigerator before serving.

COLE SLAW

Peel and grate two carrots and one-half green cabbage and place in bowl. Pour dressing over bowl and refrigerate.

SPINACH SALAD

This one is slightly more complicated, but well worth the effort if you're a bacon fan. Fry three strips of bacon until crisp and remove from pan. Remove all but one teaspoon of bacon fat from the pan. Add dressing* and bring mixture to a boil. Pour dressing over one pound of freshly washed and dried spinach. Crumble bacon and sprinkle on top of salad.

*Herbs are optional.

Now that you've learned the basics of the gluten-free diet, let's travel to Southern Italy for a delicious gluten-free meal featuring some of my favorite recipes.

CHAPTER NINE

Dinner with Dr. Fasano

"How can I describe it? Good food is like music you can taste, color you can smell. There is excellence all around you. You need only to be aware to stop and savor it."
—GUSTEAU FROM *RATATOUILLE*

LEARNING TO COOK ALONG THE AMALFI COAST

When most people think about the Costiera Amalfitana–the Amalfi Coast in Southern Italy–they think about the scenery. The 30-mile drive from Sorrento to Salerno is one of the most spectacular scenic drives in the world. With towns perched on the cliffs and the Mediterranean Sea sparkling below, it's a favorite international tourist destination.

In 1997, the United Nations Educational, Scientific and Cultural Organization added the Amalfi Coast to its list of World Heritage Sites, citing its exceptional cultural and natural scenic values. Now the world is committed to preserving the architectural and scenic wonders contained in the familiar landscape of my childhood.

In the town of Positano, a fishing fox is carved into the bas-relief panel over the doorway to the bell tower of the Church of Santa Maria Assunta. This thirteenth-century relic provides the perfect symbol for the Amalfi Coast, where people enjoy the best of both worlds from the sea and the mountains.

On the city walls of the marine republic of Amalfi these words are inscribed: "The day that the Amalfitan people go to Paradise, it will be a day just like any other day." The sentiment expresses the idea that the residents of the Amalfi Coast already live in "paradise."

Now that I live and work in the United States, I've learned how to enjoy crabs steamed in spicy Old Bay and fresh Maine lobster. For our gluten-free Italian "banchetto," however, I have chosen the fresh food from the sea and the farms of Southern Italy to create the perfect blend for our banquet.

My mother is a fantastic cook, and I've adapted some of her recipes here. In the Campania region we enjoy a wide variety of seafood, meats, and fresh dairy products. Have I mentioned that the famous mozzarella buffalo cheese, "Mozzarella di Bufala," comes from the water buffaloes of Campania?

When you combine these ingredients with the vegetables and fruits of the region, you have a heavenly cuisine that is naturally gluten free. And these meals are always combined with the appropriate wine that helps to blend the dishes as we move from one course to another at the right pace. I've given you a few suggestions here for pairing our dishes with appropriate wines. With very few exceptions, drinking beer would be a sacrilegious breach of proper Italian cuisine!

Even in its drinking etiquette, dining in Southern Italy is naturally gluten free. After this Italian meal, you won't feel "stuffed" but content with the marvelous combination of fresh ingredients and flavors. Please note: Unless otherwise specified, the quantities listed serve approximately four adults–very generously!

ARE YOUR RECIPES DIFFICULT?

Every cook likes to achieve success with his or her first attempt at a new recipe. So although you can gauge how difficult a recipe will be for you, I've created a rating system for the recipes as follows:

One fork ⅃ – *easy*
Two forks ⅃⅃ – *medium difficulty*
Three forks ⅃⅃⅃ – *more complex*

"ANTIPASTO" OR APPETIZER
"Insalata Caprese" or Capri Salad
Wine Selection: Fiano di Avellino is a strongly flavored white wine from
Campania. Wine historians trace this grape back to the ancient wines of
the Romans and Greeks.
Recipe Rating:

The region of Italy where I come from grows fantastic tomatoes—drenched with the southern summer sun. This is an extremely simple summer dish that makes a very satisfying first course. And if you've never tasted soft mozzarella cheese, you're in for a real treat. It's "delizia!" Many residents of Campania grow basil and other herbs year round. And of course, with its ancient olive trees, Campania is the undisputed champion producer of the best extra virgin olive oil in the world.

This salad is named for the Island of Capri, where Roman emperors including Augustus and Tiberius traveled to escape from the pressures of life in Rome. Perhaps they found some tranquility in the famous sea cave, the "Grotta Azzurra," or Blue Grotto, while dining on the regional delights.

Ingredients:
- 2 large fresh tomatoes
- Fresh basil
- 1/2 pound Mozzarella di Bufala di Campania (soft mozzarella cheese)
- 1 tablespoon extra virgin olive oil

Using a bread knife, slice tomatoes fairly thickly in 1/2 inch slices. Select soft mozzarella cheese packaged in water so it remains moist and flavorful (don't use the hard mozzarella used for pizza topping). Carefully slice the mozzarella cheese in 1/2 inch pieces. Place the mozzarella on top of the tomato and add a sprig of freshly washed basil on top.

At this point, you can drizzle with 1/2 teaspoon of olive oil and serve. Or if you are preparing ahead of time, refrigerate on individual plates and drizzle olive oil on top just before serving. Use one generous tomato slice per serving.

"PRIMO PIATTO" OR FIRST COURSE
"Risotto Al Funghi" or Mushroom Rice Risotto
Wine Selection: Negroamaro is a rustic red wine native to Puglia in south-eastern Italy. The grape is mainly grown in Salento or Italy's "heel."
Recipe Rating: ⚞⚞⚞

Although rice risotto is typically a Northern Italian dish, risotto is a great addition to the gluten-free diet. You can use vegetables other than mushrooms, such as zucchini, summer squash, eggplant and tomato, or a combination of vegetables. Don't be afraid to experiment. It's the secret to great cuisine as well as new scientific discoveries!

Preparing a smooth, creamy rice risotto can be a tricky business. The first step is the proper selection of the rice. I recommend Super-fine Arborio rice from Italy, which has a naturally high starch content to give it that snap when you bite into it.

Making risotto is a little like making pudding or watching a toddler. If you ignore it for just a minute to attend to something else on the stove, someone or something will quickly get into trouble. To make a smooth risotto, the basic procedure is creating a flavorful vegetable base, adding rice, and adding broth in small quantities.

Ingredients:
- 1 1/2 cups uncooked Superfino Arborio rice
- 1 large white onion, chopped fine
- 4 cups shitake mushrooms
- 1/2 glass (4 oz.) white wine
- 2 cubes gluten-free vegetable bouillon
- 2 tablespoons extra virgin olive oil

Prepare bouillon by adding 4 cups of boiling water to 2 vegetable bouillon cubes in a medium size saucepan. Turn the heat as low as possible on the bouillon to keep it simmering.

The next step is the preparation of the vegetable base. Using a sharp knife, cut the ends off of the onion, remove top layer and discard if necessary. Slice onion in half lengthwise and chop fairly fine. Heat a deep saucepan to medium heat (you'll cook the risotto in this pan). Heat the olive oil to sauté the onion.

When the oil is hot (you can tell by adding a small piece of onion first to see if it "jumps"), add onion and cook just until golden brown. Add the wine and cook on low for an additional 5 minutes. Wipe the mushrooms clean with a mushroom brush or paper towel and chop them finely. Add them to the saucepan oil and sauté until soft.

Now it's time to add the rice to the mushroom base. Stir the rice into the mushroom mixture and stir for 2–3 minutes. The next step is adding the broth. This is where true skill comes into play to make the perfect risotto. You must add the broth slowly, 1/2 cup or so at a time, so the rice can absorb the broth after each addition.

After you add the broth, continuously stir over low to medium heat. This will take about 30–40 minutes depending on the rice. You might not need to add all the broth. Start tasting the rice when you've added most of the broth. The risotto is done when the texture of the rice is a little firm with a smooth texture overall. Risotto is best eaten right off the stove—but please serve in bowls or plates—not from the pot! Serves four.

SIDE DISH OR VEGETARIAN OPTION FOR FIRST COURSE
"Parmigiana di Melenzane" or Eggplant Parmesan
Wine Selection: From the coast of Tuscany, Morellino di Scansano is another wine from a variety of red grapes from central Italy called Sangiovese or "blood of Jupiter" grapes.
Recipe Rating: ❘❘❘

This is one of my mother's favorite dishes. The main attraction of this gluten-free melanzana parmigiana is the fantastic blend of homemade tomato sauce, the sharp taste of eggplant, the smooth taste of mozzarella cheese, and the layer of parmigiana (parmesan) cheese on top. Making the sauce takes a little time, but believe me, it's definitely worth the effort.

My mother prepares melanzana parmigiana with the traditional egg and flour layer coating the eggplant. I've adapted the more traditional recipe, which comes directly from the Bourbon royal family tradition. (Make sure you use hard mozzarella cheese that is not packaged in water and not the soft mozzarella used in Insalata Caprese. It's the same mozzarella cheese that you would use for making pizza or lasagna.) This version is made without breadcrumbs or flour, a gluten-free variation popular in Campania. You'll be amazed at how satisfying this dish is without the extra gluten-filled layer.

Ingredients:
- 10 teaspoons extra virgin olive oil for sauce, plus oil as needed for frying the eggplant slices
- 1 large red onion, finely chopped
- 2 cans of 32 oz. peeled tomatoes
- 2 medium or three small eggplants
- 1 pound hard mozzarella cheese
- 1 cup freshly grated parmigiana cheese
- Sprig of fresh basil
- Pinch of salt
- My mother's secret ingredient (see below*)
- Brown paper bag from supermarket
- 11" x 17" baking dish

Sauce Preparation:

Using a sharp knife, cut the ends off of the onion, remove top layer and discard if necessary. Slice onion in half lengthwise and chop fairly fine. Heat a large skillet or frying pan to medium and add 10 teaspoons of olive oil. When the oil is hot (you can tell by adding a small piece of onion first to see if it "jumps"), add onion and cook until almost brown.

Add peeled tomatoes, bring to boil and turn heat down to low. Add a pinch or more of salt and my mother's secret ingredient* (a 1/2 teaspoon of sugar, or honey if you prefer). Cook very gently over very low heat for 1 1/2–2 hours to boil the water off of the tomatoes. Stir occasionally. It should be pretty thick. Chop the basil coarsely and stir into the sauce.

Enjoy the wonderful aroma as you get ready for the next step! You can use this time to prepare the other dishes in our gluten-free Italian feast. After the sauce is ready, you can move on to cooking the eggplant and assembling the dish.

Eggplant Preparation:

Wash the eggplant and dry with a paper towel or clean dishcloth. Cut open brown paper bag and place on top of cookie sheet or large cutting board on counter close to stove (trim paper if needed). Using a sharp knife carefully cut off both ends of the eggplant and discard. Slice the eggplant in 1/2 inch pieces. Heat a large skillet or frying pan (you can use the same one that you made the sauce in, but rinse it out and dry it thoroughly first) to medium high.

When the pan is hot, add about 4 tablespoons of olive oil and evenly distribute to cover bottom of pan. When the oil is hot, carefully add eggplant slices 3 or 4 at a time. Turn eggplant once, cooking until it is soft and lightly browned on both sides. Lift slices gently out of the pan with tongs, drain along the side of pan to remove as much oil as possible, and place on brown paper bag to drain. Repeat until eggplant is cooked.

Now you're ready to assemble your dish. Preheat the oven to 350 degrees. Slice mozzarella about 1/4–1/2 inch thick. Dot the bottom of the baking dish with tomato sauce. Add your first layer of eggplant, topped with mozzarella cheese. Try to match the sizes of eggplant slices with sizes of mozzarella cheese (it must be the laboratory scientist in me—but I like to make them uniform if possible!). Cover slices with tomato sauce and sprinkle parmigiana cheese on top. Add another layer and continue as above. At this point, you can refrigerate the dish for cooking later.

Otherwise, bake in oven for 20–25 minutes until cheese is melted and just starting to turn very lightly golden brown. (Be careful not to overdo it!) Serve on individual plates and garnish with basil. Bellissimo e buonissimo!

"SECONDO PIATTO" OR SECOND COURSE (FOR MEAT EATERS)
"Salsiccie all'agrodolce" or Spicy Italian Sausages
Wine Selection: Chianti is the classic red wine of central Tuscany. An authentic chianti must contain at least 80 percent of Sangiovese grapes.
Recipe Rating:

Ingredients:
- Spicy Italian sausage (one for each person)
- One 7 oz. jar of sliced, sweet red pepper hulls
- One 8 oz. can tomato paste

Heat a large skillet or frying pan. Add sausages and cover halfway with water. Cook over medium heat until sausages are about halfway cooked (15–20 minutes). During the process, prick the sausages with a fork to release the juices from the sausage. While sausages are cooking, place the sweet peppers in a colander and rinse off with water. Add the peppers and the tomato paste to the sausages. Cook for another 10–15 minutes, stirring occasionally, until the sauce thickens. Cut the sausages in 2-inch pieces, making sure that they are cooked all the way through.

"SECONDO PIATTO" OR SECOND COURSE (FOR NONMEAT EATERS)
"Salmone al Forno" or Salmon with Lime and Sesame Seeds
Wine Selection: Fumé Blanc, from the Napa Valley in California,
is a crisp, dry white Sauvignon blanc.
Recipe Rating: ￥￥

If you come from the South of Italy, it's part of your childhood experience to love and respect the sea and what it can provide to you and your family. Fish is an integral part of our everyday life. I began fishing with my grandfather when I was five years old. I remember helping him cast the net out and being impatient about pulling it out of the water to check the variety of fish trapped in the cul de sac.

Even if salmon is not a Mediterranean fish, it is highly appreciated in the culinary art of Campania. And some research studies suggest that the omega-3 fatty acids found in salmon may lower the risk of heart disease, and could protect against symptoms of depression, dementia, cancer, and arthritis.

Ingredients:
- 1 1/2 to 2 pounds salmon (wild caught preferred with skin on)
- Juice from 2–3 limes
- Olive oil
- Sesame seeds

Preheat oven to 350 degrees. Line a baking sheet with parchment paper and coat very lightly with olive oil. Place the salmon, skin side down, on parchment paper in pan. Squeeze the juice of 2–3 limes into bowl. Use pastry brush to coat salmon with lime juice. Coat the top of the salmon with sesame seeds. Bake for 15–20 minutes. Fish is done when it flakes easily with a fork. Be careful not to overcook!

"DOLCE" OR DESSERT
Tiramisu served with Insalata di Frutta
Wine Selection: A distinctive dessert wine from the volcanic islands off the
northeast coast of Sicily, Malvasia delle Lipari has a strong fruity flavor
and distinctive light orange color.
Recipe Rating: ⅋⅋ – ⅋⅋⅋

Although the origins of tiramisu, which translates to "lift me up" in Italian, are controversial, almost everyone agrees that this modern classic tastes delicious. This version is made with gluten-free ladyfingers, available from the Schär company.

Please note that this dish also contains raw eggs as a traditional method of preparation. My dietitian would be very distressed with me if I didn't tell you to take precautions if you choose to use raw eggs. Young children, pregnant women, and those with food sensitivities or compromised immune systems are advised not to consume raw eggs. In Italy, we like the old-fashioned method of leaving them uncooked. Otherwise, cook the egg yolks with the sugar over a double boiler for about 10 minutes, stirring constantly until the mixture is thick.

Ingredients:
- 1 1/2 cup white sugar
- 7 egg yolks
- 1 cup brewed espresso or strong coffee
- Two 8 oz. containers mascarpone cheese
- 2 teaspoons vanilla flavoring or brandy or dessert wine
- Two 8 oz. packages gluten-free ladyfingers
- 1/2 cup limoncello (Italian lemon liqueur)
- 11" x 17" baking dish

Separate the eggs, reserving the whites (see Chapter Eleven for a delicious dessert recipe to use up the extra egg whites). Beat the egg yolks with a whisk or mixer on medium speed, gradually adding sugar and continuing to beat eggs until the mixture is light yellow. Add mascarpone and vanilla flavoring and beat till smooth. Stir in the espresso or coffee until smooth.

Warm 6 cups of water with 1/2 cup of limoncello on the stove over low heat. Dip one package of the ladyfingers in the warm water and limoncello mixture and quickly place in layers in the baking dish.

Spread half of the cheese mixture over top of the ladyfingers. Dip the second package of ladyfingers, place on top of the first layer, and spread the remaining cheese mixture over the top. Cover tightly with plastic wrap and refrigerate for 4 hours or longer. Before serving, dust the top of the tiramisu with cocoa powder.

For some nutritional punch, serve with a fresh fruit salad of seasonal cut-up fruit (pineapple, apple, strawberries, melon, kiwfruit, etc.) or your favorite berries. Makes eight servings.

I hope you enjoy this delicious and easy authentic dinner from Southern Italy. In the next section, the real experts—patients and parents who implement the gluten-free diet every day—offer their insights.

PART THREE

Gluten Free for Life

CHAPTER TEN

Pregnancy and the Gluten-Free Diet

"A grand adventure is about to begin."
—Winnie the Pooh

LEARNING FROM THE EXPERTS

Feeding people on the gluten-free diet, whether they live in New Zealand, China, or Uruguay, can be a complicated business. But once you get comfortable with the foods that you can and can't eat, it does get easier—as our experts below will tell you.

Many of us think we don't have the time to cook nutritious and satisfying meals because of our fast-paced lifestyle. As a home cook trained in the delicious cuisine of Southern Italy, I disagree with that assessment. My grandmother, who was a fantastic cook, used to say, "A meal that takes more time than 20 minutes to cook is not good enough to be put on the table."

Of course there are some exceptions to this rule (for example, my tomato sauce takes several hours to achieve perfection), but if you cook with simple and fresh ingredients, you can prepare many healthy and nutritious meals for yourself and your family in a short amount of time.

But how do we implement a good dietary lifestyle to manage celiac disease once it is diagnosed? It's intuitive that the challenges and opportunities are different depending on the age of the individuals.

In Part Three, with the guidance of patient-experts and others, I focus on the gluten-free diet lifestyle throughout the different stages of life from conception, pregnancy, childhood, family life, and teenage and college years, to the "golden age" of the elderly. For people with gluten-related disorders, living an enjoyable, healthy, and balanced life on the gluten-free diet is easier than you might think.

CELIAC DISEASE AND REPRODUCTION

Of all the things that I have learned about celiac disease, one of the most surprising is how it can manifest in every system in the body. One of the most underrecognized effects of undiagnosed celiac disease is what it can do to the reproductive systems of both women and men.

In women, undiagnosed celiac disease can result in delayed menarche, early menopause, and an increased number of miscarriages. Swedish scientists determined a decrease in fertility prior to diagnosis, with an improvement in fertility in patients with celiac disease who were following a gluten-free diet. Although there is limited research on men and the effects of celiac disease on their reproductive system, some studies support the findings that couples with unexplained infertility have a higher rate of celiac disease than the general population.

While I have a lot of experience in treating patients with these challenges, I believe the best way to view what celiac disease can do to you in pregnancy is through the eyes of a person with first-hand experience. So I enlisted the aid of one of my patients, Dr. Anna Quigg. A psychologist and mother of two, Anna has celiac disease and can offer a unique perspective and some knowledgeable insights about keeping healthy during pregnancy.

TIMING OF THE CELIAC DIAGNOSIS

There are two possible scenarios to consider: A woman who has already been diagnosed with celiac disease is planning for pregnancy or a pregnant woman discovers she has celiac disease. While many considerations are the same for both patients, there are unique challenges for women who are diagnosed with celiac disease while they are pregnant.

Anna was faced with the first scenario when she and her husband planned to conceive their first child. At that time, her celiac disease was already well managed by the implementation of the gluten-free diet. She had developed a close relationship with her gastroenterologist and dietitian, which proved very beneficial during both her pregnancies.

FOLLOWING THE GLUTEN-FREE DIET

Anna's first step in planning for conception was to ensure that she was correctly following the gluten-free diet. She underwent testing for micronutrient deficiencies and appropriate levels of minerals and vitamins.

We know that a suboptimal implementation of the gluten-free diet can be enough to create intestinal damage that impairs nutrient absorption without causing clinical symptoms. So simply because you feel healthy and have no symptoms, it doesn't mean that your celiac disease is well controlled. If you have celiac disease, get tested for nutrient levels before you get pregnant.

Once the lab tests show good nutritional status and the lack of anti-tTG antibodies (confirming good compliance with the gluten-free diet), you're ready to plan for conception. Although pregnancy in a woman with celiac disease shouldn't be considered especially high risk, it's a good rule to be closely monitored throughout pregnancy to make sure you maintain proper micronutrient levels and normal anti-tTG antibodies. Even patients who are very savvy about the gluten-free diet may be exposed to cross-contamination during pregnancy.

The fact that pregnancy itself may cause symptoms such as fatigue, nausea, abdominal pain, and iron deficiency—all symptoms that can reveal the relapse of celiac disease—complicates the matter. This was the case for Anna during her second pregnancy, when she tested positive for anti-tTG antibodies during a routine test by her gastroenterologist.

A prompt diagnosis of celiac disease relapse can prevent devastating consequences that may lead to miscarriage or neonatal malformation. In the case of Anna, she had to embrace the Fasano Diet (see Chapter Five) because a clear source of gluten cross-contamination wasn't found.

WHEN THE CELIAC PANEL IS POSITIVE
By Anna Quigg

One worry you might have during pregnancy is: What if I get "glutened?" Sometimes people know right away when they've inadvertently ingested gluten because of immediate symptoms. It might not seem like it at the time, but this can be a real blessing because you've learned to avoid that food the next time around.

If you do ingest gluten, a single incident of gluten contamination is unlikely to decrease your nutritional status enough to affect your pregnancy. The stores of nutrients in your body are transferred through the placenta to the baby before being circulated throughout the mother's body. In this way, nature cares for the child first.

If symptoms of gluten in your diet are present over a longer period of time, with elevated anti-tTG antibody levels or prolonged gastrointestinal symptoms, you might begin to feel fatigued. You might also experience headaches, gastric distress, or other symptoms as the body pulls nutrients to sustain the pregnancy. If your lab results from routine testing suggest gluten reexposure, work closely with your dietitian to identify cross-contamination sources and eliminate gluten from your diet (see Chapter Five).

During the first trimester of my second pregnancy, I had been feeling poorly the entire time. When my fatigue and gastrointestinal distress didn't diminish in the second trimester, my doctor ordered a panel of celiac tests. When I found out I had an elevated tTG level, I was overwhelmed with negative feelings. I became even more careful about following the gluten-free diet. I knew the importance of providing the best possible nutritional environment for my child. I never cheated!

> When you have this overwhelming flood of emotion, paired with raging pregnancy hormones, having this strict diet to follow is the best therapy in the world. It gave me something to do. Action calmed my frayed nerves. I researched recipes, made meal plans, and went grocery shopping. I began feeling better quickly. With every meal I prepared, I knew I was protecting the health and development of my baby.

FIRST TRIMESTER

Changes in dietary habit sometimes occur during pregnancy: think about nighttime cravings for hot fudge sundaes, chocolate chip cookies, or sweet and sour chicken. This may increase your risk of exposure to unusual foodstuffs and the chance of cross-contamination. Along with your regular prenatal visits with an obstetrician, make sure you're under the care of a registered dietitian and a gastroenterologist to help you stay on the right track during your pregnancy.

This is particularly important during the first trimester, when pregnancy-related symptoms that can mimic celiac disease occur more frequently. To alleviate these symptoms, Anna relied on breakfast as her best meal of the day. "I loved to load up on eggs, bacon, and hash browns."

Applesauce, bananas, gluten-free toast, cheddar cheese, and Jell-O also helped Anna's stomach feel settled. For other women, starting the day with yogurt and fresh berries or gluten-free cereals or oats (see Chapter Seven) might be the best choice.

Anna also discovered that eating small snacks every few hours seemed to be the secret to keeping nausea at bay. She was unable to last more than two hours, after which she would become light-headed and nauseous.

She kept a variety of gluten-free cereal bars close by at her home, in her car, and at her workplace. She took her own toaster to the office to fix gluten-free toast with peanut butter. The bottom line for Anna during her first trimester was to eat whatever she could tolerate as often as she could, to take her prenatal vitamin every day, and drink as much water as she could. Anna suggests that you nap whenever you can and try to remember that this unsettled feeling will soon go away.

ANNA'S FAVORITE PICK-ME-UP
By Anna Quigg

FRESH GINGER TEA

In the early stages of pregnancy, I needed to have something in my stomach most of the time. Along with snacks and small meals, I drank fresh ginger tea, which helped settle my stomach. The great thing about this recipe is you can adjust it to your own taste for sweetness (the honey) and spice (the ginger).

To make fresh ginger tea, peel and finely grate a piece of ginger root. Use about 2 teaspoons of ginger, more or less depending on your taste.

Pour 8 ounces of boiling water over the ginger and let it steep for 3–4 minutes. You can take the ginger out at this point or leave it in (it will sink to the bottom). Add 1 teaspoon or more of honey to taste.

I like it hot, but you can also drink it chilled. In hot weather, you can pour some sparkling water into ice cube trays and add some grated ginger. Drop the cubes into your favorite cool beverage to help settle the stomach.

GLUTEN-FREE PEANUT BUTTER COOKIES

One of my favorite sweet treats during that ravenous time in my second trimester was a homemade peanut butter cookie. The recipe is so quick and easy, it's a snap!

Ingredients:
- 1 beaten egg
- 1 cup sugar
- 1 cup peanut butter

Mix well and drop on parchment paper on a cookie sheet. Bake at 375 degrees for 10 minutes until golden.

Now go put your feet up and enjoy your homemade cookies with some ginger tea!

SECOND TRIMESTER

This is the period of pregnancy when you're more at risk for excessive weight gain due to increased caloric intake and to the quality and quantity of food ingested. An increased appetite during the second trimester is generally excused by the fact that you are "eating for two." This also can contribute to a problem of increased weight. Remember that eating for two actually requires only about 500 more calories per day.

Of course, it's important to try to maintain a healthy diet with fresh fruits and vegetables, lean meats, seafood, fish, and dairy products (or alternative sources of protein including eggs, tofu, nuts, beans, and legumes) and gluten-free grain products. I've learned from Anna and other patients that it's often easier to eat well during the second trimester than in the first, when morning sickness might manipulate your appetite.

During Anna's second trimester, she loved to eat everything. She had an appetite she called "superhuman." As expected, her challenge was feeding those cravings, which included strong cravings for meat, while maintaining a healthy diet and weight.

She also developed a sweet tooth, and wanted cakes, pastries, and cookies. She craved bakery-type things that cost a lot more in the gluten-free version, which can add an economic challenge along with the nutritional one.

THIRD TRIMESTER AND DELIVERY

The baby grows exponentially during the third trimester. Your appetite might decrease as the baby rapidly gains weight and takes up more space in your midsection. Just as in the first trimester, eating small but frequent snacks is an easier way to tolerate your food.

If you've already experienced pregnancy and delivery, you know that when you're going into labor is not the time to have a relaxed or extended conversation with the hospital staff about your dietary needs. Even though the hospital stay to deliver your baby can be rather brief, ask questions beforehand to make sure that appropriate gluten-free meals will be available to you in hospital. During the prenatal tour of the facility, ask to speak with the staff dietitian, the nurses, and anyone else who will be attending to you when you arrive to deliver your baby.

Once you've packed the hospital bag that sits behind your front door, make sure to have plenty of gluten-free snacks in there just in case your gluten-free meal isn't available at the birthing center—or it really isn't gluten-free. Indeed, even though Anna had talked beforehand to everyone who would listen about her dietary needs, she found her hospital-issued food lacking in the quantity and quality department.

The first meal that she received was pancakes (sigh), eggs, and sausages. Although she notified the staff immediately that she couldn't eat the pancakes and that the other items were no longer safe to eat because of cross-contamination, it took nearly an hour before she was served a meal that was truly gluten-free.

As typically occurs in many hospital facilities, Anna filled out special diet cards every day with the details of her diet. Most of the time, the meal was delivered without gluten, but also without taste.

Anna quickly learned that the best remedy was to bring a small cooler from home with her favorite foods. She also kept a bag of nonperishable treats nearby as well, and her husband made restocking trips during her stay at the hospital. Take a tip from Anna and order meals from nearby restaurants for your family and friends to deliver as a good alternative to hospital food during your stay.

BRINGING BABY HOME

If you have a partner with good culinary skills who knows about preparing gluten-free meals, you'll be all set. You'll walk in with

your baby and be welcomed with a superb meal. But wait a minute
. . . even if your partner is a culinary genius, your partner will also
be sleep-deprived and walking around in a daze during the weeks
postpartum! If on the other hand, your significant other is not a
gourmet chef, your best option is to accept the help that your family
and friends will offer.

The way that Anna dealt with her postpartum experience was
to prepare a short list of her favorite foods and where to buy them.
People are often willing to go an extra mile for a new mom. And if
they are close friends, chances are they already know all about your
gluten-free food requirements.

But if they're new to the gluten-free world, keep it simple in
explaining your dietary needs. For example, Anna told people
that meat-and-potato meals were often the easiest to prepare. She
reminded her friends that rice, fruits, vegetables, meats, seafood,
fish, and dairy are all okay on the gluten-free diet.

A good trick of Anna's that made her homecoming more enjoyable was to prepare gluten-free foods ahead of time. She did this in
her second trimester when she had a lot of energy. She froze meals
to eat after she and the baby came home from the hospital. As you
and your baby adjust to family life again after your hospital stay,
those extra meals can go a long way in easing the transition.

Anna's final words of advice to new mothers are: "Remember to
enjoy this precious time with your new baby. Spend as much time
as you can with your little one and let other people feed you, very
carefully, as often as possible."

GLUTEN SENSITIVITY AND PREGNANCY

Of course, Anna's experience is strictly related to her celiac disease
condition. For women affected by gluten sensitivity, we have no
current evidence that gluten exposure during pregnancy has any
harmful consequences other than the reappearance of symptoms.

The fact that gluten sensitivity doesn't cause intestinal damage or malabsoprtion of nutrients and micronutrients suggests that
gluten exposure wouldn't have the same negative consequences

to the growing baby as it does in celiac disease. Because gluten sensitivity is a relatively recently described condition on the spectrum of gluten-related disorders, however, we need to generate additional information and data to establish the real impact of accidental or voluntary exposure to gluten in pregnant women affected by gluten sensitivity.

YOU'VE JUST BEEN DIAGNOSED WITH CELIAC DISEASE— AND YOU'RE PREGNANT

Developing celiac disease while you're pregnant presents additional challenges to both the mom and the baby. This scenario is not unusual, since we know that pregnancy is one of the conditions that can trigger celiac disease in genetically predisposed women.

Several hypotheses have been developed to explain why this happens. One possibility is changes in the makeup of the microbial community in the gut. (For more details on gut microbial community, see Chapter Fifteen). I believe that the change in microbiota that typically results during pregnancy from hormonal changes could be a trigger that pushes a genetically predisposed woman from latent celiac disease to active celiac disease. We need more research to fully establish this connection.

When the obstetrician's suspicion is raised by the onset of typical celiac disease symptoms, a prompt diagnosis through routine screening (blood tests and endoscopy if blood tests are positive) may help avoid complicated outcomes. These are the lucky cases.

Conversely, the absence of symptoms or symptoms confused with the typical changes experienced during the first trimester may increase the risk of malabsorption of micronutrients that are key to the proper development of the fetus. Above all, a deficit in folic acid is the most cause for concern in the area of malabsorption maladies.

PROTECTING THE EMBRYO'S DEVELOPMENT

During the embryo's development, several organs go through major maturation changes. The nervous system begins as a single sheet of cells that form a sort of flat plate. This single sheet must then fold itself into a tube as the brain develops above and the spinal cord develops below. Folic acid determines the correct folding and closure of the sheet into the tube.

Folic acid deficiency during this crucial part of the embryo's development may delay or prevent this folding and closure of the tube, which is not compatible with life. If folic acid deficiency occurs later during pregnancy, the folding of this sheet may already have occurred. The closure of the tube will remain incomplete, however, which leads to the condition known as spina bifida. Depending on the severity of the incomplete closure, a baby born with spina bifida may have problems with walking and bladder control.

I remember one case involving a nurse from our hospital. During her pregnancy, she developed severe anemia that was treated with iron supplementation. She also experienced folic acid deficiency, which was treated with vitamin supplements. Despite these nutritional deficiencies, no one thought to screen her for celiac disease. She gave birth to a baby with spina bifida. Her condition deteriorated over time, and as she developed additional symptoms, she was referred to me. I confirmed the suspected diagnosis of celiac disease.

This is the kind of story that makes me extremely sad. This story is a disturbing testimony to the fact that our failure to increase awareness of celiac disease among health-care professionals can have devastating consequences. This story also shows that there are lessons to be learned as we continue our crusade to make sure that cases like this will never happen again. Indeed, we have many patient cases with happy endings, in which the diagnosis of celiac disease was made and the patients were placed on the gluten-free diet that allowed them to complete a trouble-free pregnancy and delivery.

It's not considered cost effective right now to conduct a general screening of celiac disease in pregnant women. Some red flags that justify screening, however, are, among others, prolonged anemia that doesn't respond to iron supplements, gastrointestinal symptoms that are persistent or prolonged enough not to be strictly related to pregnancy, a history of difficulties with conception, previous miscarriage, excessive fatigue, and relatives who have been diagnosed with celiac disease.

It's my strong opinion that a lower threshold for screening pregnant women than the current threshold in the general population should be implemented to make sure we have more happy endings for mother and child.

IS BREASTFEEDING A PREVENTIVE MEASURE?

It's indisputable that breastfeeding is the best way to feed babies. According to the American Academy of Pediatrics (AAP), not breastfeeding can result in an increased risk of adverse health effects for both mother and infant. The AAP recommends that mothers breastfeed exclusively for about six months and then introduce nutritious, complementary foods while continuing to breastfeed.

This topic is particularly important for babies at risk of celiac disease since it's been reported that breastfeeding may have an impact on the onset of celiac disease later in life. Currently there are two schools of thought about breastfeeding and the risk of celiac disease development.

The first school of thought is championed by the Swedish scientific community that suggests that implementation of breastfeeding can prevent celiac disease in at-risk babies. The second school of thought proposes that breastfeeding may delay, but not prevent, celiac disease onset. This debate is still far from being settled since long-term follow-up studies need to be completed to determine which of the two theories is correct.

Our Center is coming close to the finish line of one of these studies. Dr. Carlo Catassi is completing the analysis of what will be the longest longitudinal follow-up study of infants at risk for celiac disease ever conducted. These babies have been monitored from birth until their tenth birthdays. So far the preliminary data seems to suggest that breastfeeding does not decrease the risk of developing celiac disease. It remains undisputable, however, that breastfeeding is the best nutrition practice for the first six months of life.

A similar debate revolves around the introduction of gluten-containing baby food at weaning. There is general agreement that introducing gluten too early can increase the risk of celiac disease in genetically predisposed babies.

The evidence for this theory came from an unfortunate natural experiment in the mid-1980s in Sweden. The government recommended a change in infant feeding practices that included the use of a "follow-on" formula fortified with wheat to be introduced to babies after weaning. Between 1978 and 1982, the prevalence of celiac disease was 1.7 per 1,000 live births. Between 1984 and 1996, there was a fourfold increase in the rate of celiac disease.

Previous generations of babies not exposed to the gluten-fortified formula maintained the general trend of approximately 1 percent frequency for celiac disease. When the link between the celiac disease epidemic in Sweden and this fortified formula was made, the formula was retired from the market. The next generation of babies was fed regular formula (without gluten) and returned to the expected rate of 1 percent of the population with celiac disease.

Using epidemiological tools, scientists from Umeå University in Sweden demonstrated that half of this "epidemic" was explained by the proportional increase of infants introduced to gluten after weaning. The results left little doubt about the link between the early introduction of gluten and the increased risk of development of celiac disease for infants in this unfortunate "natural experiment."

THREE SCHOOLS OF THOUGHT

Unlike the conclusive outcome in Sweden, the debate is ongoing about whether delaying the introduction of gluten in babies at risk for celiac disease has any advantages. There are three main schools of thought.

The first one suggests that it's destiny for at-risk babies to develop celiac disease, no matter how long you delay the introduction of gluten into their diet. Supporters of this theory suggest introducing gluten at the age of weaning (four to five months) to secure an early diagnosis with the onset of symptoms from early gluten exposure.

A second school of thought suggests that there's a window of opportunity between four and seven months of age during which gluten introduction may decrease the chance of developing celiac disease. This theory is supported by data generated in a limited number of at-risk babies followed for a short period after gluten introduction.

The third school of thought proposes that delaying the introduction of gluten can either prevent or strongly delay the onset of celiac disease. This theory is based on retrospective data suggesting that the frequency of celiac disease increases directly with the time of exposure to gluten in the diet. Of course, each theory has merits and flaws related to the incomplete information that we're currently examining. In Chapter Fifteen, you'll find a detailed discussion of current research on the timing of gluten exposure.

A STATE OF CONSTANT VIGILANCE
By Meghan Harrington-Patton

NINE YEARS TO MY DIAGNOSIS

I was diagnosed at age twenty-eight after nine years of not knowing what was wrong with me. My problems started three days after graduating high school, when I had sinus surgery. I had complications from too much anesthesia medication, and I was tired all summer.

By the time I entered college that fall, I had developed bowel trouble. When I went to the college's health center, the doctor said, "It's probably stress." I remember thinking, "No, I don't handle stress this way. I've been much more stressed before in my life, but I've never had these GI issues."

During the next eight years, I had three rounds of blood work, three rounds of stool sampling, and two colonoscopies. Two different primary care physicians told me it was IBS. Neither doctor ordered the simple blood test to measure the antibodies that point toward celiac disease.

I have Turner syndrome (a chromosomal abnormality affecting one in every 2,500 females), which has a higher risk factor associated with celiac disease. According to Dr. Fasano, between 4 and 8 percent of people with Turner syndrome have celiac disease compared to 1 percent of the general population. Both of my primary care physicians missed the connection between Turner syndrome and celiac disease.

Instead, each time I went in for an office visit with worsening symptoms, I was told, "Eat more fiber. Go home and have some Raisin Bran or a whole wheat bagel." Of course, these were the absolutely worst things I could eat, and I would become extremely ill with diarrhea several times a week. I also broke out in skin rashes (dermatitis herpetiformis), suffered migraines, and was fatigued. Ironically, unlike many other people with celiac disease, I could not lose weight. I was baffled and so was my personal trainer.

On my first visit to a gastroenterologist, I was finally diagnosed by an experienced nurse practitioner. As soon as she heard my story she said, "It sounds like you've got celiac disease." One simple blood test was ordered to see if I had any of the three common antibody markers found in people with celiac disease. The results were positive and the levels were incredibly high. After nine years of not understanding what was wrong, the GI nurse had me diagnosed in two days.

I was immediately scheduled for an endoscopy to confirm via biopsies of my intestinal tissue that I had celiac disease. The procedure was much easier than a colonoscopy (no yucky prep!) and painless. The results showed a lot of damage to my small intestine with classic scalloping of the mucosal folds and atrophic villi.

Through the biopsies, I was also diagnosed with gastroesophageal reflux disease or GERD, for which I had never felt consistent symptoms. This is how insidious celiac disease can be. I had what looked like "rings of fire" all along the walls of my esophagus. It's called Barrett's esophagus, and it can eventually lead to cancer if left untreated.

When I was finally diagnosed, it was just before I got married. I went completely gluten free. The toughest part was reading the labels and watching out for "modified food starch" because I didn't know if it's wheat-based (bad), soy-based (OK), or corn-based (OK). I remember standing in the grocery aisle looking at all the things I couldn't eat—things like Campbell's soups, Kraft Macaroni & Cheese—and being completely overwhelmed.

However, I gradually learned to find great gluten-free products, and how to make some myself. I immediately began to feel better after going on the gluten-free diet. The migraines and rashes quickly disappeared. And from my diagnosis in March to my wedding day in August, I lost 15 pounds with no significant change in my exercise routine.

As a final testament to how quickly I healed, I became pregnant one month after my wedding—just six months after my diagnosis. Blood work revealed that my iron, potassium, and vitamin D levels (which all had been very low) had all returned to normal within six months of being on the gluten-free diet. My 6 lb., 9 oz. daughter was born at 39 weeks without any complications.

TEN MONTHS TO MY SON'S DIAGNOSIS

I gave birth to my son nearly three years later. When I learned about the Center's baby study (see Chapter Fifteen), I got very interested and eventually enrolled Sean soon after he was born. As part of the study, when I started to feed Sean solid food at four months, I was given a powder to mix with his food. It was a "double-blind" study, which means that neither the doctors nor the parents know what the babies are getting—gluten or corn starch.

Sean must have gotten the gluten, because at about ten months, he developed symptoms. He was often in pain when he had a bowel movement. It was typically the first bowel movement of the day (about 12 hours after he had had his gluten-containing meal) that seemed to be the most painful.

When Sean began having gastrointestinal issues, Dr. Fasano decided to order an early celiac disease antibody test for Sean. The baby's results were high. The test was repeated a month later, and when the results were still high, Dr. Fasano ordered an endoscopy. Even though the surface images of the endoscopy looked good, the biopsies of the tissue samples showed damage to the intestinal villi. From then on, it was gluten free all the time for Sean.

Almost immediately, he became a happier baby. For the first time, he slept through the night on a regular basis. He also became more tolerable of diaper changes because his belly hurt less. And he was less fussy at mealtimes.

Even though there are more gluten-free products available now then when I was diagnosed, products for babies aren't labeled gluten free. I do a lot more label reading for Sean than I have to do for myself.

Since an infant can't tell you how he or she is feeling, you have to be super vigilant about cross-contamination. I know what it's like to have a celiac attack, and I don't want my child to go through that. His health is the most important thing.

One of the hardest decisions you'll have to make (unless everyone in the family has a gluten-related disorder) is whether to make your household gluten free. If you don't create a gluten-free household, then you'll have to learn how to handle cross-contamination. And in the case of babies, remember: "Crumbs fall and babies crawl!"

If he's crawling around on the floor somewhere, and there's just a breadcrumb on the floor, he could get sick just from eating that. Childcare can be really difficult, because of the risk of cross-contamination and other kids eating and running around. For example, how do you keep a toddler from eating a Goldfish cracker?

My suggestions for how to handle childcare include several options. For special occasions, you can provide snacks and meals for the school/center so that everyone eats gluten free. (This can be quite expensive.) You can provide snacks and meals for your child and insist that your child eat separately from other children. You can place your child in a small, at-home childcare center with a vigilant provider. Or you can work from home or hire a childcare provider to come to your home.

My babysitter has a daughter with celiac disease, so I'm lucky. Unlike Sean, she wasn't diagnosed until she was eighteen months old. According to her mother, she was symptomatic at nine months and emaciated at fifteen months. In contrast, Sean didn't have any of the physical characteristics or classical presentation of an infant with celiac disease. What he did have was a vigilant mother who was familiar with celiac disease and celiac attacks.

Fortunately, again, our babysitter had already been watching Sean on a regular basis, so his safe childcare was uninterrupted. Our babysitter's household is completely gluten-free, except for when the father and seven-year-old son go out for pizza together.

Since we share the household with my in-laws, we're in a different situation. Including our four-year-old daughter, we all work as a team to keep fourteen-month-old Sean away from gluten-containing products. So far, it's been a success. To our knowledge, Sean has not become cross-contaminated while at home. And at the end of the day, having a healthy, happy child is worth any sacrifice needed!

As Meghan says, having a healthy, happy child is worth any sacrifice. The next chapter takes you further along the gluten-free parenting journey, as you learn how to help your child navigate the gluten-free diet in school and other social situations.

CHAPTER ELEVEN

Gluten-Free Milestones in Childhood

*"Everyone is kneaded out of the same dough
but not baked in the same oven."*
—**YIDDISH PROVERB**

EATING SAFELY IN SCHOOL

As your infant with celiac disease develops, you're in full control of his or her dietary needs. It's only a matter of time, however—and trust me, time really does fly—that you pack his or her little backpack for their first day in prekindergarten or preschool.

Now the rules of the game change drastically. You're not the sole controller of the diet anymore. Now you have to trust people you don't know to make sure that your child won't be contaminated with gluten exposure.

Many schoolteachers have a clear understanding of the needs of kids who have food allergies to things like peanuts or dairy. But appreciating the details, and especially the importance of a gluten-free diet for kids with celiac disease and other gluten-related disorders, may be a new learning experience for the people at your child's school.

The challenge of finding the best school for your child's educational needs becomes even more complicated when you have to make sure your child's dietary needs are also met. The school's staff members need to understand that even a crumb from another child's sandwich on the lunch table can represent a frightening proposition for your child.

In other words, that first day of school signifies the shift of celiac disease from a family matter to a community matter. If you have other kids, or your memory still serves you well, you remember that along with playing together, eating together is a central activity in preschool, kindergarten, and elementary school.

Andrea Levario knows this all too well. Lawyer, lobbyist, and head of the American Celiac Disease Alliance (ACDA), Andrea has lived with a husband and son who both have celiac disease. Seeking help for her son affected by celiac disease, she initially contacted the Center in regard to his medical care. When we learned she was a lobbyist in Washington, D.C., and the FALCPA law was being formulated, we joined forces to expand the bill so that not only wheat allergy but also celiac disease would be included in the legislation (see Chapter Seven).

I turned the tables and asked Andrea for advice on how to make sure your child can eat safely at school and in other settings. She graciously shared the benefit of her experience for parents of celiac children. And according to Andrea, planning ahead is not only the first step to the successful management of the celiac child's diet—it's the key.

IDENTIFYING THE RISKS

Whether your child is dining at home, enjoying snacks with the soccer team, or eating lunch with classmates, adjustments are necessary to accommodate the gluten-free diet. Of course the modification needs to be customized based on the setting and the age of the child.

For example, Andrea used to pack an entire lunch and snacks when her young son was invited for a playdate with a friend from elementary school. As a teenager, since he had grown up on the gluten-free diet, her son was able to make his own safe food selections at a friend's home. School and organized activities at any age can present several different settings where your child's safe eating needs might need to be monitored by a knowledgeable adult.

When a child with celiac disease is ready to eat outside the home on a regular basis, parents must identify where and when their child may be sharing food with others. It's better to know ahead of time if an activity or environment poses a risk of contamination.

These settings could include birthday parties (at school, a private home, or a restaurant), sporting activities, school or group outings such as Scouts, or simply eating at school. Having a game plan for managing these adjustments ahead of time will relieve some of the fear and anxieties you might experience when your child with celiac disease or a gluten-related disorder eats away from home.

For sports and extracurricular activities, Andrea suggests you call the coach or teacher. Even better, she says, is to give them a detailed letter explaining your child's medical condition, along with a list of snacks he or she can eat. A face-to-face meeting with the person in charge of your child's meals or snacks gives you the chance to ask questions and provide some guidance on the do's and don'ts of the gluten-free diet.

This proactive measure of communicating information about your child's needs beforehand provides vital safety information that can help minimize issues down the road. It can be used or modified for different purposes in school or other settings.

NAVIGATING THE SCHOOL SETTING

Of all the situations for which she had to prepare her celiac child, going to school was the most challenging one for Andrea. Her questions included:

- Are schools required to provide gluten-free lunches?
- How will we navigate class parties or other special celebrations?
- What about class projects incorporating foodstuffs such as pasta, which contain gluten?

She realized immediately that even with the best preplanning and communication, one size does not fit all when it comes to working with teachers, principals, or food service staff. At school, Andrea focused her attention in the following areas in terms of keeping her child safe:

- Birthday and other celebrations
- Tactile or sensory activities that include food in the classroom setting
- Field trips or extracurricular activities
- School lunch
- Access to the bathroom
- Emergency evacuations

Andrea also quickly learned that sharing experiences with other parents of children with celiac disease or food allergies was always helpful. Her child's pediatrician was a good sounding board for socialization and developmental concerns, with recommendations of ways for parent and child to navigate difficult or unexpected situations.

Once Andrea gathered this information, she drafted a school plan, making sure to solicit input from her son whenever possible. After all, it was ultimately her son who needed to learn how to manage this significant part of his daily life.

KNOW YOUR CHILD'S RIGHTS

When you're faced with decisions about school, it's vital to consider what resources are available to help your child succeed in the educational environment. Many parents of children newly diagnosed, or even those whose kids were diagnosed years ago, are not aware that federal laws that guarantee equal access to programs and services apply to people with celiac disease.

Here is where Andrea's background as a lawyer comes to the fore and helps us navigate the legal jargon. For example, I learned through Andrea that the National School Lunch Act, and its program of the same name, makes it possible for students with celiac disease to participate in this "major activity" within the school community. For those students with celiac disease who are eligible for free or reduced-cost breakfast or lunch, the availability of such meals means they don't have to go hungry.

SCHOOL LUNCH OR BROWN BAG?

Will your child buy lunch at school? Andrea advises that this is one of the most difficult decisions for parents of kids with celiac disease. Being among friends at lunch and sharing the experience of the communal table is an important part of the school day.

Some parents or teenagers might prefer having control over the gluten-free diet and pack a lunch from home each day. But if your child wants to buy lunch, Andrea says, "Make it happen!" School officials may try to dissuade you, as Andrea and many other parents have found, but don't be discouraged.

Federal law requires dietary accommodations to be made, but the school food service program doesn't receive additional funding to cover costs incurred to provide medically required meals. The cost of gluten-free bread, pasta, or crackers, which exceeds that of wheat-based products, has to be absorbed by the school district.

My lawyer-friend Andrea informed me that the Healthy Hunger-Free Kids Act, which was signed into law in December 2010, increases the amount of money schools receive per meal. This measure might make it more financially feasible for schools to serve students with special dietary needs.

DOING THE PAPERWORK

As you might expect, and as Andrea found out when enrolling her son at school, the route to a seat at the gluten-free school lunch table begins with documentation of need. The school requires the parent or guardian to submit a written medical statement for special dietary accommodations. Each school district has its own form or one that is provided through its state Department of Education. Ask your school for its copy or look for it on the school district's website (see "Other References" at end of book).

A physician or other recognized medical professional must complete the form (as I did for my patient, Andrea's son) detailing that the child has a documented disability (celiac disease) and requires a medically prescribed diet. There is a space on the form for foods that can and cannot be eaten.

I was very surprised to learn from Andrea that, according to the United States Department of Agriculture, celiac disease is considered a disability. This means that requests for gluten-free meals must be accommodated or legal action can be initiated if the requests are not met. Currently other gluten-related disorders are not defined as disabilities and, therefore, the mandatory obligation of the school to provide a gluten-free meal plan in these cases may not apply.

The medical statement essentially serves as the gluten-free diet prescription. It must provide details of which foods are safe for your child. School food service personnel may not alter or change that prescription. The gluten-free meals are required to meet the same nutritional standards as the regular lunch, but they do not have to be identical, even though parents sometimes expect the latter.

For example, if pizza is on the regular menu, your child may or may not be offered a gluten-free version. Although this is slowly changing with the growing awareness of gluten-related disorders, few schools will dedicate the resources to make that happen. They are required only to make "reasonable accommodations" to be in compliance with the law. Most meet this standard by establishing multiweek meal patterns with different selections offered during that time frame.

WALKING THE LUNCH LINE

If you decide to pursue gluten-free lunches, Andrea says that a visit to the cafeteria and food service supervisor is mandatory. There you can assess the knowledge of those charged with overseeing the food service. Have the supervisor walk you through the lunch line and explain how your child will be identified to the staff, and how your child will make his or her meal selections.

Based on her experience, Andrea says, "Ask a lot of questions as you walk through the line." Questions such as: "Will the child be handed a preprepared plate?" or "Will he or she make a selection from predetermined gluten-free options?" Ask if a registered dietitian is on staff, and if that person is trained in the gluten-free diet.

Don't feel shy about asking if the food service supervisor is familiar with celiac disease or other gluten-related disorders. You might be surprised at the response. With the growing awareness of gluten-related disorders, the supervisor might tell you that the school food service staff members have served a number of students affected by these conditions and are prepared to accommodate your child.

To answer questions about preparing meal plans, altering menus, or checking the nutritional adequacy of the gluten-free meals, you have a great resource at celiac centers around the country. Andrea is grateful to our registered dietitian, Pam Cureton, who is well known for guiding food service staffs and preparing meal options to ensure our young patients can safely join their friends in the lunch line. Registered dietitians from celiac centers around the country regularly respond to questions and even help in adjusting meals when needed.

CREATING AN ACTION PLAN FOR SCHOOL
By Andrea Levario, J.D.

Once you've carefully considered the lunch alternatives and have decided to purchase meals, the first step is to outline a plan, which includes your ideas for minimizing or responding to accidental ingestions of gluten. (This plan also can be followed in situations other than the school environment in which your child may come into contact with food.)

The second step is to request a letter from your physician explaining that your child has celiac disease and detailing what actions may be necessary to ensure his or her safety at school. The third step is to schedule appointments with the school principal or other administrator and the school nurse to discuss your child's needs. Give copies of the letter from your physician (make sure you keep a copy!) to administrators, teachers, health-care staff members, and school food service supervisors and staff.

Remember that old adage: "An ounce of prevention is worth a pound of cure?" If your child has already been assigned to a homeroom, meet with the homeroom or primary teacher. Identify potential problems and discuss the best solutions ahead of time.

During your meeting, take notes on the teacher's comments and suggestions. Follow the same steps for specialty teachers in subjects like art, where food or supplies made with wheat pose contamination risks.

Finally, after all the meetings and consultations, see if you feel confident that the practices and procedures, along with a firm commitment from the school staff members, will ensure a safe environment for your child. If the answer is yes, then incorporate any additional notes or safeguards into a written school action plan.

Be sure to highlight your willingness to make adjustments and your availability to discuss concerns should they arise. Make copies and distribute your school action plan to all the people you met with previously, along with other teachers or appropriate staff members.

WHEN THE ACTION PLAN ISN'T ENOUGH

The relative simplicity and flexibility makes this approach attractive to many families. In fact, variations on the school action plan are widely used by parents of students with celiac disease and other gluten-related disorders.

This type of plan, however, lacks any guarantee that the actions will be carried out. In these circumstances, parents might become regular visitors at the school or on the phone, checking to make sure promises are kept. For this reason, parents may opt for an alternative approach, and pursue a 504 plan.

The plan name refers to the section of the Rehabilitation Act of 1973 that prohibits discrimination based on disability. Like the former approach, the plan is tailored to the individual child and his or her needs, but the 504 plan comes with a means of accountability. If the school fails to comply with the requirements of the plan, the penalty could be the loss of federal funding. In the absence of a 504 plan, there may be no documentation of the school's responsibility to meet the student's needs.

The ACDA collaborated with the Disability Rights Education and Defense Fund (DREDF) in developing a model 504 plan for students with celiac disease. Among the specific provisions in the ACDA/DREDF model plan are requirements for:

- Staff members involved in the care and education of the student to receive training in the management of celiac disease and how to identify symptoms of gluten ingestion
- Gluten-free foods to be prepared in a separate area, cooked in separate pans and served with clean gloves
- School food service personnel to develop a system for identifying the student when moving through the cafeteria line so that a member of the staff can ensure the selected food is safe
- Unrestricted bathroom access and ready access to hand-washing facilities
- Each substitute teacher and substitute school nurse to be provided with written instructions regarding the student's celiac disease care
- Notice in advance of food-related activities held in the class or otherwise attended by the general school population
- Parents/guardians shall provide the school with a 3-day emergency supply of nonperishable gluten-free foods
- Emergency notification procedures in the event of accidental ingestion

The plan provides specific requirements; school personnel are assigned responsibility for the actions for which they are accountable. To view the plan, go to http://americanceliac.org/wp-content/uploads/2009/08/ACDA-Model-504-plan.pdf.

A student must qualify for a 504 plan. The process begins when a parent or guardian makes a written request to the school for accommodations or services under Section 504.

Once the school receives the request, the school will set a time for the evaluation and send notice of the meeting time and place to the parent or guardian. At the meeting, a multidisciplinary team composed of persons knowledgeable about the student, the disability, and possible accommodations, including the parent(s) or guardian(s), will evaluate the medical information and other data to determine whether the student is eligible for a 504 plan.

Although parent participation isn't mandatory, it's highly recommended that you attend as an advocate for your child. If your child is eligible, the 504 team members will create a plan to address what is needed to allow the student equal access to accommodations and related services. The plan will then be distributed to all the teachers and others who need to implement it.

All 504 plans must be monitored, which occurs in part through annual reviews. The 504 team members will meet to determine if adjustments are necessary, whether the student's disability status has changed, or if eligibility should be continued.

Knowing that there is a defined process—a roadmap with signals for meeting the needs of your student with celiac disease—is what leads parents to choose this option. Accountability is a strong enticement and one that shouldn't be shortchanged.

In the end, parents will have to decide which school plan approach is best, based on the needs of the student with celiac disease and the family. Whether flexible or formal, remember that it's vitally important that there is a plan that identifies potential problem areas and management strategies before any difficulties arise.

HELPING YOUR CHILD BECOME INDEPENDENT

Early on, Andrea realized that she was the best advocate for her child. And she wants other parents to benefit from her experience. To ensure that the school environment is safe, she urges parents or guardians to maintain a positive attitude when working with teachers, administrators, and food service staff members.

Whether it's your three-year-old attending nursery school or your nineteen-year-old going away to college, preplanning and good communication are the key components that will ensure your child will be able eat safely in different environments. Andrea and I agree that an important part of a parent's job is to prepare our children to become independent and secure as they develop their gifts and move into the wider world.

Whether our children have a gluten-related disorder, another limiting condition, or have no eating or health restrictions, it's important to encourage our children to make healthy and safe decisions about their dietary habits. In the case of celiac disease—it's not just important—it's vital.

GREAT GLUTEN-FREE DESSERT
(AND DINNER TOO) FOR KIDS OF ALL AGES

PAVLOVA
From Helen Allan, Christchurch, New Zealand

For your next birthday party, make a "pavlova"—a delicious meringue shell filled with whipped cream and topped with fresh fruit. With its sweet, fluffy interior and crunchy crust, meringue is a favorite with kids of all ages. The dessert, which is claimed by both New Zealand and Australia, was created for the great imperial Russian ballerina, Anna Pavlova, during her world tour in the 1920s.

Ingredients:
- 4 egg whites
- 1 cup fine granulated sugar (castor sugar)
- 1 teaspoon white vinegar
- 2 teaspoons cornstarch
- 1 teaspoon vanilla extract
- 1 cup heavy whipping cream
- 1 tablespoon powdered sugar (if desired)
- 1 teaspoon vanilla extract
- Strawberries and kiwi fruit

Preheat oven to 250 degrees. Beat egg whites on high speed until they look like ribbons when dropped from the beater. Add sugar, one tablespoon at a time, beating after each addition.

Beat meringue mixture until it forms stiff peaks, but isn't dry.

Fold vinegar, cornstarch, and vanilla into mixture. Using parchment paper on a cookie sheet, spoon meringue mixture into a circle on sheet about six to eight inches in diameter (a rubber spatula really helps with this step).

Bake for 1 1/2 hours. Turn oven off and open door, leaving meringue in oven to cool. The meringue shell will fall as it cools, but this is okay—that's what the whipped cream is for!

When the meringue shell is cool, whip the cream in a mixing bowl until it thickens. If desired, add sugar and vanilla to cream. Don't overbeat cream or it will clump. Cover meringue with whipped cream and sliced fruit. You might want to make two—this is a very popular dessert! One pavlova serves six to eight people.

And just in case you'd like the kids to eat dinner before dessert, try this traditional New Zealand family dinner one weekend.

NEW ZEALAND SUNDAY DINNER:
ROAST LEG OF LAMB AND VEGETABLES
From Helen Allan, Christchurch, New Zealand

Ingredients:
- 4–5 lb. leg of lamb
- 2 tablespoons cornstarch or white sugar (to help gravy brown)
- 1 to 2 tablespoons olive oil
- 1/4 cup cornstarch or gluten-free flour
- 1 to 2 cups wine, stock, or warm water

Preheat oven to 450 degrees. Sprinkle lamb with salt and olive oil. Rub flour or sugar over lamb and place on metal rack in roasting pan. Cook uncovered for 15 minutes, turn over and cook for 15 more minutes. Turn oven down to 325 degrees and cook meat uncovered for 2–3 more hours, depending on how well you like your meat cooked. (Use a meat thermometer to test for doneness).

To make gravy, drain fat from pan and add thickening: Mix 1/4 cup corn flour or gluten-free flour with 1 to 2 cups or so of wine, stock, or water, using a wire whisk to get rid of any lumps before you add to pan juices. Bring to slow boil, stirring all the time. Take off heat when it thickens. Serves eight.

SIMPLE MINT SAUCE

Ingredients:
- 1/2 cup fresh mint
- 1 cup vinegar (add more or less to taste)
- 1 cup hot water
- 1/4 cup white sugar (add more or less to taste)

Wash and finely chop mint. Mix sugar into hot water and add vinegar. Add mint and serve with roast lamb and gravy. You'll find that a little goes a long way. Or you can really make it special with mint chutney.

AUNTIE HELEN'S FAVORITE MINT CHUTNEY

Ingredients:
- 2 cups fresh mint
- 1 pound onions
- 1 pound apples
- 4 cups white vinegar
- 1 teaspoon salt
- 1 pound sugar
- 1 tablespoon mustard

Put ingredients through mincer or food processor. Bring vinegar, salt, sugar, and mustard to boil. Cook on low boil for 5 minutes, cool, add mint mixture, and pour in bottle.

Vegetable Options: You can cut up root vegetables (potatoes, sweet potatoes, turnips, parsnips, onions, and others) and put in the roasting pan about 1 hour before the roast is due to come out of the oven. This is a really delicious way to roast vegetables, but you'll lose all your lovely pan juices for the gravy.

An alternate would be to roast the vegetables in olive oil and a "wee" bit of butter and cornstarch for browning. But for a traditional New Zealand dinner, serve the leg of lamb with fresh peas (with a sprig of mint) and boiled new potatoes in their jackets.

DEFINING A DISABILITY

As a final note from Andrea, it's worth pointing out that Section 504 of the Rehabilitation Act of 1973 as amended, and the Americans with Disabilities Acts amended, prohibit discrimination on the basis of a disability in educational programs or institutions, or in programs receiving federal funding.

While celiac disease is not specifically identified in these laws, an individual with the conditions meets the statutory test and regulatory requirements that qualify him or her as having a "disability." Although parents are sometimes uncomfortable with the condition known as celiac disease being classified as a disability, it's important to understand that these statutes are all about ensuring equal access and opportunity to all academic and nonacademic activities and programs, including extracurricular programs.

A related concern, which Andrea tells us is commonly shared by parents at support group meetings or national conferences, is whether the disability determination will affect the child's future educational opportunities, for example, college admissions or scholarships. Andrea assures us that it will not. In addition, the information regarding a student's disability is considered confidential, and is not part of the student's academic record.

A CAUTIONARY TALE

As I learned, however, every rule has its exception. Several years ago (before many of the laws mentioned by Andrea were implemented), I received a heartbreaking e-mail from a very nice young man. He explained to me that his lifelong desire was to join the U.S. Navy. Since childhood, he had a dream of wearing the white uniform of a U.S. Navy midshipman and attending the U.S. Naval Academy.

He worked very hard toward his goal. He took all the appropriate classes in middle and high school. He participated in a variety of extracurricular activities to beef up his portfolio. He doubled up his math and science classes to become as competitive as possible in those areas. He scored exceptionally well in his SAT exams.

And he finished in the top one percentile of his high-school class.

When it came time to submit all the admission paperwork to the Naval Academy, he had all the attributes of an ideal candidate. But reality hit hard for this young man when, during his physical exam, they discovered that he had celiac disease. For this reason, and this reason alone, they planned to dismiss his application.

He contacted me as his last hope to attain his goal of becoming a midshipman It was a dream that had taken him years of hard work, which he had lost in a matter of minutes. His message sincerely broke my heart, despite the fact that I never met the young man, nor did I have a clear understanding at the time how much it meant to him to become part of the U.S. Navy.

THE CELIAC "CONDITION"

I was outraged by the fact that he was singled out as not fit for admission to the Naval Academy based on a "disability" that involved only his special dietary needs. Indeed, I never grow tired of telling people that the term celiac "disease" is becoming obsolete. The concept of "disease" involves a malady or something that is wrong—something that is malfunctioning.

This can be the case for a person with celiac disease who is exposed to gluten and suffering from symptoms. But once the gluten-free diet is implemented, and the symptoms go away, the autoimmune insult of the intestine goes away, and the autoantibodies go away, this individual is now indistinguishable from any other healthy person. Therefore celiac "condition" rather than celiac "disease" would be a more appropriate term.

I explained all this to the Navy commander who took my call when I advocated for this young man to be reconsidered for admission to the Naval Academy. His response was very cold and matter of fact. "We cannot accommodate special dietary needs when our soldiers are deployed. Therefore, we cannot accept this young man into our Academy." So despite laws protecting the equal rights of people with disabilities, the application of this young man was dismissed without a chance of appeal.

We've made tremendous progress in easing the transition of children with celiac disease from safe and supportive home and family settings to similar school and community settings. But we still have a great deal of work to do before these children are treated in the same manner as their peers. It is their right, and it is our moral obligation to continue fighting so that the sky is the only limit they will face in pursuing their dreams.

PARENTING A TEENAGER WITH CELIAC DISEASE

For those of you with children who have gone through the teenage years—or for the younger readership who remembers this critical time of life—it's no surprise that this can be one of the toughest transitions for both parents and kids.

Indeed, this is the time of cutting the umbilical cord from the family as the center of the child's universe. Your child is moving toward his or her peer group as the most influential world that dictates your child's day-to-day lifestyle.

As a parent who has experienced this transition three times, when it happened I had this recurring feeling that my IQ had dropped about 150 points overnight. As the parent of a teenager, suddenly, how can I know what life is all about or what real life is supposed to be? I'm not cool anymore, and I live in the past.

These are the words you might hear from the same kids who not so long before loved to spend time with you, playing or working or traveling together. But when your child hits that crucial crossroad of the teenage years, just thinking about going out to dinner with his or her parents goes against the teenage mindset.

BLENDING IN WITH PEERS

Now, if you turn 180 degrees to see this transition from the perspective of a teenager, your main goal is to blend in with your peers. If you don't look like your friends, if you don't act like them, if you don't think like them, and if you don't dress like them, you could become an object of bullying and discrimination.

Therefore, it should come as no surprise that teenagers with celiac disease live this daily dichotomy of blending in with their peers on one hand and eating differently because of their celiac condition. Imagine yourself as a celiac teenager. You go to school, pack your lunch, and sit with your friends with whom you want to share everything. But you have to act differently when it comes to one of the most important activities at school: sharing food in the cafeteria.

And imagine how a teenager with celiac might react when their friend asks why they eat in such a weird way. What would you do about it? Stand up and explain that you have celiac disease and you need to be different in the way you eat? Or would you make an effort to blend in with your peers and give in to the offer of sharing food that contains gluten? It's a tough choice here; particularly if your parents made you follow a gluten-free diet. Try to remember what you thought about your parents when you were a teenager.

Just as facing up to a school bully takes a strong personality, similarly only strong and mature teenagers may go through these experiences without giving in or compromising their diet. To complicate matters, as children enter puberty, interest often shifts into engaging in one of the most romantic activities of this age: dating. How would you manage your celiac disease on your first date? Would you talk about it, or would you ignore it and just go with the flow?

WHEN SYMPTOMS RETURN

I remember the case of a young man who came to the clinic because, after years of being on a gluten-free diet, he relapsed into symptoms that included stomachache and diarrhea. His parents were rightly concerned and brought him to the Center for a general assessment. As we typically do in these cases, we ran his celiac panel of blood tests and sure enough, it was positive.

There was no doubt that the symptoms returned because he had been reexposed to gluten. Our registered dietitian spent an excruciatingly long time examining the diet of the boy without finding the source of cross-contamination. In the end, I asked the parents to give me a few minutes alone with the young man.

I opened up a heart-to-heart discussion with the young man. I told him there was no way that he was experiencing the relapse of celiac disease without being reexposed to gluten. I said that this was the time to share with me, without any reservation, if there was anything that he was doing to create the situation.

He told me there was indeed something. He was dating this girl that he liked very much. A few months before his visit to our Center, he asked her out to the mall, where they had dinner. When the time came to order their meals, he was too shy to explain his dietary needs. He decided to go along with what she was going to order, and they shared a pizza. He knew that he was going to get sick, but to his major surprise, days passed by and nothing happened.

So he started to question if indeed he really had celiac disease or if the disease had gone away. He wondered if he should be forced to stay on a gluten-free diet. He didn't fully realize that since celiac disease is an autoimmune disease, it's not like a food allergy in which the ingestion of the offending foodstuff is immediately followed by the onset of symptoms. Unlike a true food allergy, the complex machinery of an autoimmune reaction can take weeks, if not months or years in some cases, to become fully operational.

Not realizing the damage he was causing when eating out with this girl, he continued eating an unrestricted diet, until—sure enough—his symptoms came back. They became so severe that his parents brought him to our Center. After listening to his story, I told him that I fully understood the rationale for what he did. And honestly, if I was in his shoes, I'm not sure how I would have reacted.

I also pointed out, however, that there is nothing more important than your state of health so you can truly enjoy a normal life with your family, friends, and sweetheart. I told him that if this girl really cared about him, she would definitely accept and respect his dietary needs. In his case, these needs are a medical necessity.

He told me that he'd learned his lesson. He went back on a gluten-free diet, and as expected, his symptoms resolved. And as far as I know, he's still dating the same girl.

CHAPTER TWELVE

Navigating Gluten-Free Family Life

"As a pediatrician, and even more so as the father of three children, I like to stress how beneficial it is for families to share healthy meals together in a relaxed atmosphere. Nutrition plus nurture is a very powerful tool for successful and happy children."
—**ALESSIO FASANO, M.D.**

FACING CHALLENGES OFF THE FIELD

Statistics show that the custom of American families sharing a meal and conversation around the dinner table each night has dropped dramatically during the last two decades. With the busy schedules of many families, it can be tough to make connections over good food and family gatherings. But for some families, the challenge of going gluten free can lead to a deeper awareness of good nutrition and healthy eating habits, and a deeper intimacy develops as family members prepare healthy gluten-free meals together.

One family sharing that experience is that of Rich and Shelley Gannon and their daughters, Alexis and Danielle. At the Center for Celiac Research, we first became acquainted with the Gannons through the generosity of Rich, a former football superstar and Most Valuable Player for the National Football League in 2002.

In 1998, when Rich was a rising quarterback for the Kansas City Chiefs, his younger daughter, Danielle, was diagnosed with celiac disease after a very difficult first year of life. The struggles that the Gannons faced to get a correct diagnosis and adjust to the gluten-free diet made them passionate about helping others who face the same challenges (see Foreword).

When Rich and Shelley learned about the advocacy work of the Center, they became two of our strongest supporters. Rich stepped forward to act as a national spokesperson to advance awareness of celiac disease. Shelley's enthusiasm and Rich's celebrity status have helped us raise awareness of gluten-related disorders.

Danielle later became a patient as the Gannons continued to look for the right answers about celiac disease and gluten sensitivity. Despite carrying the genetic profile for celiac disease, Shelley and Alexis didn't develop the condition, but they were diagnosed with gluten sensitivity. I've followed thousands of families who handle celiac disease as part of daily life. I chose the Gannon family to share their story because of our long journey together and what the Gannons share with the Center—the goal of improving the quality of life of people affected by gluten-related disorders.

With Rich often needed on the football field, Shelley took the lead in this journey toward safe gluten-free living for their infant daughter. You will appreciate hearing directly from her perspective what family life with celiac disease and gluten sensitivity is all about. Her story begins before I met Rich and Shelley, just after their first daughter was born.

DANIELLE'S DIAGNOSIS

Shelley Gannon: Danielle was born in April 1997 and was just constantly sick. As an infant, she had a lot of upper respiratory infections. That was the start of many illnesses and ear infections, and of course, she was put on loads of antibiotics. When she got really sick, the scariest part was staying awake to watch her to see if she was still breathing.

So that first year was rough. As almost anyone with a child with undiagnosed celiac disease knows, getting answers can really be tough. The doctors said, "Your baby's fine. We'll just give her antibiotics, and that will take care of it." Well, it didn't take care of it. One doctor told me Danielle was sick because I was a stressed out mom since my husband played football. I didn't go back to his office again.

By Danielle's first birthday, we were really struggling to figure out what was wrong with her. She had a bloated belly—the same thing you see in old medical textbooks showing typical kids with celiac disease. She had diarrhea and vomiting and was always fussy. Rich had just joined the Kansas City Chiefs, and we moved from Minnesota to Kansas City in August 1998. Of course, she got sick when we moved, and we had no doctors in Kansas City. I still have this terrible memory of driving around unfamiliar streets with a screaming baby trying to find an emergency room.

We were sent to a gastroenterologist at Children's Hospital in Minnesota for a battery of different tests. Meanwhile, Rich was at training camp in Wisconsin, and Danielle was going downhill fast. He left training camp to be with her in Minnesota. It was a huge news story in the Kansas City papers that the new star quarterback had left in the middle of training camp.

Finally we went to a pediatric gastroenterologist at Children's Hospital in Minneapolis who said, "I think I might know what's wrong with your daughter." He stopped all the screenings and did an endoscopy. "She's got celiac disease," he said. We said, "What's that?" We had never heard of it; we had no idea what gluten was. But still, after months of sickness and frustration, it was a great relief to know that we could help her. That was in 1998. It had taken 14 months for Danielle to receive the correct diagnosis.

LIFE WITHOUT GLUTEN

Dr. Fasano: I think many of our readers will feel a sense of déjà vu hearing this story. I'm sure that many of you with a child diagnosed with celiac disease may have experienced the same struggles, the same fears, the same uncertainties, and finally the same relief that Shelley shared with us in describing how the family was initiated into the celiac community.

The next step is also common ground for patients making a lifestyle transition once they have been diagnosed with celiac disease—learning how to eat safely on the gluten-free diet.

Shelley Gannon: At first, learning to feed Danielle on the gluten-free diet was a pretty rocky learning curve. After Danielle was diagnosed, we met with the hospital dietitian for half an hour. She gave us a two-page list of what we could feed the baby.

Meanwhile, Danielle was eating her last meal before being discharged after being diagnosed with celiac disease. They gave her corn flakes, which have gluten. Awareness about celiac disease and information on the gluten-free diet were practically nonexistent back then—even at the hospital.

We left the dietitian's office, and Rich had to travel back to training camp. There I was, driving home with Alexis, who was three years old at the time, and Danielle, who promptly threw up all over herself and her car seat. And I had to find some kind of safe food for her. I stopped at a local food co-op and asked them where they kept the gluten-free food. They had no idea how to help me. Boy, did I have a lot to learn.

At first, it felt really scary not to know what was safe and what wasn't. If the health-care professionals at the hospital didn't know, and the people at the local food co-op didn't know, how would I be able to find out? I remember thinking, "What am I going to feed my kid?"

Well, I thought, maybe the labels on food would show me what was safe for Danielle. That didn't work either. This was long before the Food Allergen Labeling and Consumer Protection Act was passed in 2004. After trying to make sense out of the food labels at the supermarket to find food safe for Danielle—a task that took hours—I was even more confused and frustrated. I remember Rich calling me one afternoon and asking me if I was still at the grocery store. I had spent three hours reading labels.

The saving grace came when Danielle's doctor connected me with another mom whose son had been diagnosed a month before Danielle. The two of us met with another mother and started the R.O.C.K. (Raising Our Celiac Kids) group. From those humble beginnings, it's grown into a great support and advocacy group for nearly 200 families in Minnesota and thousands of other families in chapters around the country. I'm not sure I would have been able to treat Danielle successfully without the early support I found through R.O.C.K.

I also called the Celiac Society Association (CSA). They were helpful with the basics of the diet: fruits, vegetables, meat, rice, and potatoes. They also made me realize how strict I would have to be about Danielle's diet—it was pretty scary. I called a lot of food companies and read a lot of labels. There were no Internet listings of gluten-free brands back then. You couldn't Google "gluten-free" or use a phone app to find a gluten-free restaurant.

So I learned a lot the hard way, which meant calling the toll-free numbers on packages and trying to find someone who knew what gluten-free meant. It also meant relying on other parents of children with celiac disease for information and using the trial and error method to find the sources of hidden gluten.

We put Danielle back on her bottle, and I fed her semi-solid foods by making a bigger hole in the nipple. She was so lacking in nutrients, we were doing whatever we could to get nutrition in her. And she sucked those meals down like nobody's business. She ate a lot of potatoes and chicken that first year.

SHELLEY AND ALEXIS GO GLUTEN FREE

Dr. Fasano: There are two approaches that families with a member recently diagnosed with celiac disease take in terms of food habits. Either accommodations are made for the person newly diagnosed with celiac disease while the remainder of the household continues consuming gluten-containing foods—or the entire household embraces the gluten-free diet. The Gannons decided to go for the second option. And surprise, surprise . . .

Shelley Gannon: With Danielle's diagnosis, I had to rethink about how our family ate. I began to cook like my grandmother used to cook, making everything from scratch. Danielle would still get sick, and I'd have to solve the mystery of where the gluten contamination was coming from. One time it turned out to be from a gluten-free flour mix that had "gluten-free" stamped all over it. I later learned that the mix had been cross-contaminated during production.

There were lots of frustrating things like that. I kept a log of what I fed Danielle. When something like that happened, I would go back and look for clues about why she was suddenly fussy and keeping us up at night. Now I can laugh and say that it was like a CSI mystery series–find the missing gluten. But back then, it really became overwhelming at times.

In the kitchen, I made all the usual changes, like getting a separate toaster, and utensils and pots and pans for cooking and serving Danielle's food. In the first few years we kept things separate, and I was careful about cross-contamination. As time went on, I discovered that I had problems with gluten and was eventually diagnosed with gluten sensitivity, but not celiac disease. Alexis also had trouble with gluten after a bout of strep throat in third grade. We both carry the DQ8 gene for celiac, but endoscopies showed no intestinal damage, hence the gluten sensitivity diagnosis.

Consequently, our kitchen became a gluten-free zone, except for Rich's cereal and breads. Even though Rich has three family members with celiac disease, he doesn't have it. We both wished that we had known more about celiac disease earlier; especially that it's genetic, since we have extended family members with the condition. We then would have known what to look for when Danielle was so sick, and she could have been diagnosed sooner. It's so important to let your whole family know about any genetic disorders so they can get tested and be aware of potential risks.

Since Danielle's diagnosis, our extended family members have been fantastic about learning about the diet and making sure we have gluten-free options available whenever we get together. When they saw how sick Danielle was, there was never any question about their support.

In those early days, it took me about six months to get a really good grasp of the basics of the diet. Not only was there little information available, but I was also a very inexperienced cook. Eventually, I learned to cook like grandma, but it was a full year before Danielle was really thriving after going on the gluten-free diet. And when she was fussy, she loved to be held. And of course, her favorite spot was when her dad held her in the football hold.

SUPER BOWL CHILI
From Shelley Gannon

Ingredients:
- 1 pound lean ground beef or turkey
- 1 large onion, diced
- 1 cup celery, diced
- 1 green pepper, diced
- 2 cloves garlic, chopped
- 1 large or 2 16 oz. cans kidney beans or beans of choice
- 1 large can of tomato juice (I like V8)
- 1 small can of tomato sauce
- 1 large can whole tomatoes, diced
- 2 packages chili seasoning
- Salt, pepper, and garlic salt to taste
- Worcestershire sauce, several shakes
- 1 package gluten-free pasta, cooked per package instructions
- Sharp cheddar cheese, grated
- Green onions, chopped

Brown hamburger in a heavy skillet, then add garlic, onion, celery, and green peppers. Cook on medium heat until ingredients are soft. Add all other ingredients and stir, and then simmer for at least 20 minutes. Cook gluten-free pasta according to directions on box. Serve chili over pasta; top with grated cheese and green onions. Serves four to six.

TEACHING HEALTHY HABITS EARLY

Dr. Fasano: Like many other people who go on the gluten-free diet, the Gannons enjoyed a healthier diet because they made many of their own meals from fresh ingredients. As the children got older, they joined Shelley in the kitchen, making gluten-free food preparation a real family affair.

Shelley Gannon: As I became more experienced with the gluten-free diet, I learned how little we know about what goes into our food.

Suddenly, when your child's life depends on it, the ingredients list takes on a whole new meaning. At first, I was shocked at the long list of mostly unpronounceable ingredients on many food labels. I then got a label-reading book from CSA; it really was like learning another language. On the gluten-free diet, our eating habits became much healthier, which was a bonus for the professional athlete in the family.

As Danielle began to grow, she became interested in food and cooking at a very early age. I encouraged both my girls to "get messy" in the kitchen. It's important to teach kids with gluten-related disorders how to eat safely–at home and away from home. And for us, that started very early in our family kitchen.

ROY'S MELTING CHOCOLATE SOUFFLÉ
(A FLOURLESS CHOCOLATE CAKE)

Ingredients:
- 6 tablespoons unsalted butter
- 4 oz. semisweet chocolate
- 1/2 cup sugar
- 1 1/2 tablespoons cornstarch
- 2 eggs plus 2 egg yolks

In a saucepan over low heat, melt butter and chocolate together. Set aside. In a mixing bowl, combine the sugar and cornstarch. In a separate bowl, whisk the eggs and yolks together. Add the melted butter/chocolate mixture to the sugar mixture and combine thoroughly with a wire whisk. Stir in the eggs and whisk until just smooth. Place in the refrigerator overnight.

Preheat the oven to 400 degrees. Divide the mixture evenly into four buttered and sugared baking cups or ramekins (approximately 2 inches in diameter by 3 inches tall). Scoop the mixture into the molds so they are two-thirds full.

Place cups or ramekins on a cookie sheet and bake on the top oven rack for 20 minutes. Using oven mitts or potholders, remove from the oven and turn molds upside down to release the soufflés to individual plates. Add a scoop of vanilla ice cream and a sprinkle of powdered sugar.

I'd wrap Danielle in a big apron, put her on a chair, give her a mixing bowl with a big wooden spoon and some ingredients, and she was happy for hours. We watched shows from the cooking network, and she loved to experiment with baking. Now her experiments with gluten-free baking are some of the best things we've tasted—and we've tasted a lot of gluten-free food!

We soon learned that, unlike baking with gluten flour, gluten-free baking has more variables for things to go wrong: the amount of liquid, shortening, or oil in the recipe, and even the oven temperature can be critical to success. One of Danielle's most spectacular flops was a molten chocolate lava cake based on the delicious recipe from a fantastic restaurant called Roy's Honolulu. The first few times she tried it, it was a delicious chocolate mess. But she persevered, and it's become one of the family favorites for special occasions.

Both the girls are pretty careful about what they eat, and they've been responsible for their own diet at high school. They pack their lunches most of the time, which makes it much easier. The risky part at school is the treats and candies in the classroom. Candy bars and licorice are only two candy sources that could contain gluten. When possible, always check the ingredients of what your children might consume at school (see Chapter Eleven).

Of course, no kindergarten student is able to do that, so it's good to give your child's teacher a small treat jar for your child to have a safe treat when the other children are eating something (birthday cupcakes are a temptation) that contains gluten. The school environment was more challenging for Alexis, who was diagnosed at age eight with gluten sensitivity. She had already tasted real birthday cake. It was easier with Danielle, who had been treated with the gluten-free diet from infancy.

One way to ensure healthy eating is to take existing recipes and make them gluten-free, and it's a fun family activity. We like to convert recipes for Mexican and Italian food (think corn tortillas and gluten-free pasta). Danielle also makes a killer gluten-free pizza—that's another family favorite. We've tried many gluten-free pizzas, and none of them are as good as Danielle's. She likes to use Chebe mixes and gets the dough really thin. She adds sauce, cheese, and our favorite toppings of fresh basil (you can grow this fragrant herb in your window), onions, peppers, and sausage. Gluten-free banana bread is another favorite that we often bake for gifts. We converted this recipe from Danielle's grandmother's to a delicious gluten-free version.

NANA KAY'S BANANA BREAD
From Shelley Gannon

We replace the flour in this recipe with Pamela's gluten-free baking mix. Pamela's baking mix includes xanthan gum, baking soda, salt, and baking powder. You have to add these ingredients if you are using plain gluten-free flour that does not have them already added.

Ingredients:
- 3 cups gluten-free flour*
- 2 1/2 teaspoons xanthan gum
- 1 teaspoon cider vinegar
- 2 teaspoons baking soda
- 1 teaspoon salt
- 2 cups mashed bananas (3–4 very ripe bananas)
- 2 cups sugar
- 1/2 cup vegetable oil
- 4 eggs
- 1 bag chocolate chips

* Or use Pamela's baking mix and eliminate next four ingredients

Heat oven to 350 degrees and grease bottoms of two 9 x 5 x 3 loaf pans. If not using premade baking mix, combine flour, xanthan gum, cider vinegar, baking soda, and salt in a mixing bowl; blend well with an electric mixer on low speed. Beat bananas separately in a large mixing bowl, then add all the ingredients except chocolate chips to the bananas and beat on low speed for 1 minute.

Fold in chocolate chips and pour mixture evenly into pans. Bake for about 50–60 minutes or until a wooden toothpick comes out clean. Cool for 10 minutes then remove from pans to cool completely. If you are making muffins, bake for 20 minutes, testing doneness with toothpick. Makes two loaves or 12 muffins.

FACING MORE GLUTEN CHALLENGES

Dr. Fasano: From Shelley's story, it seems that everything is pretty straightforward and easy. The problem was identified, the solution was implemented, and the return on investment came not only with the resolution of Danielle's celiac disease, but also for Shelley's and Alexis's gluten sensitivity. So putting the entire house on a gluten-free diet (with the exception of Rich's items) was not such a complicated enterprise after all.

Wait a minute . . . not so fast!

Shelley Gannon: Even though we've got things under control at home, sometimes it can be tough when you're eating on the road. And of course, there are things that we still miss. When we go out to eat at a restaurant, we still miss digging into the breadbasket. Even though the breads are improving all the time, it's hard to replicate that soft, moist, "gluteny" texture. Going out to eat when Danielle was young was pretty tough. I'd have to call the restaurant manager ahead of time, and I would worry constantly about cross-contamination.

That's still a major concern if we're traveling or dining out, but it's much easier now with tasty gluten-free options in many restaurants. And with gluten-free cell phone apps and texting, I can look up menus and options and share them with the girls while they are away at camp or traveling.

Our lives are so busy, now the challenge is keeping the food packed for the car. With the girls' activities, sometimes that's where they have their meals. It does get harder to have a sit-down meal when they're in high school, but we still make that a priority as often as we can. If we can't, I try to make quality time with them while we're getting from place to place. And sometimes, that's when we get hit with an accidental gluten exposure–if I'm rushing and I buy something that I'm not sure about. Gluten-free apps and Internet research can help here, too.

FROM OUR FAMILY TO YOURS

Dr. Fasano: Based on what Shelley has shared with us so far, it's pretty obvious we're dealing with a pro in the gluten-free world. Just as Shelley learned from the experience of another mother of a child with celiac disease early in her journey, Shelley shares her words of wisdom with other parents and family members.

Shelley Gannon: My number one thing is to tell you to listen to your "gut" instincts. You're the parent and you know your baby or child. You know when something isn't right. With infants, you have to pay attention to the number of diapers they go through, the amount of liquid they drink, and their moods.

You also need to know what they might have put in their mouth, which is crucial information for a child with celiac disease. And their symptoms and behavior might not be caused by a reaction to gluten; it could be another food allergy or something altogether different. But if you suspect celiac disease or a gluten reaction, make sure you get your whole family tested.

The second thing is not to let a doctor or health-care professional brush you off. Remember that you can never ask too many questions. If you hit a brick wall, go around it, and never stop advocating for your child. There are many more gluten-free options available now and much greater awareness of celiac disease and gluten sensitivity. It's a lot easier at school and social events than it used to be.

My third piece of advice is to join a support group. It's invaluable to have help from people who are facing the same issues that you are. I'm not sure what I would have done without the mothers from R.O.C.K. Then once you have a good grasp of the diet and everyone is healthy, get involved with the Center for Celiac Research. Give back by participating in the Center's annual walk to raise funds for awareness and research about celiac disease and other gluten-related disorders.

That way, you can bring hope to other families facing the same challenges that we have. We've been incredibly lucky. Even though Danielle wasn't diagnosed for some time, she has recovered completely. Other families aren't so lucky, and children and adults can suffer unnecessarily from years of misdiagnosed or undiagnosed celiac disease.

The last thing I want to stress is how important it is to keep a positive attitude. Even though it was especially hard in the early years, I never saw giving up gluten as a hardship. Instead, as I learned more about all the wonderful–and healthy–gluten-free options, I began to see it as a chance to improve our family's health. Now we view eating delicious gluten-free food as an adventure–and we're happy to share the adventure with others along the way.

Dr. Fasano: I think that in discussing family lifestyle, I would not be able to do justice to the topic as Shelley was able to do so eloquently. Her daughter Danielle, now a high-school student in Minnesota, has also come a long way from her early experiments in the kitchen. The gluten-free lifestyle is as natural to her as breathing, and she's always happy to share it with family members and new friends.

"TIME OUT" IN THE KITCHEN
by Danielle Gannon

My Favorite Things to Eat

I have lots of favorite foods. For snacks, I used to love Fritos, but now it's popcorn—and a peanut butter and jelly sandwich on gluten-free bread with grapes on the side. And of course, I like pizza.

My mom always let me cook, even when I was little. Now I make my own pizza crust. I like to knead it and roll it really thin. We've had lots of gluten-free pizza in different places, but my mom says my crust is the best she's ever tasted.

Our family likes Mexican and Italian food. When we lived in California, we ate a lot of Mexican food. One of my favorite meals is just a corn tortilla heated in a pan over the grill or stove and cheese melted in the middle—or you can add chicken, onions, olives, and salsa—whatever you feel like!

My Favorite Things to Make

I like baking stuff like muffins and cakes and cupcakes—and decorating the cupcakes. Two of my favorite cooking shows are *The Cake Boss* and the *Ace of Cakes*. We always try to experiment with regular recipes for things like scones and cookies to make them gluten free. Sometimes it takes a while to get them perfect using gluten-free ingredients. My mom has a really good gluten-free banana bread recipe (see above).

I like desserts and sweet things, and I like to make "puppy chow" for my friends.

DANIELLE'S "PUPPY CHOW"

Ingredients:
- 1/2 stick (4 tablespoons) butter
- 1/2 cup smooth peanut butter
- 3/4 cup semisweet chocolate chips
- 2 cups Rice Chex
- 1/2 cup (add more if needed to coat) powdered sugar

Melt the butter, peanut butter, and chocolate chips in a glass bowl in the microwave. Melt in 30-second increments and stir thoroughly. This can be tricky, depending on your microwave's output, so go slowly. Add powdered sugar to the melted mix and stir. Put Rice Chex in the melted mixture and stir it gently. I use a wooden spoon to drop the "puppy chow" pieces onto waxed paper.

How I Eat at School

Even when I was little, I knew what I could and couldn't eat. Most of the kids at my school pack lunches, so staying away from gluten at school is pretty easy. And my mom came with me the first day and told everybody about my celiac disease. It's really no big deal to me. Everybody has something that they're dealing with, like lactose intolerance or a learning disability or something like that, mine is celiac disease.

One of my good friends at my school has celiac disease. We both pack our lunches and go out to eat together, too. It's great that she can come over to my house and be able to eat anything she wants. When she first came to school, I helped her get used to things like the cafeteria and the lunch line. The local news reporter came to our school and did a television story on us.

Fancy or Simple Food?

One of the best meals I ever had was at the MGM Grand Hotel & Casino in Las Vegas. It was pretty simple, but really delicious. The chef came out and talked to us about what he could make gluten free. We had homemade Angus burgers and homemade steak fries with homemade ketchup, followed with sorbet for dessert, and it was all gluten free. Yum!

So I guess I like pretty simple stuff, like a salad with grilled chicken for lunch. But sometimes when I bake, I like to get fancy. One year when my dad was in the Pro Bowl, we had this amazing chocolate soufflé cake in Hawaii (see recipe above). My neighbor and I had a lot of fun figuring out how to make it. You make the batter the day before, and you have to make sure everything is just right—like the oven temperature and the timing—before you bake it. I had to make that cake a couple of times to get it right. Now we love it for special occasions.

Looking at the Future

Well, I really like to cook. I like French and Italian cooking, and I like watching Emeril and the *Barefoot Contessa*. Our whole family watches Gordon Ramsay and *Hell's Kitchen*. I might see where my cooking interest takes me. But I really like science too—especially biology. I guess I'll see what happens!

CHAPTER THIRTEEN

Getting Through College Gluten Free

"Never fall out with your bread and butter."
—ENGLISH PROVERB

FOLLOW ADVICE FROM THE EXPERTS

Although I had many people and families to choose from, I knew from the earliest days of brainstorming this book who the best person would be to help us navigate the college years on a gluten-free diet. A close friend and former colleague from the University of Maryland Dr. Mary McKenna is one the world's foremost researchers on developmental brain injury. She also knows firsthand about celiac disease.

A licensed nutritionist, Mary shares the disease with her son, John Mink, a recent college graduate. They also happen to be patients of mine. We've discussed the challenges of living the gluten-free life at college on many occasions.

With guidance from his mom and assistance from others, John traveled his way safely through a gluten-free path at two different colleges. Mother and son both learned—sometimes the hard way—how to make the most out of the college dining experience while remaining gluten free. In this chapter, they share advice on how to plan your college visits, how to interact with food service employees, and how to evaluate the food and dining services at each college or university you visit.

Communicating with various campuses—early and often—is one of the keys to a successful gluten-free college experience. Mary and

John provide detailed information on what offices you might need to talk with, including student health services, special accommodations services, residence life, and others. They share experiences unique to a transfer student and discuss the pros and cons of dorm living versus apartment living.

Since John graduated from college, there has been a positive movement toward improved conditions in college and university dining halls, driven by demand and also recent legislation. In 2012, Lesley University in Cambridge, Massachusetts, faced a lawsuit brought by several students about the lack of gluten-free options and safe food conditions for students with food allergies in the dining halls. The university reached an out-of-court settlement with the Department of Justice in a ruling passed under the Americans with Disabilities Act (ADA). As discussed in Chapter Eleven, ADA prohibits discrimination against individuals with disabilities by public accommodations, including colleges and universities, "in their full and equal enjoyment of goods, services, and facilities."

From the proverbial gluten-free chicken gumbo to dry-roasted almonds (soup to nuts), this mother-and-son team provides a comprehensive list of food and supplies to take to school along with helpful books, websites, college food service links, and some great downloadable apps. By following Mary and John's guidance, the college student in your family can focus on learning and having fun at school while Mom and Dad can rest a little easier about their student eating safely in a new environment.

Their insights are powerful, and their firsthand experiences are unique, so I asked them to share those experiences with you here.

THE COLLEGE YEARS
by Dr. Mary C. McKenna and John M. Mink

STAYING SAFE WHILE STUDYING

Attending college or university should be an exciting time of expanding horizons where a student grows personally as well as intellectually and socially. The most important goal is to find the college or university with excellent academic programs in your area of interest and the type of campus environment that's right for you. After that decision is made, it's time to tackle the gluten-free part of the academic equation.

As John can attest, someone with celiac disease can attend any college or university and, depending on the environment, with a little or a lot of effort, eat safely. It's getting easier every day to eat healthy gluten-free meals on U.S. campuses. But doing your gluten-free homework ahead of time will make an enormous difference in your adjustment and your parents' peace of mind.

Planning ahead is the key to both a successful college search and safe gluten-free eating at the college or university that you ultimately choose. Along with your high school guidance office, many websites and books provide advice on the selection process.

Some colleges and universities list gluten-free and other dining services options on their websites and offer gluten-free, vegetarian, vegan, and dairy-free alternatives on their menus. With major media outlets like *The Wall Street Journal* writing about dining options in colleges, the list has really expanded. The Internet is a great initial resource to determine the "gluten-free climate" on campus, but there's no substitute for visiting the dining hall unannounced. Once you have narrowed down your choice of colleges, you're ready for your first campus visit.

STEPS TO TAKE AFTER SELECTING YOUR SCHOOL

This is a very exciting time for you and your family. But remember how important it is to deal proactively with offices in student services to make sure your needs are met. And the earlier you set your gluten-free wheels in motion, the easier your transition will be.

But first some words of caution for the parents: Don't expect the housing office to know about your student's need for a gluten-free diet. Because of HIPPA regulations, student health services cannot share medical information about your student with the housing office or disability office or dining services. It's up to you and your student to make sure these offices are aware of your needs.

- Send an e-mail to dining services advising them that you will be attending. Tell them the exact dates (an overnight visit or orientation, etc.). Thank them in advance for their help with your needs.
- Send in health forms with information about your celiac disease and a list of any gluten-free medications that you take to student health services. Include information from your physician with documentation of celiac disease or gluten intolerance.
- Provide the office for students with disabilities with your information. This office may help facilitate matters and help to ensure that accommodations are made.
- Make sure to send in your housing form early—this is very important! If you have a choice of dorms on a large campus, choose a dorm near a specific dining hall if necessary. Certain dining halls might be better equipped to deal with special dietary needs, or gluten-free food supplies might be stored in a specific dining hall.
- Prepare yourself to deal with many different offices and people at the college or university including dining services, health services, the disability office, residence life, coordinator of student visits, catering, student orientation organizers, orientation counselors, and RA (Resident Assistant) in the dorm (think pizza parties, ice cream, etc.). Be patient and polite, but firm and insistent about your needs.
- Document all of your correspondence. Send a follow-up e-mail after phone conversations to ensure that everyone is on the same page.
- Send both a hard copy and a PDF listing your gluten-free foods and gluten-free medications to the health services office.

- Some institutions might require a "504 plan" to be filed with the health services office. To qualify for a 504 plan (see Chapter Eleven), the student needs a letter from the doctor confirming the diagnosis of celiac disease or other gluten-related disorder. A 504 plan outlines specifically what the college or university must do to accommodate the student's medical dietary needs.
- Don't accept something that will create a problem (e.g., off-campus housing for transfer students). Be prepared to explain, explain again, and again until the people you are dealing with understand the nature of the problem.
- Post a question on the Celiac List Serv celiac@listserv. icors.org to get feedback about the food at your college.
- Make friends with the people in dining services and always say "thank you."

CHECKING OUT GLUTEN-FREE OPTIONS

You'll need to know if safe, healthy, and gluten-free food is available at the schools you've chosen to visit—something that might not be as easy as it sounds. Meeting with members of the dining services staff and assessing the current and future status of gluten-free dining on campus should be an integral part of each campus visit.

If you're really interested in a particular college, find out if obtaining gluten-free food will be a problem at that particular school. The willingness and support of the dining services staff in supplying gluten-free dining options can affect your decision about that particular college. Make sure you do your research!

It's a good idea to visit the college during a regular visiting day or open house program. These structured programs usually have meals, so sign up and request your gluten-free meal or meals beforehand if possible. You can test the waters to see what kind of feedback you get in response to your request. If the college cannot accommodate your request for a gluten-free meal, this could be your first red flag.

It may not be a deal breaker, however, as there are two important points to consider: 1) Have you given them adequate notice that you need a special meal? Arranging for open house days is complicated; you need to request a special meal at least a week in advance. 2) Meals for open house events often are catered and not prepared by the regular dining services. Make sure to ask about this because you may need to deal with both offices during your visit. And remember to check with whoever has prepared your meal to make sure it really is gluten free.

During your visit, try to eat in the dining hall. This is particularly important if the meals during your visit have been catered. The dining hall is where your student will eat every day, and the quality of the food is important. Arrange ahead of time to meet with the director of dining services, a dietician, and food service staff member who will deal with your student on a daily basis. Be sure to thank them for their help, and remember to send a follow-up e-mail thanking them for providing gluten-free food during your visit.

DOING THE DINING HALL

For people with gluten-related disorders, eating safely means getting down to the details of storage, food preparation, and brand names. You and your student must be prepared to do whatever it takes to makes sure he or she is eating safely.

Find out how many dining halls the school has, and which ones offer gluten-free food. It seems like a simple question, but it's a really important one. You don't want the dorm to be very far from where you and your friends eat.

If necessary, when you put in your housing request, ask for specific dorms close to the dining hall. This can be listed as "special consideration" or "needs-based housing," which most likely has priority over standard housing. This is especially important on large campuses with limited housing.

QUESTIONS FOR THE DINING SERVICES STAFF MEMBERS

1. How many students, if any, are currently served gluten-free meals?
2. What kinds of meals do they feed the students?
3. Do they have a sample menu you can see?
4. Ask to see where gluten-free foods are kept and check the following:

   - Where do they store special food items for students with gluten-free needs?
   - Check for dry, cold, and frozen storage. Can the students have access to the storage spaces?
   - Have there ever been any problems with food storage? (For example, do items ever disappear or become contaminated?)
   - How do they supply gluten-free bread and can students order gluten-free baked goods or other items?
   - Do they have a dedicated toaster for gluten-free breads in a safe area separate from nongluten-free breads?
   - Do you need to talk to a particular person at mealtimes? Do you need to call ahead for special meals?
   - Can students get gluten-free pizza? Do they need to order it a day ahead?
   - What kind of condiments and salad dressings do they use?
   - What beverages are usually offered? Do they have Lactaid milk?
   - Ask to see brands of specific products (for example, bacon, cold cuts, and other products).
   - What kind of eggs are used, and are they powdered or pasteurized?
   - Who prepares the eggs and how are they taught about gluten-free foods and preventing cross-contamination?

- What's on the gluten-free dessert menu? Is the ice cream gluten free? Check out the setup to see if there is risk of cross-contamination. For example, how easy is it for another college student to use the scoop from the cookie dough bin on the vanilla ice cream?
- What kind of potato chips, taco chips, and salsa do they serve?
- How often do they change food suppliers? (Insist that you be told ahead of time if they do.)
- What would they prepare for an "emergency meal?"
- Can you bring specific products that you like to eat? (If they say no, ask why not.)
- What do they do for holidays or special meals? (Homecoming or Family Weekend, for example)
- Is there a set menu (pick from your list of a dozen items) or do you follow the normal menu? If you want something other than the set menu, how long will it take to prepare?

MAKING SENSE OF MEAL PLANS

Most colleges have several meal plan options that students can select. Usually these are a combination of a certain number of meals at the dining hall (for example, 1–3 meals/day) plus a fixed amount of money for eating at other places on campus (for example, $100–$500). Many colleges require students to purchase meal plans, especially for the first year, but meal plans are optional at some colleges.

Initially, you have to make an educated guess as to which meal plan will work best for your student. It is important to ask if they can change their option if they select the wrong plan. You can often change plans in the first few weeks of a term, and most colleges allow students to change every term.

Specific questions to ask about meals and meal plans include:

- If you're on a sports team or traveling band, etc., ask what provisions are made for meals during trips.
- What are meal options in a fraternity or sorority house?
- What are the meal options for students in over-flow housing?

  This is a very important question as some overflow housing can be in hotels several miles from the campus. You need to determine if the food service capabilities and food storage capacity and security are adequate in the over-flow housing location. You also need to con-sider the additional complication and issues of dealing with more than one food service office. For instance, when John transferred to a large university, we had to lobby and negotiate for two weeks to have him housed in a dorm on campus.

EXPLORE OFF-CAMPUS EATING OPTIONS

Most colleges have several types of places to eat in addition to the traditional dining halls. These may include fast-food options, coffee shops, and stores (convenience, bookstores, etc.). Take a quick look around at these places to see what food options are available. You might be pleasantly surprised. We found several kinds of frozen gluten-free meals on each campus John attended.

Look to see what other gluten-free food options are close to campus, or where students can eat apart from the food offered on campus. After four or five years of eating the same food, your student will need a break.

ON-CAMPUS OR OFF-CAMPUS?

Living in a dormitory is a big part of the college experience. Many colleges and universities require first-year students or even all undergraduates to live in campus housing. Since different schools have different policies, we have suggestions below on how to assess the housing.

Tour the dorms and check what facilities they have for cooking and what appliances students can have in their rooms. It is important to tour several dorms as the cooking facilities can be quite different in newer and older buildings. Dorms usually have a kitchen with a refrigerator, stove, and microwave. Students can usually have small refrigerators and microwaves in their dorm rooms. Toaster ovens are not allowed in dorm rooms because they are a fire hazard.

We recommend that you buy a minifridge with a separate freezer to store frozen meals and pizzas. A larger minifridge (approximately 7 cubic feet) with room to store bread etc. might be a better fit for your room. Some campuses have a rental program. If you are considering a rental, be sure to determine if the minifridges available provide enough freezer space for storing some gluten-free food.

EASY FOOD FOR DORM DINING

Gluten-free frozen entrees and cornbread, cake, and waffle mixes all can be cooked in the microwave; gluten-free microwave popcorn, cheese, fruit, cereal, milk, and power bars are other popular choices.

Dealing with celiac disease or your gluten-related disorder is important, but your overall goal is to live your life as a college student. Along with eating and dining, also consider the life experiences you'll have in a dorm versus an apartment.

The upside of living in a dorm is that you'll probably be closer to the dining hall. The downside is that meal plans are often mandatory, and you might have limited storage space for gluten-free foods in your dorm room.

With apartment living, you'll have more control over your food (putting roommate issues aside). The downside is that you might need to drive a car, ride a bike, or take public transportation to get your groceries. You'll also have to educate your roommates about the dangers of cross-contamination.

Good meals take time to prepare. Planning ahead in your shopping and cooking will help to ensure nutritious and safe gluten-free eating in your apartment. Chapter Eight has helpful tips on shopping and setting up a separate gluten-free kitchen area.

GETTING STARTED

Remember that even if a dining hall provides gluten-free food, some of the items may be different from what you usually eat. There will probably be some items that you don't like. We found that it was helpful to bring a startup package to ease the transition to dining hall food and to give food service personnel an idea of what you like to eat.

We initially brought the following gluten-free items: salad dressing, hot sauce, bread, waffles, maple syrup, gluten-free English muffins, breakfast cereal, bars, cookies, and frozen pizza. It's very important to label all of your food products and containers with your name and "gluten-free food."

Be sure to bring a variety of good storage containers, clips, and some sandwich bags so that any items opened can be closed securely and protected from contamination. One of the colleges John attended gave him two milk crates for storage, one for dry items and one for items stored in the walk-in freezer.

KEEPING YOUR STUDENT HAPPY AND WELL-FED

Parents: Be sure to check with your student about the safety and quality of the food, and if food service is meeting his or her needs. If your student is having any problems with the food, be sure to encourage him or her to address any problems right away. Lend your assistance if your student is unable to address the problem alone. Lack of variety can be a problem at some colleges. And if chicken is the default dining hall meal, serve something other than chicken to your student on the first return visit home!

Send care packages with your student's favorite gluten-free foods and gift cards for restaurants that have gluten-free menus (e.g. Outback Steakhouse, P.F. Chang's, Uno Chicago Grill, and others).

Find a great restaurant for your student's birthday and your visits. Get recommendations from other parents, students, and people you've met on campus.

A smart phone can help you to stay gluten free. Some college towns will have great stores like Whole Foods, Trader Joe's, Wegmans, or Giant Food with great gluten-free selections and supermarket brand gluten-free products. In other stores a smartphone app can scan the bar code and determine if the item is gluten free, making shopping much easier. (See Appendix at the end of the book for a selection of helpful apps.)

College can be one of the most wonderful and exciting times in a young adult's life. Look for the colleges and universities that fit your particular profile—academic, social, geographic, and other areas of interest—and then find out how well they will feed you. It's getting easier every day to obtain gluten-free meals almost everywhere.

As awareness continues to increase and labeling improves, it will become even easier. Check frequently for new smartphone apps to find products and places that make your life easier and more enjoyable. If you do your homework before going off to college, this will ease your transition and help to ensure your success.

CHAPTER FOURTEEN

Gluten in Your Golden Years

"Old age is no place for sissies."
—BETTE DAVIS

CELIAC DISEASE STRIKES ALL AGES

We've been through the timeline of celiac disease development from the prenatal stage to adulthood and have kept the best for last–the golden age. As previously mentioned, during my training in medical school it was an indisputable dogma that celiac disease was a pediatric condition. Now we've learned more about the mechanisms involved in the onset of the disease, and we diagnose people at all stages of life. It's pretty obvious that there is no age spared by this condition.

As we mentioned at the beginning of this section, however, our current knowledge suggests that celiac disease can really start at any age. Therefore, you can be a senior citizen with celiac disease, either because you were diagnosed as a child, or because you developed the disease in your elder years.

SAVING LIVES WITH BANANAS

As a pediatric gastroenterologist, I have a lot of respect for that most humble of fruits–the banana. As every caretaker of small children knows, banana slices, mashed banana, or banana puree are all foods that you can almost always get your child to eat when nothing else will go down.

The banana is the headliner in the familiar "BRAT" diet of banana, rice, applesauce, and toast that used to be a vital tool in every pediatrician's black bag. Although the BRAT diet might not be as popular with pediatricians—and the "T" component of toast is a definite no-no for anyone on a gluten-free diet—the humble banana continues to be a staple ingredient in both the gluten-free diet and the rehabilitative diet for digestive disorders.

Intertwined with the history of celiac disease, bananas were used long before Willem-Karel Dicke identified gluten as the offending foodstuff in the development of celiac disease. In the era when celiac disease was considered only a childhood disease, bananas were sometimes the only food given to babies in the hope of saving the lives of some of these desperately ill children.

As a medical student at the University of Naples, I learned about Dr. Sidney Haas and the "banana diet" he developed in the 1920s to treat children in his pediatric office in New York City (see Chapter One). His paper, "The value of the banana in the treatment of celiac disease," published in 1924 listed the following approved foods for a child with celiac disease: albumin milk, pot cheese, bananas (as many as the child would eat: four to eight each day), oranges, vegetables, gelatin, and meat.

Interestingly, the diet also excluded bread, crackers, potatoes, and all cereals. Dr. Haas's successful treatment of eight children and the publication of his paper gained the diet a wide popularity for treating children diagnosed with celiac disease.

While learning about the famous treatment that no doubt saved the lives of many children, little did I suspect I would soon meet one of the "banana babies," as these childhood survivors of celiac disease came to be called. A few of these hardy individuals are still alive today, even though many of them spent years on a regular diet.

At that time, it was believed that celiac disease was a temporary problem, and the affected children would outgrow it over time. Now we know that once it is diagnosed, celiac disease is a lifelong condition. We also know that it's a disorder that is increasingly diagnosed among the elderly.

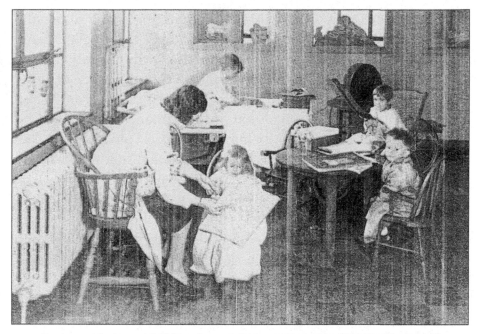

Barbara Hudson (child in center) being treated at the University of
Maryland hospital in the 1930s. (Courtesy of *The Baltimore Sun*)

BARBARA HUDSON AND THE UNIVERSITY OF MARYLAND

In 2006 as we celebrated the tenth anniversary of the Center for
Celiac Research, I had to choose the ideal spokesperson to capture
the essence of our Center's mission to improve the quality of life
for people with gluten-related disorders. I had no doubt about who
would make the ideal candidate. In my view, Barbara Hudson was
the quintessential example of the long road that the Center had
traveled and the amazing achievements we had made in such a
short period of time.

One of the first "banana babies" admitted to the hospital at the
University of Maryland in the 1930s, Barbara is probably one of the
last survivors of this generation of banana babies. When she came
to our Center for a consultation many years later, she brought me
a yellowed page from the University Hospital newsletter. It told
the story of these very ill children along with her picture as a little,
blond baby being cared for by a compassionate nurse.

One of the most remarkable comments she made about the article was that the nurse, now in her late nineties, lives in the same retirement community where Barbara's sister, who is also affected by celiac disease, now lives. The typical clinical history of these banana babies is going from being extremely sick as an infant, being admitted to the hospital, fed on the banana diet, discharged as "cured" of celiac disease, being placed back on a regular diet only to be rediagnosed in later life. I realized that sharing Barbara's story, which follows this trajectory, would be like shrinking 70 years of celiac disease history in the United States into a few minutes.

When I mentioned my idea to Barbara, I thought she seemed quite nervous about it (I was wrong!). I told her that if she would speak from her heart, she would do a marvelous job. And people would be mesmerized by how far the celiac community had come from those early times. Here is (slightly adapted with Barbara's permission) the transcript from the speech Barbara Hudson gave in 2006 in the conference facility of Davidge Hall, the oldest medical building still in continuous use for teaching in the United States on the campus of the University of Maryland School of Medicine.

THE STORY OF A "BANANA BABY" FROM BALTIMORE
By Barbara Hudson

I weighed 8 pounds and 2 ounces when I was born on Valentine's Day, Feb. 14, 1936. According to my mother, I was a very healthy baby until I got the measles in April of 1937. They thought the measles were the problem. Because after that, I started not "to thrive," which is the quote from my baby book.

But it really coincided with the fact that I was now eating table foods—that was the real problem. Our family doctor told my parents to take me to a pediatrician in Baltimore. On July 4, 1937, my parents brought me to University Hospital in Baltimore, where I stayed for ten days. But I didn't get better. On Sept. 21, 1937, my mother dropped me off at the hospital again and was told not to come see me for six weeks. I don't think they thought

I was going to survive. But my mother did. She said she never doubted that I would come home.

Of course, eventually I came home, but not until June 28, 1938. I ended up staying in the hospital for nine months and one week. One of my earliest memories is standing in a crib and looking through a window at nurses working at a desk on the other side.

Dr. Loring Joslin was my pediatrician, and he diagnosed my problem as celiac disease. We don't know how he did that at that time. But my diet became baked bananas and Bulgarian buttermilk, which I think also contained dehydrated banana powder. There was another little boy in the hospital at the same time I was there. We were called the "banana babies."

In Dr. Joslin's obituary in 1958 in *The Baltimore Sun*, he was credited with being the first physician to show the "value of pectin and dehydrated banana powder in the treatment of diarrhea in infants and children." I lived on baked bananas and Bulgarian buttermilk for two or three years. Bananas were hard to find back then when you lived 20 miles north of the city. A family friend or family member would have to go into Baltimore to buy the weekly supply of twenty-one bananas.

My mother said the stuff looked so terrible she never had the heart to taste it, and I certainly don't remember what it tasted like either. My mother was told that I would outgrow this condition, so other foods were gradually added to my diet, and I seemed to be able to tolerate them. Dairy products were the last things to be added, and I could finally eat ice cream when I was six years old. That was a real landmark!

During elementary and high school, I had diarrhea many times, but nobody connected it to celiac disease. In spite of that, I thought I was cured from celiac disease because they had said that I would outgrow it. After college, I married. I taught kindergarten. I had four sons, and I had no problems during any of the pregnancies. But in 1963, at the University of Michigan hospital in Ann Arbor, Michigan, I was diagnosed with dermatitis herpetiformis.

Back then, drugs were used to control it, not diet. And none of the doctors made the connection to celiac disease. As an adult the diarrhea would reoccur, and in 1968 I had it for two months. Again the doctors made no connection to my early history of celiac disease. I could never be further away from a bathroom than ten minutes. My sister did all my Christmas shopping that year because I couldn't leave the house long enough. With no answers, the doctors said my problem was probably from "nerves."

In 1984, while living in Connecticut, I had a physical, and my doctor said I was very anemic. And I said, "I've been anemic all my life." And so she said, "Really, your blood cells look awfully funny also." So she sent me to a gastroenterologist. He asked me my medical history. I gave him my whole medical history, and he said, "You couldn't have had celiac disease, the test for that wasn't invented until the 1970s!"

He did a biopsy. And sure enough, I had celiac disease. The villi in my small intestine were as flat as flat. I never went back to see that doctor again. And later, after that, I had a skin biopsy that showed that I also had dermatitis herpetiformis. So after more than forty years, I was rediagnosed as a celiac and put back on a gluten-free diet that I've followed ever since.

My skin cleared up and my gastrointestinal tract is much better. My sister was diagnosed with celiac disease in 1976 at Union Memorial Hospital in Baltimore. At the time, my mother was relieved that it wasn't cancer. She was sure that it was cancer because my sister was so sick.

It wasn't easy for either of us to find gluten-free food back then. She lived in Maryland, and I lived in Connecticut. We were on the phone all the time, sharing our ideas of various things we could eat. Back then, there were no support groups in Connecticut. We lived out in the country, where I became a support group for other people with celiac disease in the neighborhood.

One night a woman came to my house in tears. She said her eight-year-old daughter had just been diagnosed with celiac disease. Her daughter was so upset because she could never again have an Oreo cookie. I said, 'Yes, that's right. She can never have another Oreo cookie, but there are lots of things she could eat.' And we talked about those things. I also said, 'There are a lot of diseases that are a lot worse than celiac disease.' And by the time the mother left, she had a new confidence about her daughter and the gluten-free diet.

It's so much easier now to eat a gluten-free diet. There are gluten-free things in every grocery store around. But I still do a lot of my own cooking—especially soups. It's true that sometimes this disease can be a real pain in the neck. I try to always carry something with me to eat if I'm going to be away at mealtime—especially when I'm traveling. On the other hand, I've enjoyed long trips without any problems related to diet.

I know that if you have celiac disease, you can have a good life. I'm healthier than many of my friends of the same age. My husband of more than 50 years, my four sons, and my 12 grandchildren know that I've had a good life, even though I started out all those years ago as a banana baby in Baltimore."

REAL SOUPS FOR THE CELIAC SOUL
From Margaret Flaherty, Sudlersville, Maryland

Soup makes a wonderfully restorative meal any time of year. But these two gluten-free recipes from Margaret Jane Flaherty (mother of Susie Flaherty), are a real treat in the cold winter months. Serve with gluten-free crackers, bread, or muffins of your choice.

MARGARET JANE'S CHICKEN SOUP WITH RICE

Ingredients:
- 4–5 pieces chicken (breast, thigh, or leg)
- 6 cups gluten-free chicken broth (homemade or Swanson's; low or no sodium)
- 1/2 large onion, chopped
- 2 large carrots, peeled and chopped
- 2 large sticks celery, chopped
- 1 1/2 cup uncooked rice (Arborio is a good choice)
- 1/2 teaspoon poultry seasoning or sage

- Salt and pepper, as desired
- 1 teaspoon sugar
- 1 teaspoon lemon juice
- 1 tablespoon butter (optional)
- Fresh parsley

Place uncooked chicken pieces in large pot and cover with chicken broth. Bring to boil and simmer until meat is cooked (approximately 30–40 minutes). Remove chicken and cool. Strain the broth through a fine mesh strainer into clean container and place stock in refrigerator. Cool until fat comes to top, and remove fat with spoon. Remove meat from chicken, discard skin, bones, and gristle, and cut meat in pieces.

Place stock on stove, add vegetables and seasonings and cook over medium heat just until soft. Add rice, cover, and simmer until rice is cooked. Add sugar, lemon juice, and chicken pieces and heat through. Adjust seasonings to taste. If desired, add butter for a flavor boost and garnish with fresh sprigs of parsley before serving. Serves six.

MARGARET JANE'S SPLIT PEA SOUP WITH HAM

Ingredients:
- Meaty ham bone or ham hocks (ask butcher if you're not sure what to buy)
- 6 cups gluten-free chicken broth (homemade or Swanson's; low or no sodium)
- 1 medium onion, chopped
- 2 large carrots, peeled and chopped
- 2 large celery sticks, peeled and chopped
- 2 cups dried split peas
- 1 bay leaf
- 1/2 teaspoon dried thyme
- 1/4 teaspoon dried basil
- 1 teaspoon sugar
- Salt and pepper, as desired
- 1 tablespoon butter (if desired)
- Fresh thyme

Cover ham bone with chicken stock, bring to boil, and simmer for 45 minutes to 1 hour. Remove ham bone and strain stock through fine mesh strainer into another container. Place stock in refrigerator and cool until fat comes to top. Remove fat with spoon, place stock on stove, and add peas. Bring to boil, reduce to simmer, and cook peas for 45 minutes to 1 hour until peas are soft.

While peas are cooking, cut up ham into small pieces, discarding fat and gristle. When peas are soft, add vegetables, seasonings, and sugar, and cook until soft. Add ham and correct the seasonings for best flavor. Add butter if desired. Garnish with fresh sprigs of thyme. Serves six.

THE WORST-CASE SCENARIO

Barbara's story has a happy ending. Unfortunately, there are many other untold stories that have a very different outcome. These people are not around anymore to tell us about their experiences, but I feel obligated to give voice to one of those stories.

This is the story of another woman. We'll call her Helen, even though it's not her real name. Just like Barbara, she developed celiac disease in her early childhood and was later told that she had outgrown the condition. In the late 1970s, her mother followed the physician's recommended instructions and put Helen back on a regular diet. She thrived and had a healthy adult life. She married and gave birth to two children with no problems.

Suddenly, when she was in her early forties, she developed severe abdominal symptoms and was transported from her rural home to the emergency room of a major hospital in Pennsylvania. To the emergency room doctor, it was immediately obvious that Helen was suffering from an intestinal occlusion, which means that the intestine was closed to the passage of foodstuff and gas.

This is one of the most frightening scenarios that a physician can face, since the consequences of such conditions can be devastating if not promptly treated. Even more concerning is the fact that these obstructions generally are caused by severe conditions like tumors. Sure enough, Helen was diagnosed with intestinal lymphoma, an extremely rare and the most severe complication that a celiac patient can face. This condition is seen in adults who have had non-responsive celiac disease for more than 20 to 30 years.

By the time Helen was admitted, the intestinal lymphoma had caused complete obstruction of the intestine. It was too late to intervene. Nevertheless, when she learned of the diagnosis, she asked to be transferred to our Center. Unfortunately, besides confirming the diagnosis originally made by my colleagues in Pennsylvania, I had very little to offer Helen.

I spent hours listening to her story and answering her many questions, including her greatest fear that she had developed intestinal lymphoma because she had been reexposed to gluten for so many years. Of course, unfortunately, there was no way for me to ease her fears by telling her it was "destiny" that she would develop intestinal lymphoma. We're still not completely sure what would eventually cause this unfortunate outcome, even if a specific genetic predisposition seems to play a role.

Helen knew that she was going to die. She made me promise that what had happened to her would never happen again—starting with her family. Of course, I screened her family members and sure enough, her daughter was diagnosed with celiac disease.

Helen was relieved by the fact that her family would be in good hands. Her story taught me that mission statements like the one of our Center—to improve the quality of life with people with gluten-related disorders—are not merely abstract words, but for the people for whom we care and their families, it really does exemplify the healing power that health-care professionals have the privilege to be entrusted with.

Ever since Helen passed on, my colleagues and I have worked extremely hard to increase the awareness of celiac disease and the importance of a prompt diagnosis, so that lymphomas can be detected at an early stage and stories like Helen's will not happen again. I know that Helen would be pleased with the remarkable progress we've made, since nowadays celiac disease, gluten sensitivity, and the gluten-free diet have gained much greater recognition by health-care professionals and the general population. Another dramatic story of a patient who was diagnosed with celiac disease at age sixty-five had a very different outcome.

CELIAC DISEASE CAN STRIKE AT ANY AGE

Financial controller Tom Hopper is very good at managing numbers. With late-onset celiac disease diagnosed at age sixty-five, Hopper is now an expert at managing his health on the gluten-free diet—and he feels better than he has in years. But it took months of agonizing gastrointestinal attacks, several emergency room visits, more doctors than he can remember (including at least seven gastroenterologists), and an emergency evacuation from Logan airport in Boston before his health took a turn for the better. I asked Tom to share his story and his tips on sticking to the gluten-free diet.

"EVERYTHING IS NOT A VIRUS"
By Tom Hopper

"I'm not leaving here until you figure out what's wrong with me." These were my words to the doctors at Massachusetts General Hospital, after I'd been there for five days. I was now on my second team of doctors with still no answers to the debilitating condition that had disrupted my life for almost six months.

My attacks—as I called them—always began with cramping in my legs. Soon I would begin vomiting and then suffering from severe diarrhea. I also suffered from debilitating leg cramps that had me holding onto the top of the bathroom door at times. Hours later, I would be drained and exhausted from the ordeal.

The first attack on September 25, 2007, lasted seven hours and landed me at the Howard County General Hospital (HCGH) emergency room in Howard County, Maryland. They replenished me with fluids, made sure my vital signs were OK, and sent me home.

On October 3, I was back at the same ER with the same complaint. This time they admitted me for three days and ran lots of tests, including MRIs and ultrasound exams. The hospital results reflected a possible "systemic viral infection causing abnormal liver function tests." An abdominal ultrasound showed some gallbladder sludge that could affect the bile duct, but otherwise everything was normal. No blockages. They couldn't find anything really wrong.

Meanwhile, on October 11, I had another series of attacks and landed back at HCGH for another four days. I had MRIs again, CT (computer tomography) scans, an upper GI endoscopy, and a colonoscopy. The hospital results reflected improved liver enzymes, but one gastroenterologist wrote, "I would like to rule out celiac disease, especially given the elevated transaminases. Celiac disease has been associated with gastrointestinal complaints and elevated transaminases."

Transaminases are enzymes in the liver that—as this savvy physician pointed out—can become elevated if you've got celiac disease. For some unknown reason, celiac disease was not pursued, much to my later anguish. Finally, the gastroenterologists reported that both the esophageal and colonic mucosal linings were normal. Three gastroenterologists had examined me.

(Note from Dr. Fasano: When Tom shared this information with me, I was puzzled by the fact that they didn't find anything wrong as a result of the endoscopy. Nevertheless, the chance exists that if the person performing the endoscopy didn't see any gross inflammation in Tom's intestine, he or she might have decided not to perform a biopsy. Sometimes the intestinal damage of celiac disease can be characterized by an intestine that appears grossly intact, but the biopsy reveals a totally destroyed gut mucosa. Therefore, the rule should be that if celiac disease is suspected, an intestinal biopsy should be conducted irrespective of how healthy the intestine appears during the endoscopy.)

As follow-up, the physicians from HCGH sent me to a hematologist who confirmed on October 19 that I was anemic—a condition I had known about for years. He said, "Let's just keep an eye on this."

Later in December, I followed up with one of the gastroenterologists, and as a result of that meeting (after an attack that I self-managed), I underwent a capsule endoscopy. I swallowed an electronic pill and wore a monitor for 24 hours. No abnormal results and blockages were detected.

But then on February 2, 2008, I had an attack and another emergency room visit. Once more, the diagnosis was viral irritation of the stomach and intestinal tract. The ER doctor told me not to eat peanut butter or chocolate. The doctor couldn't really give me a reason why I couldn't eat these favorite foods of mine—but said it might help.

At this point, my wife was becoming very frustrated that no one could figure out what was going on. She contacted the founder of a medical practice that specializes in digestive diseases, and I went to see him on February 6. He recommended that I have a procedure called an ERCP (endoscopic retrograde cholangiopancreatography) with a sphincterotomy. I had another attack the next day, and the ER doctor agreed that I should have the ERCP.

In an ERCP, a thin, flexible tube with a camera on the end is passed down through your stomach and into the upper part of your small intestine to the opening of your bile duct. The specialist said they would examine the entrance to the bile duct and enlarge it if necessary by shaving a little bit off of the muscle.

I had the outpatient procedure performed on Tuesday, February 26, 2008. The surgeon visited me in the recovery room. He said everything went well. He also told me, "You'll never have to see another doctor the rest of your life."

IN DISTRESS AT LOGAN AIRPORT

After the ERCP, I thought the worst of it was over, but I was wrong—the worst was yet to come. I began eating soft foods and working my way back to a normal diet. I had some nausea on Wednesday, which I was told might happen after the procedure.

In the meantime, I had an out-of-town business meeting scheduled on Friday, February 29, to interview candidates for my company. I went to BWI (Baltimore Washington International Thurgood Marshall Airport) for a 6:30 A.M. flight to Boston. I ate an egg sandwich and some orange juice before I got on the plane.

As soon as I boarded the plane, the attacks started again and I began to vomit. I was in the restroom when it was time for takeoff. The stewardess asked me to take my seat; I was on my fourth airsick bag when we landed. Just as it had been with all my other attacks, the diarrhea started during the vomiting and the lower leg cramps continued. I was in the airplane restroom after we landed. They couldn't board anyone while I was still on the plane—not even the cleaners could come on board.

I had a little break and got off the plane. But I spent the next hour and a half in the restroom at Logan airport. I knew there was a 12:30 P.M. flight back to Baltimore, and I wanted to get back home and get some help. I went to see an airline agent, but I was so weak I couldn't stand up in the line.

I was down on one knee when an airline representative came up to me and asked if I needed medical assistance. The airport emergency team called an ambulance, and I was transported to Massachusetts General Hospital (MGH).

At the hospital, the attacks of vomiting and diarrhea continued until I brought up green bile. I knew that would eventually happen and then the attack would end—just as it had happened every time when I had visited the ER at HCGH. It was the exact same pattern that happened before the ERCP.

All this time, no one in my office knew what was going on, and my wife didn't know where I was either. Eventually the company found out and flew my wife up to Boston and arranged for her to stay at a hotel nearby. They also arranged for her transportation to and from the hospital. They were terrific!

LOOKING FOR ANSWERS AT MGH

I was assigned a team of doctors and given blood tests to start. I told them I'd just had this ERCP procedure done, but I was back to having the same issues that had started six months before. And then after five days, my case was kicked up a notch. Meanwhile my hospital records had been faxed up to MGH, and I received a new primary physician.

The doctors had done a lot of tests and analyses. They

replenished my fluids and put me back on a regular diet. The attacks started again, and we went through the same thing. After the attack stopped, they restored me with fluids, put me back on a regular diet, and started again.

At one point, a bone marrow test was performed to measure the quantity and quality of my blood cells. But, with this pattern, it dawned on the doctors that it might be something in the diet that was causing my attacks. It still took a while to figure out what it was.

Now it had been seven days since my admission. My primary doctor came in with some associates and started asking me all these questions: Has anyone else in your family had gastrointestinal issues? (My father's father passed away on vacation in Maine in 1940 after coming down with some type of gastrointestinal bacteria.) Where are your ancestors from? (My father's side was Dutch—my mother's side was English.) He said, "Ah, Northern European—that's good." And I told him my father had cancer of the bladder and liver.

My wife was quite puzzled and asked him what it was all about. He said, "We think you might have something called celiac disease." He went on to explain about the condition and said they wanted to screen me to see if I was susceptible to celiac disease. In the meantime, they would put me on a liquid diet.

At this point, I told him I wasn't leaving the hospital until they proved to me that I was OK. You can probably guess what's coming next. They did a DNA blood-screening test for a celiac gene marker and received results from an upper endoscopy with biopsy to check for damage to my intestinal nodes and villi. Both tests came back positive.

They told me I had celiac disease. I was sixty-five years old. So many different tests and procedures had been done, there were certainly some that should have shown it earlier, and there were so many digestive disease doctors involved.

A young nutritionist came and sat on the edge of my bed as she explained what gluten is, and that I couldn't have items with wheat, barley, oats (if cross-contaminated), or rye. I asked her if

I could have peanut butter "Of course," she said. I asked her if I could have chocolate milk. I was relieved when she told me I could eat dairy products, too.

My wife spent the next two days in the Whole Foods grocery store close to the hospital checking out the gluten-free food aisles. I was started on a gluten-free diet. My condition stabilized, and on March 11, 2008, I was discharged back to Baltimore.

The surgeon who did the upper endoscopy that confirmed celiac disease told me I should have a follow-up in two months to see if my intestines were healing. I asked her, "Are you going to do it?"

I flew back to Boston on May 6 for the procedure, which showed my intestinal nodes and villi were healing. As I was coming out of anesthesia, I opened my eyes and my primary doctor was standing by my bed. "I just wanted to see how you were doing," he said. I was so grateful. What a surprise.

LEARNING ABOUT THE CENTER FOR CELIAC RESEARCH

So I stayed on the gluten-free diet and did quite well, except for a couple of attacks when I accidentally ate gluten and became contaminated. On August 12, 2010, I had a really bad attack, and my wife called my primary doctor from MGH. He recommended that I find a celiac specialist in my area for follow-up. My wife did some research, and we were surprised to find we had a world expert on gluten-related disorders and celiac disease right here in Baltimore.

I began seeing Dr. Fasano for my maintenance visits that September. After learning about the great work at the Center for Celiac Research, I became an advocate for teaching people about celiac disease. Dr. Fasano and the Center are an amazing medical team. Their support activities are top-notch.

I don't want anyone to go through the horrible time that I had before finding out what was causing all my distress. I have been privileged to help raise awareness about celiac disease and the Center's work by sharing my story with *Allergic Living* and AARP magazines, and on National Public Radio, CNN, and

MEDSTAR Television productions.

I probably feel better now from food that I eat than I felt five years ago. Although I had lost weight because my nodes and villi were not providing nutrients to my blood stream, I have tried to keep my gains under control now that my digestive tract is functioning properly again.

Understanding what your limits are and accepting that fact is the first step to managing your health. With my wife and daughter's support, I learned to eat gluten free—I couldn't have done it without them.

Sure, I miss a few things—especially when I'm eating out at restaurants, but I don't have any regrets about what I have to do in my food selection. So much has improved in four years. We like to have friends over for dinner, and they will often say—"I really felt good after I ate dinner at your house." No gluten!

My advice for people just starting on the gluten-free diet is to "pay more attention and read labels and ingredients." Even though I'd been on the diet for four years, I had a gluten "attack" at Easter in 2012 just because I wasn't really thinking about what I was eating.

My wife Leeda is Armenian, and every Easter we have a traditional apostolic meal with her family. Part of the ritual is to break off a small piece of Armenian blessed bread and put it in your wine glass before you drink the toast.

Well, I didn't even think about the fact that it was bread—I was thinking about it in the sense of the traditional meal and the religious meaning. There was enough gluten in there to set me off for an eight-hour attack the following Monday. You must always be thinking!

My advice to older people in general is to get yourself checked out if you feel like you have any symptoms that could be related to gluten or celiac disease and have the respective tests performed. You learn to understand what your body is saying to you. People who have gluten sensitivity, which is different from celiac disease with intestinal damage, often suffer from bloating and nausea. Remember—everything is not a virus!

SOLVING THE MYSTERY OF GLUTEN REACTIONS

While Barbara and Tom share the joy of gluten-free living in their golden years, you should appreciate by now that they got to their final destination following two completely different paths. Barbara had celiac disease for most of her life, but was incorrectly told that she would outgrow the disease. Therefore, she was rediagnosed in her forties. Tom was healthy most of his life and developed celiac disease in his sixties.

Why do some people develop it at age two and others at age seventy-two? Why does celiac disease lapse in some people when they go back onto a regular diet, only to resurface years later with either a manageable outcome like Barbara's or with devastating consequences like Helen's? Why is the inflammation and therefore the symptoms in some people confined to the intestine, while in others it spreads to other parts of their bodies?

We have no definitive answers to these questions, but in Part Four we'll offer some plausible hypotheses based on a series of recent breakthroughs in related research. These will give us a hint of what the future of celiac disease and other gluten-related disorders will look like. One thing I know for sure: By the time we celebrate the 25th anniversary of the founding of the Center (2021), our understanding of gluten-related disorders and the balance between health and disease, and treatment and prevention, will present a very different scenario.

RETIREMENT LIVING AND THE GLUTEN-FREE DIET

Depending on your circumstances, there are several considerations facing a person with celiac disease in the retirement community. If you have had celiac disease for a long time, you'll be familiar with the diet and will be able to assess any retirement community or shared living situation.

If you're newly diagnosed, review the information from Chapter Eight on dining out and traveling and Chapter Thirteen on eating safely in college, which offers good advice for dealing with food service offices and institutions. If you're partaking in community meals, talk to the administration and dining services staff about what they offer in terms of gluten-free cuisine.

The same basic rules to avoid cross-contamination in any outside setting apply to eating safely in situations other than your own kitchen. Other special circumstances that might affect elderly patients include the number of medications they might be taking. Check with the pharmacist, and if necessary the drug manufacturer, to make sure your medications are gluten free (see Chapter Seven). If someone else does your grocery shopping, make sure that they have a list of the do's and don'ts for a good gluten-free shopping experience (see Chapter Eight).

If you are the caretaker for an elderly person on a gluten-free diet, make sure you're familiar with the gluten-free diet and accompany the patient to his or her physician and dietitian visits. If he or she is in a retirement community or group home, make sure that the gluten-free diet is adhered to in meal preparations. If necessary, talk to the administrator, nurse, dietitian, or dining services staff at the retirement home. Watch for cross-contamination symptoms that can include diarrhea, sudden weight loss, or loss of appetite.

Keep in mind that elderly patients can be diagnosed with celiac disease at any time. Red flags that indicate testing for celiac disease that should be considered include gastrointestinal distress, sudden weight loss, and anemia. Sometimes dementia or Alzheimer's-like symptoms can be the result of celiac disease (see Chapter Six). They can also be caused by other factors, such as a deficiency of vitamin B12. It's important for elderly patients with gluten-related disorders to be tested regularly for vitamin deficiencies and work with their registered dietitian to maintain good nutrition.

PART FOUR

Going Beyond Gluten

CHAPTER FIFTEEN

Preventing Gluten-Related Disorders

"We may not be able to get certainty, but we can get probability, and half a loaf is better than no bread."
—C. S. LEWIS

LOOKING FOR ALTERNATIVE ANSWERS

When I conducted my informal survey of celiac patients in 1994 (remember Aladdin's lamp from the Introduction?) I realized that the most popular wish for patients with celiac disease was to go back to a regular diet. At the time, I thought that this was just wishful thinking that would never come to pass.

Little did I know then about the extraordinary breakthroughs we would make in the next two decades, some of which occurred in our Center. Elsewhere in this book, I've noted that the other two wishes, avoiding a biopsy and increasing awareness of celiac disease and other gluten-related disorders, have been achieved. We've been able to make those wishes come true through a lot of hard work. But the hard work was inspired by listening to the needs of the people in the celiac community.

So where do we stand with treatment alternatives to the gluten-free diet? Even just eight years ago, this would have made a very short chapter. There was nothing on the horizon to give celiac patients hope of something other than complete abstinence from food and food products that contained gluten.

Treatment and Prevention Alternatives to the Gluten-Free Diet

Treatment	Method	Status
Zonulin Inhibitor	Block zonulin and reduce intestinal permeability or "leaky gut"	Successfully completed Phase IIb clinical trials with plans for Phase III trials under way by Alba Therapeutics.
Break down indigestible gluten fragments to keep them from generating immune response	Treatment with drug ALV003	ALV003: Promising results in several clinical trials including recently completed Phase IIa trials by Alvine Pharmaceuticals
Tissue Transglutaminase Inhibitors	Keep tTGs from interacting with gluten to keep autoimmune process at bay	Various trials under way at different locations
Therapeutic Vaccine	Develop tolerance to gluten by vaccinating with selected gluten fragments	Nexvax2: Clinical trials under way in U.S., Australia, and New Zealand
Prevention	Method	Status
Delay Gluten Introduction	Delay introduction of gluten to infants until one year of age	No drug: Promising results from small separate studies done at University of Maryland, Baltimore, and Università Politecnica delle Marche, Italy; large study in recruitment phase
Modify Gluten Introduction	Introduce small quantities of gluten to genetically predisposed children during breastfeeding period	PREVENTCD: International project sponsored by European Union 6th Framework Programme to investigate hypothesis of developing early tolerance to gluten

The breakthrough for me came at an international meeting in Florence, Italy, in 2005. At that meeting, I was asked to elaborate on the possibility of a novel treatment for celiac disease. We were working on the technology to inhibit zonulin, which is responsible for increased leakiness in the gut (see Chapter Four). Alba Therapeutics had been formed to investigate the promising compound AT-1001 (now called Larazotide acetate) for the treatment of celiac disease. The way my colleagues responded to my lecture was another déjà vu moment.

It was similar to the skeptical and cold reaction to my earlier assertion that celiac disease existed but was overlooked in the United States. I received very doubtful feedback from many of my peers. Indeed, they considered that any alternative treatments to the gluten-free diet were unthinkable, unfeasible, and unattainable.

In only nine years, however, we've seen a steady increase in clinical trials evaluating several technologies for alternative treatments for celiac disease. Once again, even my more skeptical colleagues have accepted the concept that with our increased knowledge of gluten-related disorders, alternative or integrative treatments are a real possibility.

Since 2005, more than 75 clinical trials related to gluten in various ways, from treating Autism Spectrum Disorder to a potential vaccine or treatment with hookworm, have been registered (see www.clinicaltrials.gov). What's the science behind all this? What have we learned that makes this third wish, if not possible, at least plausible? To provide the rationale for all these studies, we need to look at some key findings that made these investigations possible.

YOU ARE WHAT YOU EAT

My grandfather used to say, "Tell me what you eat, and I'll tell you who you are." When I was young, his words didn't make much sense to me. Now I deeply appreciate the philosophy behind his simple statement.

During the past twenty years, our knowledge of human health and disease has enjoyed an extraordinary shift in some basic scientific paradigms. Ancient Greek and Roman physician/philosophers identified four basic elements—air, fire, earth, and water—that dictated the balance between health and disease. They believed that when these elements were out of balance, disease occurred. By putting these elements back into balance through herbs, diet, or other means, the patient would be cured, according to these ancient healers.

Since the days of the Greek and Roman physicians, and up until twenty years ago, very little progress had been made in understanding the basis of human health or what makes a person retain or lose that healthy balance. But the era of "omics," or the study of something in its entirety, began almost two decades ago, and the pace of discovery about the balance between the state of human health and disease has grown exponentially since then.

CRACKING THE HUMAN GENOME

With the development of genomics, scientists and physicians alike were convinced that deciphering the human genome would be the key to paving the way to understanding and eradicating all human diseases. Even though it was a daunting exercise to crack the code of the human genome, two major efforts began along parallel tracks.

The first one was supported by the federal government under the leadership of Francis Collins, head of the National Human Genome Research Institute of the National Institutes of Health. The second was supported by private industry under the leadership of a visionary but controversial scientist named Craig Venter. The race involved hundreds of scientists and several billion dollars.

President Bill Clinton, flanked by Francis Collins and Craig Venter, announced the results at a press conference on June 26, 2000. The first comprehensive survey of the human genome had been completed. And on that day, several of my basic scientific assumptions flew out the window as I contemplated the announcement that heralded the new era of "personalized medicine."

I was shocked to learn that humans are genetically fairly rudimental beings. In 2004, scientists from The International Human Genome Sequencing Consortium revised their estimate of 35,000 human protein-encoding genes downward to between 20,000 and 25,000. The remaining 80 percent of our genetic material was considered useless, just junk DNA, the leftover material of evolutionary mistakes. Now our gene pair numbers are almost on a par with those of the common garden earthworm.

On the other hand, scientists from the University of Georgia projected a conservative estimate of between 164,000 and 334,000 protein-encoding genes in the genome of wheat. With numbers like those, it seems like we're at the bottom of the genetic scale of sophistication.

With the decoding of the human genome, the concept of one gene controlling one disease no longer held true. We learned that many genes could be involved in the evolution of a disease. Once we began to appreciate that genomics was not a simple answer to end all disease, the second era of discovery began.

SOLVING THE PROTEOMIC PUZZLE

Focused on the expression of proteins, "proteomics" became the next nexus of our scientific universe. If the paradigm of one gene for one disease wasn't true, we had to find another answer. Could one gene determine the expression of several proteins, which in turn dictate the color of our skin, our eyes, and our hair along with our height, and according to some scientists, even our intelligence?

But once again, just as with genomics, the study of the proteins expressed in health and disease (proteomics) did not give us simple answers to our complicated questions. So we've gone even more microscopic, in a paradoxical search for very small organisms in a vastly diverse universe. Through "microbiomics" we're looking at the human microbiota in the gut for answers to questions about the balance between health and disease.

Recent discoveries seem to go along with my grandfather's sentiment that we are what we eat—literally! Technological advances have given us the research tools to study the composition of the bacteria that live in symbiosis with us from birth to death. In great detail, we can examine this parallel civilization, called the microbiome, which seems to have a great deal of influence on the balance between health and disease.

Based on what we're learning about the microbiome of the gut, I'm now convinced that humankind is made up of two genomes. The first one is the human genome. That's the one we've known about for a long time that we inherit from our parents. Sometimes these genes are defective. If their information is translated into the production of proteins, they can increase the risk of disease. This genome is fixed. It doesn't change over time and is transmitted on to our progeny.

The second, and probably more important genome, is the one expressed by the multitudes of bacteria that live with us. They collectively contain one hundred times more genes than we do.

If we're lucky enough, we inherit this second genome from our mothers during natural delivery in childbirth. If we inherit the good bacteria selected by our mothers to live peacefully with their genes, it's likely that these bacteria will also live peacefully with our genes. After all, half of our genes come from our mothers.

If, on the other hand, we're born by Caesarean section, then all visitors, namely good bacteria and bad bacteria, can inhabit our intestines. This scenario can increase the chance of switching from a state of health to a state of disease. This theory is already supported by many observations in the literature suggesting that the risk of developing autoimmune diseases, including celiac disease, is much higher in babies born by Caesarean section.

Unlike the human genome, the human microbiome can change over time. It's influenced by many environmental factors including diet, infections, surgeries, and antibiotic use, to name only a few. In my opinion, the result of this interplay between the human genome and the human microbiome ultimately holds the key to the answer of how to maintain the yin and yang between health and disease.

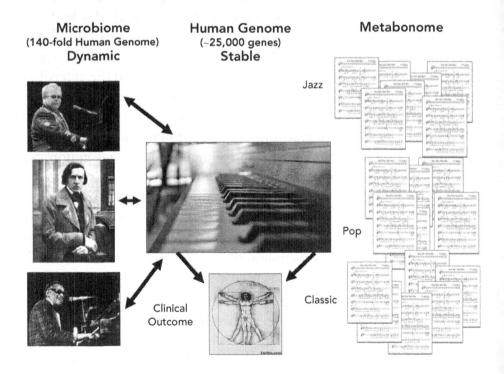

PLAYING THE "PIANO" OF THE HUMAN GENOME

To better clarify this concept, let's assume the human genome can be compared to a piano with 20,000 notes, and each note corresponds to a gene. Let's also assume that to develop complex diseases like celiac disease, more than a single gene should be defective to increase the genetic predisposition.

Just as with any piano, even the "human genome piano" will remain silent unless a piano player strikes the keys. In my view, it's the microbiome that's responsible for playing the human genome piano. And because the microbiome can change over time, the music being played also can change.

What makes the story even more fascinating is the very recent discovery, which is the result of more than 10 years of work by 440 researchers worldwide, that what was considered junk DNA is not junk after all! Indeed these tiny pieces of DNA are control stations through which environmental factors, including the microbiome, dictate if and when notes (i.e., genes) are played (i.e., expressed).

Let's say that to play the music of celiac disease, two hundred of the 20,000 notes need to be struck. A good microbiome, one that lives peacefully with us and is conducive to a good state of health, may only touch a proportion of these two hundred notes. Therefore, the genetic predisposition to develop celiac disease doesn't necessarily result in the manifestation of the disease.

If we're exposed, however, to one of the environmental factors named above that can change the microbiome, the new composition of the bacteria may lead to the expression of all two hundred genes needed to develop celiac disease. This theory is supported by several observations that came from our Center. Indeed, we've discovered that the microbiome of infants at risk of celiac disease is different from the microbiome of infants who aren't at risk.

We've also answered another seemingly inexplicable question related to a dogma that I previously considered a pillar of celiac disease autoimmunity. If celiac disease resulted from the interplay between the genes we inherit from our parents and gluten (the indisputable environmental trigger of celiac disease), we thought the disease would have to begin with the introduction of gluten into your diet. That happens almost universally in the first year of your life with the introduction of solid foods.

So how did we explain the onset of celiac disease in adulthood? Researchers thought the immune system of these individuals was less aggressive. They thought the intestinal damage characteristic of celiac disease started with gluten introduction in the diet. They also thought that for those patients who developed symptoms later in life that the critical mass of damage that causes symptoms occurred throughout a period of years. This contrasted with infant cases of celiac disease with intestinal damage and diagnosis within the first two years of life.

It was shocking for us to learn otherwise. A study we published in 2010 followed more than 3,000 healthy adults for a period of 50 years during their lifespan. As so often seems to occur in these studies, the main scope of our study was very different from its final outcome.

DEVELOPING CELIAC DISEASE LATE IN LIFE

Before this study, I believed that the game of celiac disease was over when genes interact with the baby's first taste of gluten. Our goal in this study of seemingly healthy adults from Washington County, Maryland, was to find out how asymptomatic celiacs (people who hadn't been diagnosed with celiac disease but who had typical intestinal damage without visible symptoms such as gastrointestinal distress) would develop clinical symptoms over time.

To my astonishment, we discovered that in this group of blood samples from more than 3,000 seemingly healthy individuals, the incidence of celiac disease doubled every 15 years. It was one in 500 in the 1970s, one in 250 in the late 1980s, and nearly one in 100 in the early 2000s. Among the subjects who eventually developed celiac disease, there were many who had been able to eat gluten safely for decades. Then after such a long period of time (for some people it was more than 70 years), they lost the luxury of tolerating gluten and developed celiac disease.

These shocking findings raised two interesting and key questions. What kind of physiological tricks did their bodies employ to tolerate what was the indisputable trigger (gluten) for so long? I'm convinced that whoever is able to answer this question will have the key to unlocking the secret behind many diseases affecting human-kind, including many cancers, autoimmune diseases, and degenerative diseases like Alzheimer's and dementia.

The second key question is: What happens to these individuals to make them switch from tolerance to the immune response that leads to celiac disease? I believe that the answer to this second question is indeed related to changes in the microbiome.

I think this is the only way to explain the apparent dichotomy of people developing celiac disease at different ages. What's even more intriguing is the discrepancy of celiac disease between identical twins. Even though identical twins share the same genes and are both exposed to gluten, we know that in 25 percent of cases of identical twins, one will develop celiac disease and one will not.

Keeping these things in mind, let's look at two key avenues being explored as alternatives to the gluten-free diet: 1) prevention for those at risk of celiac disease but who haven't yet developed it and 2) treatment for those who already have the condition, which is described in the final chapter. Let's start with prevention.

EATING FOR GOOD HEALTH

So, to bring us back to my grandfather's philosophy, it's well known that diet, together with the use and abuse of antibiotics, is the most influential environmental factor dictating the microbiome in the gut. This might also partially explain why we have experienced an epidemic of immune-related diseases during the past 50 years.

With the rise of industrialization and our increasingly fast-paced lifestyles, many people don't take the time to cook meals on a regular basis. We often rely on pre-packaged foods, which have a very different composition compared to the food that humans have consumed during the millennia of our evolution.

Growing up in Southern Italy some time ago, I belong to a generation that still remembers the seasonality of produce. Strawberries were available only in the summer and exotic fruits were not available at all. There was only a short window of the year when you could enjoy certain fresh vegetables such as tomatoes, cucumbers, zucchini, and sweet corn.

Now all these produce items, and many more, are available year-round. They can be genetically modified to be virus resistant, insect resistant, and herbicide resistant. For marketing reasons, they're sometimes modified to be a uniform color free from blemishes. And in the case of watermelons, some even have their seeds genetically removed for our eating convenience.

Having year-round access to fresh fruits and vegetables and a wide variety of other foodstuffs can contribute greatly to both our health and our sense of well-being. As every nutritionist (and many mothers) know, eating a variety of foods is key to good nutrition. Nonetheless, it's hard for me to believe that these sudden and fairly drastic changes in our eating habits would have no consequences on the composition of our microbiome and therefore on our health and well-being.

IT'S ALL A MATTER OF BALANCE

So what's my message to you as a result of our current research and the state of our grocery stores? One very exciting lesson that I learned from these studies at the Center for Celiac Research is that you are not born with celiac disease. It's not destiny that you will develop celiac disease just because you're genetically predisposed.

That tells me that there must be a way to twist destiny by making sure that the good bacteria, the ones that live in peace with us, will stay there. If they're disturbed by a change in lifestyle, including dietary changes, the use of antibiotics, and abuse of prepackaged and highly processed foods with many preservatives and unnecessary fillers, this is something that you should try to minimize as much as possible.

For every person, and for every person's gut, it seems the balance between health and disease is a very individual matter. As we map more of the microbiome and learn how to distinguish more carefully between friendly and unfriendly microorganisms, we hope to move closer to learning about how to create that balance in such a complex world. To close this gap, three major prospective studies have been launched in Europe and the United States.

"PREVENTCD" STUDY

The "PreventCD" study, supported by a European consortium, enrolled 1,000 infants who were randomized to either receive traces of gluten (about 100 mg) early in their infancy or to remain gluten free until they were weaned between four and seven months of age.

Some researchers think that very early exposure to minimal amounts of gluten may induce tolerance and therefore prevent the immune system from reacting to later exposure to gluten with the onset of celiac disease. It's a similar concept to the preventive effect of vaccination. Right now, no information is available on the efficacy of this intervention in preventing celiac disease due to the fact that the study has not been unblinded yet.

THE ITALIAN CELIAC DISEASE PREVENTIVE STUDY

In collaboration with a consortium of Italian colleagues and under the leadership of its co-director, Dr. Carlo Catassi, the Center for Celiac Research collaborated in an ongoing study started in 2004 involving more than 700 at-risk infants. One group of babies was introduced to gluten at the time recommended by the American Academy of Pediatrics (from four to seven months). Another group of babies did not receive gluten until twelve months of age.

After almost ten years of follow up, outcomes from the study suggest that late introduction of gluten in the diet will delay the onset of the disease, but it seems to make no difference in preventing the disease, at least in the ten years' time interval. This age limit may increase as the children grow older. One important lesson learned through this study is that children who missed the often-recommended window of opportunity for gluten introduction from four to seven months of age did not have an increased risk of developing celiac disease.

If this data is confirmed through longer follow-up studies, a delay in the introduction of gluten may be considered. That way, quality of life might be improved by shortening the period needed to follow a gluten-free diet. The delayed introduction of gluten can be even more rewarding for those children with two copies of the HLA-DQ2 genes who seem to be at a much higher risk of developing the disease (see Chapter Five). Based on our research findings that people can develop celiac disease at any age, the children from this study need to be closely monitored for the onset of celiac disease later in their lives.

Another lesson learned from this study is that the level of antibodies can fluctuate over time. A subgroup of these infants may initially present with the appearance of the anti-tTG antibodies, a typical sign of loss of tolerance to gluten that leads to the autoimmune intestinal insult typical of celiac disease. But that loss of tolerance isn't necessarily permanent, meaning that the destiny of these kids to absolutely develop celiac disease over time isn't signed, sealed, and delivered.

Ninety-six of the children in the study had positive blood tests, and 72 showed intestinal damage after endoscopies. The other 24 children had no damage. They had the antibodies and potential for celiac disease, but not the enteropathy.

We thought it was only a matter of time before all these children developed celiac disease. But something more puzzling occurred. After we retested them, 21 had developed negative antibodies over time even though they were on a regular diet. Of the remaining three with positive antibodies, one infant developed celiac disease and the other two infants had fluctuating antibodies for the next two years.

This means that the yin and yang between tolerance and immune response to gluten is not a one-way street. Sometimes these kids can lose the battle, but not the war. This fascinating highway of gluten tolerance and gluten immune response becomes another opportunity to learn how to reverse a process that we believed irreversible—that of immune attack causing autoimmune disease.

CENTER FOR CELIAC RESEARCH STUDY

The third and final study has been designed by our Center to recruit approximately 500 at-risk infants who will be followed for five years without any dietary intervention. What we want to learn with this new study is the natural history of celiac disease, how its onset is related to the feeding regimen (breastfeeding vs. formula feeding), and how the use of antibiotics can have an impact on the loss of tolerance to gluten.

We're also looking at what specific microbiome composition carries the risk of triggering celiac disease in genetically predisposed infants, and, most important, if we can identify specific molecules (called metabolites) that can predict who is at risk of losing tolerance to gluten later on in life.

In an earlier proof-of-concept study, we recruited approximately 60 babies. In that study, we learned that the microbiome of infants at risk for celiac disease is different when compared to the microbiome of infants who are not at risk of developing celiac disease.

We also learned a lesson that could have remarkable consequences for the future management of autoimmune diseases. Indeed, in this pilot study, we were able to identify a metabolite called "lactate" produced by a specific group of bacteria called lactobacilli.

The number of these bacteria present in the microbiome peaked months before the onset of autoimmunity, and then dropped just before the infants developed their diseases. If the decline is the sign of the onset of celiac disease, maybe we can keep these children in a constant state of tolerance by maintaining the number of lactobacilla in their microbiota at high levels so that their lactate levels will not drop over time.

Interestingly enough, we saw this trend in an infant who developed celiac disease and an infant who developed type 1 diabetes. Given the comorbidity between these two autoimmune diseases, it should not be surprising that infants at risk for celiac disease may develop type 1 diabetes.

If these findings are confirmed in large numbers, these results could represent the classic crystal ball to look into the future of children who will eventually develop autoimmune diseases. If indeed, we can confirm that lactate and its changes over time can be the red flag for future autoimmune evolution in at-risk babies, we may eventually intervene to maintain lactate production at a higher level. This way, we can keep these babies in a perennial state of tolerance to gluten and therefore, we may be able to avoid the onset of celiac disease.

In other words, we would have the ability to know which infant is on the verge of losing the war that leads to autoimmunity. In these cases, we could intervene by reestablishing a friendly microbiome to keep him or her in a state of perennial tolerance. Assuming that these preliminary findings hold true, there is a chance that in a few years from now, we might be looking at a major paradigm shift of prevention instead of treatment of autoimmune disorders.

In our pilot study, one of the babies in the group who received gluten early (at four months) developed celiac disease at ten months. Although his mother and grandmother both have celiac disease, his four-year-old sister doesn't even have the genetic markers. His mother, Meghan, manifested celiac disease after surgery, a stressor that can activate the switch from tolerance to autoimmunity.

You might remember her story from Chapter Ten, where she also shares tips about looking after an infant with celiac disease. Looking ahead to Chapter Sixteen, we will explore promising new treatments and therapies as alternatives to the gluten-free diet.

New Treatments and Therapies

"You don't miss your water till your well runs dry."
—**WILLIAM BELL**

TAKING A CHANCE ON A CLINICAL TRIAL

Several years ago, Roberto Concepción was a very good soccer player. (His name and identifying characteristics have been changed for patient confidentiality). He started playing at an early age and enjoyed success throughout his school years. A quick and aggressive center forward, he moved up the ranks until he was on a national side playing in international matches around the world.

By international sporting standards, Roberto had achieved a great deal of success. He retired in his late twenties to set up one of the most competitive soccer training camps in the United States. He remained active and in shape by teaching a new generation of soccer players on the field. But as he approached his thirtieth birthday, Roberto noticed that he didn't seem to have the same energy and drive that had propelled him into the competitive world of international soccer. He began experiencing gastrointestinal distress and noticed that he became fatigued more easily than he had in the past.

After talking with his team doctor and dietitian, Roberto underwent an exhaustive series of tests for conditions that might be causing his symptoms. After the tests came back negative, the doctor and the dietitian were stumped. But as a professional athlete, Roberto knew his body very well. He knew that he wasn't performing up to his ability. One thing he noticed was that when he stopped eating products containing gluten, he experienced some relief from bloating, cramping, and fatigue.

Roberto's physician sent him to a gastroenterologist, who recommended blood tests for celiac disease. The results came back positive. The next step was an endoscopy to look at the intestinal tissue and take biopsies to examine the microscopic villi in the intestine. Sure enough, Roberto showed the classic intestinal damage that results from untreated celiac disease. He went on the gluten-free diet, but the antibody levels in his blood remained elevated.

Roberto was traveling a lot and his compliance to the gluten-free diet was not ideal, which led to persistent symptoms and elevated antibody levels. He came to the Center to see what help we could give him. Our dietitian worked with Roberto to implement a strict gluten-free diet for three months. He still suffered from symptoms and had elevated antibody tests.

Roberto was a very good candidate for clinical trials of the new zonulin-inhibiting compound—Larazotide acetate (see Chapter Four). He enrolled in the trials that were being conducted by Alba Therapeutics, Inc., in Baltimore, Maryland.

In the double-blind, placebo-controlled trials, neither the researchers nor the subjects knew who was receiving the drug and who was not. So I didn't know whether Roberto was receiving Larazotide acetate or not. The clinical trial lasted only a few weeks and did not help Roberto resolve his problem.

The next step for Roberto was the Fasano Diet (see Chapter Five), which is a very restrictive version of the gluten-free diet. We put Roberto on the Fasano Diet for several months and his antibody levels finally dropped for the first time since he had been receiving blood tests. He went back on a less-restrictive gluten-free diet, and his antibody levels became elevated again and his symptoms returned.

So it was back to the Fasano Diet for Roberto, which he has been following for a few months now. With his travel schedule and exposure to cross-contamination in a variety of settings, an alternative treatment for celiac disease such as Larazotide acetate would be a real benefit for Roberto.

I've been a soccer fan all of my life, and I wouldn't care to place a wager on which team will win the next World Cup—it's such an exciting and volatile game. And even though Roberto knew that the clinical trial would not be the current solution to his problems, he was willing to take a risk for the sake of science. He played a small but important part in the Center's mission "to increase the awareness of celiac disease and other gluten-related disorders in order to provide better care, better quality of life, and more adequate support for the celiac disease community."

NEW IDEAS ABOUT HOW DISEASE BEGINS

The mission described in the preceding sentence came about as a result of my Aladdin's lamp experiment when I asked patients with celiac disease what their top three wishes were. You might remember that the number one wish was to be able to eat anything they wanted with absolutely no restrictions on gluten consumption.

At the time it was a laughable proposition, since no one could even imagine exploring alternatives to the gluten-free diet, one of the safest and most effective ways to treat an autoimmune disorder. But discoveries in the late 1990s and early 2000s in the fields of cell and molecular biology and immunology changed how we defined and diagnosed not only celiac disease but also autoimmunity in general.

We developed a diagnostic tool for testing tTG autoantibody levels, now implemented across the United States, at the Center in the late 1990s. In 2000, our research team discovered zonulin, an intriguing protein that pops up in some unexpected places. You've met zonulin elsewhere in this book. It appears to be involved in disease onset through the role it plays in the development of a leaky gut (see Chapter Four).

With these discoveries and others like them, scientists have created new concepts of pathophysiology that offer possible targets for treatment alternatives like Larazotide acetate to the gluten-free diet. As we expand our understanding of the complex molecular mechanisms of gluten-related disorders, and learn more about the fascinating miniature universe called the microbiome, research into alternative treatments for celiac disease and other gluten-related disorders is growing at a rapid and promising pace.

DO WE REALLY NEED AN ALTERNATIVE?

No more gluten—period. That's the cornerstone of the treatment for celiac disease. It sounds simple enough, right? But in many countries, gluten is a common (and not always labeled) ingredient in the diet of most humans.

This presents a huge challenge for patients. Gluten-free products are not always widely available, and they are more expensive than their gluten-containing counterparts. And, as in Roberto's case, dietary compliance is not always the best solution for a large proportion of patients.

Research shows that more than 50 percent of people who adopt a diet for medical reasons (for example, high blood pressure, high cholesterol, diabetes, kidney failure, and others) fail to comply over time. This makes any diet therapy a high-risk proposition.

Furthermore, even when compliance isn't an issue, a high percentage of celiac disease patients on a gluten-free diet show persistent intestinal damage, even when they are symptom free with negative blood tests. In other words, although it's the safest alternative we have right now, the gluten-free diet is not a foolproof method to prevent damage from celiac disease developing in susceptible individuals.

GLUTEN CONTAMINATION: HOW MUCH IS TOO MUCH?

A diet completely devoid of gluten is often unrealistic. People with celiac disease and gluten sensitivity are exposed to products containing trace amounts of gluten, even when the products are sold as naturally "gluten-free." For instance, oats and even rice, which are both naturally gluten-free, can become cross-contaminated with wheat, barley, or rye if they aren't handled properly during processing.

To estimate a safe threshold for daily gluten intake, let's take a look at both the residual gluten in gluten-free products and the total intake of gluten-free foods. If you consume a variety of gluten-free products and your clinical symptoms and intestinal damage both resolve, then we can assume that the gluten level is acceptable.

Most gluten-free products that are made with wheat starch contain trace amounts of gluten (see Chapter Seven). In a prospective controlled study, these products were verified to be safe. In other words, whether patients ate naturally gluten-free products or wheat-starch-based gluten-free products, there was no difference in the health of their intestinal tissue health, their blood tests for autoantibodies, or their quality of life.

We don't have much available research on the minimal levels of gluten that will affect sensitive individuals. To find out more about what these acceptable levels might look like, the Center for Celiac Research collaborated with the Italian Celiac Association. We evaluated the effects of gluten exposure of either 10 or 50 mg of purified gluten per day for three months.

Results published in 2007 from the 49 individuals in the double-blind placebo-controlled trial showed that minimal mucosal abnormalities occur even when patients followed a strict gluten-free diet. We also proved that although both 10 and 50 mg of daily gluten are clinically well tolerated, there's a trend for mucosal changes to occur at the 50 mg dose. The results proved to me that we need safe and effective therapeutic alternatives to the gluten-free diet.

A more recent study conducted with European patients with celiac disease on their consumption of manufactured gluten-free products (bread, pasta, cookies, cakes, etc.) showed minimal to no risk for cross-contamination that can lead to problems for people with celiac disease. This is good news for consumers in the United States, where gluten-free manufacturing is catching up to the advances made in Europe.

THE MATHEMATICS OF TREATMENT

As a physician, when I treat someone to correct an unwelcome condition or disorder, I'm either taking something away to prevent a reaction or I'm adding something to create some kind of reaction in the body. For example, with wheat or dairy or peanut allergy, we take only those items out of the diet. With celiac disease, patients eliminate all gluten from their diet. So we've got the subtraction part of the equation pretty well figured out in the treatment of gluten-related disorders.

Now we're working on alternative therapies, many of which add something to either generate or prevent a particular reaction in the patient's metabolism. In the last two decades, we've learned a lot about the cellular and molecular mechanisms of celiac disease. We're just starting to distinguish the different molecular mechanisms that make up celiac disease, gluten sensitivity, and wheat allergy.

By developing pharmacological compounds and enzymes, researchers are trying to figure out how to manipulate what we've learned to create new therapeutic targets.

BORDER GUARDS OF THE BODY

For many years, we thought the primary function of the intestine was limited to the digestion and absorption of foodstuffs. But by looking more closely at the anatomical and functional arrangement of the gastrointestinal tract, we learned that there's a lot more going on than we ever realized.

As we discussed in Chapter Four, along with digestion and absorption, the intestine regulates the traffic of molecules between the gut lumen and your body. Acting like a guard at a gatehouse, the intestine with its tight junctions, controls what goes in and out of the complex world of your gut.

The control of this trafficking is really at the heart of the balance between tolerance (state of health) and immune response (disease). When this finely tuned traffic control of molecules is lost, as happens when zonulin is overproduced, immune-mediated diseases can develop in genetically susceptible individuals (for more details, see Chapter Four).

TAKING A "CELIAC PILL"

As discussed in Part One, the development of the zonulin-inhibitor Larazotide acetate opened up the possibility of approaching the treatment of autoimmune diseases by correcting intestinal barrier defects. This possibility has already been successfully explored in an animal model of autoimmunity.

Following these proof-of-concept experiments, Larazotide acetate was tested in double-blind, placebo-controlled human clinical trials by Alba Therapeutics. Almost 800 patients who have been exposed to Larazotide acetate (as compared to the placebo) experienced no adverse effects. Following acute gluten exposure, gastrointestinal symptoms were significantly more frequent among patients of the group exposed to gluten alone when compared with the gluten plus Larazotide acetate and the placebo groups.

Combined, the data suggests that Larazotide acetate is well tolerated and appears to be effective in preventing the symptoms triggered by gluten ingestion by people with celiac disease. Alba Therapeutics recently successfully concluded a Phase IIB double-blind, placebo-controlled study to evaluate the efficacy of Larazotide acetate in people who fail to respond to a gluten-free diet.

Plans for a Phase III study are under way. If Phase III is successfully completed, the most likely next step is approval from the FDA for use in the general population. With the "Fast Track" designation of Larazotide acetate by the FDA, this development could come about in the near future.

TAKING THE TOXIC OUT OF WHEAT

First it was nature, then it was early farmers, and later it was scientists who hybridized wheat by combining different genetic varieties to obtain characteristics such as greater yield or shorter growing time. In another subtractive application of my therapeutic treatment equation, one proposal is to eliminate the toxic peptides from wheat. It sounds like a simple enough solution, but unfortunately it's not.

Unraveling the puzzle of DNA in the twentieth century eventually led to the development of transgenic technology. It's a highly precise method of introducing a new gene into a living organism to make permanent changes in the next generation. While this method has led to widespread genetically engineered crops of soybeans, corn, and cotton, its application to wheat has been especially controversial, although some trials have been conducted in Europe and Australia.

These transgenic trials, however, are not designed to remove the toxic gluten peptides from wheat, which is a very daunting prospect. While gliadin is the major potentially toxic peptide in wheat that seems to be responsible for the vast majority of the immune response leading to celiac disease, there are still several other toxic gluten fragments (up to 50!) that can theoretically turn on inflammation in genetically susceptible individuals.

A new approach to revive ancient grains in which gluten content is much lower than what is present in modern-day wheat might be more appealing. Several companies are exploring this approach to develop grains with minimal amounts of gluten without changing the taste, color, odor, and sensation of the grain.

Because people with celiac disease must avoid gluten completely, however, this revival of old grains can be useful only to those individuals affected by gluten sensitivity in which a minimal amount of gluten is harmless. Enzyme treatments, like the ones described below, might also be applied to these grains to reduce gluten exposure.

ENZYME THERAPY

The gliadin peptides found in the prolamin protein in gluten are highly resistant to the digestive enzymes of our pancreas. Enzyme supplement therapy with the use of bacterial-derived enzymes that can digest gliadin has been proposed as a way for humans to completely digest the potentially toxic proteins found in wheat, barley, and rye. These enzymes would break down the gliadin fragments and render them invisible to the immune cells that set off the autoimmune process typical of celiac disease. We need more research to see whether this intervention can detoxify these peptides in the small intestine.

Another method to reduce gluten toxicity is to pretreat whole gluten or gluten-containing foods with bacterial-derived enzymes. Gluten detoxification through enzyme therapy could be an effective method for producing more palatable gluten-free products and possibly treating celiac disease and other gluten-related disorders. Finally, enzyme treatment can be even more effective when performed on ancient grains with low gluten content.

WHEN IS A T-CELL LIKE A T-SHIRT?

T-shirts are the basic building block of many wardrobes for males and females of all ages. At the initial stage of manufacture, it's the same basic design—hence the name "T-shirt." But when the designer and the production printer get together—anything goes. From fake fur to metallic gold and every color available, T-shirt design is a basic human expression around the world. Think of the many different T-shirts that you've owned, and you'll have an idea of how many different T-cells are present in the human body.

Part of the sophisticated adaptive immune system, T-cells are as versatile and potentially complex as the humble T-shirt. The first step in the manufacture of T-cells is in the bone marrow facility. After immature cells develop here, they migrate to the thymus gland in the neck. (The "T" stands for thymus.) At this manufacturing facility, the basic T-cells get their own custom printing to respond to whatever threat or invasion the body is fighting.

Immunologists are still trying to identify the functions of the many different types of mature T-cells. Some T-cells join with other cells and release "cytokines," which are typically designed to fight infections. A special type of T-cell called T-helper binds to the antigen (a foreign invader, which is gluten in the case of celiac disease) and produces antibodies resulting in inflammation. Continued research on T-cells and the role they play in autoimmunity could lead to targeted therapies for conditions such as celiac disease.

CHANGING THE EQUATION AT THE MOLECULAR LEVEL

When you eat gluten, gluten causes leakage at the cellular level of the intestine. This happens when zonulin opens up the gates in between cells allowing gluten to gain access beneath the layer of epithelial cells. Since gluten isn't welcome in this part of the body, the immune system goes after the enemy, which causes inflammation.

The inflammation creates collateral damage by destroying cells, which makes contents leak out of the cell. Among the many substances expressed within a cell, there is a very special enzyme called tissue transglutaminase (tTG) that we met in Chapter Five. We typically use this enzyme to repair wounds by linking two proteins together. tTG does this by changing the composition of these proteins so that they become sticky and join together.

Using the same trick, this enzyme is also able to modify gluten in such a way that the gluten molecule will fit perfectly on the docking station of the DQ2 and DQ8 proteins, which are present on the surface of specialized immune cells called antigen-presenting cells. The landing of gluten on this docking station initiates a cascade of events leading to the autoimmune process typical of celiac disease. This tTG enzyme is crucial to the onset of celiac disease and intestinal damage.

Gluten on the docking station is presented to the immune cells called the T-cells. Under normal circumstances, and in people without celiac disease, the T-cells would clean up this enemy—no problem. These helper T-cells are like very efficient janitors. They do exactly what they are supposed to do with great efficiency and no deviations.

In people with celiac disease, the T-cells are more like very lethargic janitors. Rather than clean up the mess, they start to produce chemicals (called cytokines) that create the collateral damage known as inflammation that specifically targets the intestinal cells and ultimately results in the autoimmune damage typical of celiac disease.

DEVELOPING A THERAPEUTIC VACCINE

A vaccine for celiac disease would change the mindset of the lethargic janitor to the efficient janitor, but it's a very difficult operation. By supplying the offending enemy (three potentially toxic peptides: gliadin in wheat, hordein in barley, and secalin in rye) in small quantities, it might be possible to reprogram the immune cells to do their job in an efficient and timely manner.

But it's more likely that it might be just like my research so many years ago with the potential cholera vaccine. It looked very good on paper, but it didn't work out very well in testing.

Although a vaccine for celiac disease would be the "holy grail" for an alternative to the gluten-free diet, I think this approach would take the longest time to become available to people compared to other alternative treatments we've discussed. It would also only be effective in 90 to 92 percent of people with celiac disease, since the vaccine is specific only for those individuals who carry the DQ2 gene. At this time, research is under way only for a vaccine candidate for DQ2-positive individuals.

Along with modifying tTG, modifying other components of the complex cellular network of the immune system might provide alternative tools for promoting tolerance. Recent research shows that gluten toxicity might not be dependent only on T-cells for recognition. Other members of the immune army, including antibodies to Interleukin-15, are being investigated for their role in refractory celiac disease.

TREATMENTS OF THE FUTURE

This overview is a brief testimony to how much we've achieved in understanding celiac disease and developing potential treatment alternatives in such a short period of time. The field is so dynamic, and the pace of new knowledge so fast, that I wouldn't be shocked if this new generation of celiac disease patients sees one or more of these technologies become reality in the near future.

Even so, I personally believe that the gluten-free diet will remain the pillar of the treatment for celiac disease. But these alternatives, or even more appropriately named integrated or complementary treatments to the gluten-free diet, could represent a safety net for celiac disease patients. That way, when our patients travel, attend public events, eat out at restaurants or visit friends and family—in other words, whenever they eat outside their homes—they will have peace of mind about staying safe.

For people with gluten sensitivity, the same alternative approach developed for celiac disease may benefit them as well. But let's remember, some patients with gluten sensitivity might have a higher sensitivity threshold for gluten. Therefore, the return to ancient grains with a lesser gluten content or grains with no gluten content could be a valuable approach for some of these people.

Only time will tell if this treatment or others that will evolve from subsequent developments later in the research pipeline will be safe and effective enough to serve as a substitute to the gluten-free diet.

Epilogue

Making Wishes Come True

Do you recall my story about Aladdin's lamp and the three wishes of patients with celiac disease from the Introduction? In large part, the work performed by people at the Center for Celiac Research has made those dreams come true.

Starting with the second wish, we've increased awareness of gluten-related disorders among physicians and other health-care professionals and the general population. For the third wish, it's now possible to diagnose celiac disease, especially in children, without the need for multiple biopsies (see Chapter Five).

And the first and most repeated wish, the ability to eat whatever you would like without worrying about gluten or cross-contamination, is coming closer to reality. Promising clinical trials of a pharmacological compound and other developments featured in Chapter Sixteen are bringing discoveries made at the Center's lab bench one step closer to treatments at the patient's bedside.

MAJOR RESEARCH DISCOVERIES

We started with the basic question about the existence of celiac disease in the United States, which we answered in 2003. Even though we were seen by many other scientists and physicians as being totally out of touch, the facts showed that celiac disease affects about one in every 133 Americans.

Another example of the pioneering research models we've created at the Center is the development of the diagnostic tTG auto-antibody blood test. This test has helped to reduce the number of biopsies needed for diagnosis of celiac disease.

We followed our diagnostic innovation of the tTG test with a proposition for a promising alternative treatment, Larazotide acetate, based on our new understanding of zonulin and leaky gut. And again our new ideas were criticized, but the role of increased intestinal permeability in autoimmune diseases, including celiac disease, is now an accepted concept, and early clinical trials are promising.

Now we're advancing the study of gluten sensitivity, and how it differs from celiac disease, to find ways to diagnose and possibly prevent the response of this second cousin on the spectrum of gluten-related disorders. And once again, we've been met with some skepticism, even in the face of scientific research that demonstrates the basic molecular differences in the two conditions.

Of course we've made many mistakes along the way; no scientist can be correct or completely accurate 100 percent of the time. And we rely on our peers to contribute to the healthy atmosphere of debate that defines good science. If I become discouraged, I remember that our primary goal is improving the quality of life for people with gluten-related disorders, and I focus on the evidence that points to how we can achieve that goal.

After eighteen years, we're looking forward to the next phase of discovery for the Center for Celiac Research. In 2013, we moved the Center to a new home in Boston at MassGeneral Hospital *for* Children. Along with providing care for adults and children with gluten-related disorders, we are also working in partnership with colleagues at the Celiac Center at Beth Israel Deaconess Medical Center and Boston Children's Hospital through the combined Celiac Program at Harvard Medical School. We'll continue our tradition of training fellows and physicians to treat gluten-related disorders and collaborating with researchers around the world to advance the understanding and treatment of autoimmune disorders.

In this new collegial and collaborative atmosphere, exciting new milestones lie ahead of us that we can't even visualize. Ultimately, people all over the globe will be the beneficiaries of discoveries made through the Celiac Program at Harvard Medical School in collaboration with national and international researchers.

MEDIEVAL CONVENT BECOMES BIOMEDICAL CENTER

Another international project close to my heart, and very close to where I grew up, is the restoration of the San Nicola della Palma convent in Salerno, Italy, into a modern biomedical research institute. The site of the former convent began life as a Benedictine monastery in 1060 and has now become part of a successful and highly sophisticated urban renewal project.

In 2007 I began working with the mayor of Salerno, Vincenzo DeLuca, to set in motion the process of taking a completely destroyed building and resurrecting it into a premier research institute for scientists from all over the globe. In a timeline most untypical for an Italian enterprise, and in partnership with MassGeneral Hospital *for* Children and other supporters, we achieved this goal in only five years.

In October 2013, the European Biomedical Research Institute of Salerno (EBRIS) was officially opened. In a marvelous conjunction of ancient and modern, the remains of the ancient church are available for visitors to view beneath the glass floor under their feet.

The "Fondazione Scuola Medica Salernitana" or the Salerno Medical School Foundation, in partnership with the Massachusetts General Hospital *for* Children now houses a research and teaching facility that echoes the progressive and enlightened atmosphere that brought scholars—both men and women—from all over the medieval world to study and teach at Salerno. With the building's recent restoration as part of the Umberto I Institute, EBRIS has joined the cultural and scientific renaissance of Salerno.

In some ways, I feel that my life, along with this book, has arrived full circle as my two worlds—America and Italy—merge. The first phase has included eighteen years of promoting the treatment and awareness of gluten-related disorders to the U.S. community and bringing together knowledge and understanding from the deep European experience with celiac disease. At the new institute, by joining European expertise with American innovation in an open-minded atmosphere, new advances not only in gluten-related disorders, but also in the treatment of autoimmune disorders and other areas will also emerge.

BUILDING ON SUPPORT FROM THE CELIAC COMMUNITY

"Dear Dr. Fasano, I miss you very much. You were a very good doctor. Good luck with your pill. When you have done with it, will you come back and take care of your patients? Lots of love, Lucia."

This letter, a treasured souvenir from one of my younger patients written as a farewell message when I left the University of Maryland, has a place of pride in my crowded office. It reminds me of the unwavering support that members of the celiac community have given the Center since its inception. From the 25-cent donation from brothers and sisters of children with celiac disease to larger gifts that have made our discoveries possible, we value every single donation and donor.

In our new environment at Massachusetts General Hospital in Boston, we're working on some exciting projects: 1) finding a biomarker (a molecular "red flag") that we can use to develop a diagnostic tool for gluten sensitivity, 2) searching for differences in the gut microbiota of children with Autism Spectrum Disorder, 3) exploring the well-established connection between gluten sensitivity and a subgroup of people with schizophrenia, 4) looking for the best time to introduce gluten into an infant's diet; and other research topics.

COLLABORATION HAS ALWAYS BEEN KEY

When I embarked on this project of writing a book about gluten-related disorders as viewed through the prism of the Center for Celiac Research, I had many reservations. I've written many scientific articles and books, but I had never tried to tell the real story of the Center for Celiac Research. I knew that it wouldn't be an easy task.

But I'm so very glad that I've completed it. This exercise forced me to revisit eighteen years of my professional career. In that process, I've remembered many details that resurfaced as I was trying to identify the winding path that brought us to our current position.

But I don't want to leave the reader with the impression that this has been a one-man journey. By revisiting this history, it shows how remarkable the dedication of so many members of the Center for Celiac Research family has been in bringing celiac disease and other gluten-related disorders to center stage in the position of the medical community.

USING YOUR HEART AND SOUL

If someone had placed me in a time machine eighteen years ago and transported me to the present time, I would most definitely conclude that we must have taken a detour. There's no way that I thought we could have made so much progress in such a short span of time.

This reflective journey has made me recall a great lesson that I learned many, many years ago from my grandfather as I enjoyed my youth. My grandfather, a visionary physicist born in 1901 but with a mind belonging to the twenty-first century, taught me that nothing is impossible in life provided that your heart and soul are ready for it.

With inventions that were way ahead of his time, he reminded me very much of Leonardo da Vinci. Growing up with my grandfather gave me the conviction to stand by my ideas if I was genuinely convinced that they would lead to transformational outcomes.

These words spoken by the 26th president of the United States in Paris more than 103 years ago have proved just as inspiring to me as the words of my grandfather.

It is not the critic who counts, not the man who points out how the strong man stumbled; nor where the doer of deeds could have done better. The credit belongs to the man who is actually in the arena; whose face is marred by dust and sweat and blood;

who strives valiantly; who errs and comes up short again and again; who knows the great enthusiasms, the great devotions, and spends himself in a worthy cause; who, at best, knows in the end the triumph of high achievements; and who, at worst, if he fails, at least fails while daring greatly, so that his place shall never be with those cold and timid souls who know neither victory nor defeat.

—THEODORE ROOSEVELT

Now it is time for me to return to work: to experience another day in the clinic with my patients, another day in the lab with my students, and another day with my colleagues as we work together to solve the intricate puzzles of science by looking at them one piece at a time.

Appendix

Apps for Mobile Phones

AllergyFree Passport Apps
Offers different apps that people with celiac disease, as well as those with food allergies (dairy, eggs, fish, peanuts, shellfish, soy, etc.), can customize to search for restaurants and menu items.
www.allergyfreepassport.com/apps/

Celiac Feed
Discover gluten-free venues nearby and in other cities with the iPhone. Join the community and Q&A to share knowledge about the gluten-free diet and celiac disease.
www.celiacfeed.com

Find Me Gluten Free
This app has addresses, phone numbers, and menus for restaurants "near me" or "near address" or cities.
www.findmeglutenfree.com/

Gluten-Free App Reviews (Academy of Nutrition and Dietetics)
www.eatright.org/media/content.aspx?id=6442467101

Gluten Free Detective (Academy of Nutrition and Dietetics)
http://tunes.apple.com/in/app/the-gluten-detective/id529788037?mt=8

Gluten Free Registry
An app for iPhone, Android Smart phones, and iPads with a searchable database of more than 23,400+ gluten-free friendly business locations in U.S. and international locations.
www.glutenfreeregistry.com

Gluten Free Restaurant Cards (free)
Provides 40 card images from CeliacTravel.com in many languages that can be used in restaurants and shown to wait staff or chefs to explain the gluten-free diet.
www.celiactravel.com/cards/

Is that Gluten Free? (iPad and iPhone/iTouch app)
This app includes 23,000 manufacturer-verified gluten-free products and more than 510 brands. You can search by brand, product name, or category with searchable ingredient tabs.
midlifecrisisapps.com/is-that-gluten-free-eating-out/

Whole Foods Market Recipes App
Free iPhone, iPod Touch, or iPad app that filters through recipes by categories and special diets such as gluten free, vegetarian, low-fat, and more. It can also find recipes that use ingredients you already have and gives the option to build shopping lists.
www.wholefoodsmarket.com/apps/index.php

(Special thanks to Dr. Mary McKenna and John M. Mink for phone apps)

Recommended Reading

In the last decade, the number of resources (books, articles, and websites), along with support groups and other advocacy organizations for people with celiac disease and gluten sensitivity, has greatly expanded. This short selection is only a starting point; many authors listed below have other books and resources for people with gluten-related disorders.

BOOKS ON CELIAC DISEASE, THE GLUTEN-FREE DIET, AND RELATED TOPICS

Adamson, E., Thompson, T. *The Complete Idiot's Guide to Gluten-Free Eating*. New York: Penguin. 2007.

Blumer, I., Crowe, S. *Celiac Disease for Dummies*. Mississauga, Ontario: John Wiley & Sons Canada. 2010.

Bower, S. *Celiac Disease: A Guide to Living with Gluten Intolerance*. New York: Demos Medical Publishing, 2007.

Brown, M. *Gluten-Free Hassle-Free: A Simple, Sane, Dietitian-Approved Program for Eating Your Way Back to Health*. New York: Demos Medical Publishing. 2013.

Canadian Celiac Association. *Acceptability of Foods and Food Ingredients for the Gluten-Free Diet Pocket Dictionary*. www.celiac.ca.

Case, S. *Gluten-Free Diet. A Comprehensive Resource Guide.* Regina, Saskatchewan: Case Nutrition Consulting. 2010.

Cavalli-Sforza, L., Menozzi, P., Piazza, A. *The History and Geography of Human Genes.* Princeton, NJ: Princeton University Press. 1994.

Dennis, M., Leffler, D. *Real Life with Celiac Disease: Troubleshooting and Thriving Gluten Free.* Bethesda, MD: AGA Press. 2010.

The Essential Gluten-Free Grocery Guide and The Essential Gluten-free Restaurant Guide from www.triumphdining.com.

Fasano, A. (ed.) *Clinical Guide to Gluten-Related Disorders.* Philadelphia, PA: Lippincott, Williams & Wilkins. 2013.

Fasano, A., Troncone, R., Branski. "Frontiers in Celiac Disease." *Pediatric and Adolescent Medicine,* Vol. 12. Basel, Switzerland: Karger. 2008.

Fenster, C. *1,000 Gluten-Free Recipes.* Hoboken, NJ: John Wiley & Sons. 2008.

Green, P. H. R., Jones, R. *Celiac Disease: A Hidden Epidemic.* 2nd ed. New York: HarperCollins. 2010.

Holmes, G., Catassi, C., Fasano, A. *Fast Facts: Celiac Disease.* 2nd ed. Oxford, UK: Health Press. 2009.

Koeller, K., LaFrance, R. *Let's Eat Out Around the World, Gluten Free and Allergy Free.* 4th ed. New York, NY: Demos Health. 2013.

Korn, D. *Living Gluten-Free for Dummies.* 2nd ed. Hoboken, NJ: John Wiley & Sons. 2010.

National Institutes of Health Consensus Development Conference on Celiac Disease. Bethesda, MD: 2004. U.S. Department of Health & Human Services.

Packaged Facts. *Gluten-free Food and Beverage Guide in the U.S.* 4th ed. Rockville, MD: Market Research Group, LLC. 2012.

Ramazzini, B. *De Morbis Artificum Diatriba (Diseases of Workers).* Padua, Italy. 1713.

Shepard, J. D. *The First Year: Celiac Disease and Living Gluten-Free: An Essential Guide for the Newly Diagnosed.* Cambridge, MA: Perseus Books. 2008.

Staton, H., Leichter, A., Bousvaros, A. *Amy Goes Gluten Free: A Young Person's Guide to Celiac Disease.* Children's Hospital, Boston, MA. 2009.

Thompson, Tricia. *The Gluten-Free Nutrition Guide.*
www.glutenfreedietitian.com

MAGAZINES

Allergic Living Magazine
www.allergicliving.com

Delight Gluten Free
www.delightgfmagazine.com

Easy Eats
www.easyeats.com

Gluten-Free Living Magazine
www.glutenfreeliving.com

Living Without Magazine
www.livingwithout.com

Simply Gluten Free Magazine

SELECTED PEER-REVIEWED ARTICLES, REVIEWS, EDITORIALS, AND GUIDELINES

Bai, J. C., Fried, M., Corazza, G. R., Schuppan, D., Farthing, M., Catassi, C., Greco, L., Cohen, H., Ciacci, C., Eliakim, R., Fasano, A., Gonzalez, A., Krabshuis, J. H., LeMair, A., World Gastroenterology Organization. "World Gastroenterology Organisation global guidelines on celiac disease." *J Clin Gastroenterol.* 2013: 47(2): 121–126.

Barada, K., Abu Daya, H., Rostami, K., Catassi, C. "Celiac disease in the developing world." *Gastrointest Endosc Clin N Am.* 2012: 22(4): 773–796.

Barg, W., Wolancyk-Medrala, A., Obojski, A., Wytrychowski, K., Panaszek, B., Medrala, W. "Food-dependent exercise-induced anaphylaxis: possible impact of increased basophil histamine releasability in hyperosmolar conditions." *J Investig Allergol Clin Immunol.* 2008: 18(4): 312–315.

Branski, D., Fasano, A., Troncone, R. "Latest developments in the pathogenesis and treatment of celiac disease." *J Pediatr.* 2006: 149(3): 295–300.

Cascella, N. G., Santora, D., Gregory, P., Kelly, D. L., Fasano, A., Eaton, W. W. "Increased prevalence of transglutaminase 6 antibodies in sera from schizophrenia patients." *Schizophr Bull.* 2012: 39(4): 867–871.

Cascella, N. G., Kryszak, D., Bhatti, B., Gregory, P., Kelly, D. L., Mc Evoy, J. P., Fasano, A., Eaton, W. W. "Prevalence of celiac disease and gluten sensitivity in the United States antipsychotic trials of intervention effectiveness study population." *Schizophr Bull.* 2011: 37(1): 94–100.

Catassi, C., Bai, J. C., Bonaz, B., Bouma, G., Calabro, A., Carroccio, A., Castillejo, G., Ciacci, C., Cristofori, F., Dolinsek, J., Francavilla, R., Elli, L., Green, P., Holtmeier, W., Koehler, P., Koletzko, S., Meinhold, C., Sanders, D., Schumann, M., Schuppan, D., Ullrich, R., Vecsei, A., Volta, U., Zevallos, V., Sapone, A., Fasano, A. "Non-celiac gluten sensitivity: the new frontier of gluten related disorders." *Nutrients.* 2013: 5(10): 3839–3853.

Catassi, C., Lionetti, E. "Case finding for celiac disease is okay, but is it enough?" *J Pediatr Gastroenterol Nutr.* 2013: 57(4): 415–417.

Catassi, C., Anderson, R. P., Hill, I. D., Koletzko, S., Lionetti, E., Mouane, N., Schumann, M., Yachha, S. K. "World perspective on celiac disease." *J Pediatr Gastroenterol Nutr.* 2012: 55(5): 494–499.

Catassi, C. Editorial: "Celiac disease in Turkey: lessons from the fertile crescent." *Am J Gastroenterol.* 2011: 106(8): 1518–1520.

Catassi, C., Kryszak, D., Bhatti, B., Sturgeon, C., Helzlsouer, K., Clipp, S. L., Gelfond, D., Puppa, E., Sferuzza, A., Fasano, A. "Natural history of celiac disease autoimmunity in a USA cohort followed since 1974." *Ann Med.* 2010: 25(1): 530–538.

Catassi, C., Fasano, A. "Celiac disease diagnosis: simple rules are better than complicated algorithms." *Am J Med.* 2010: 123(8): 691–693.

Catassi, C., Fasano, A. "Celiac disease." *Curr Opin Gastroenterol.* 2008: 24(6): 687–691.

Catassi, C., Fasano, A. "Is this really celiac disease? Pitfalls in diagnosis." *Curr Gastroenterol Rep.* 2008: 10(5): 466–472.

Catassi, C., Kryszak, D., Louis-Jacques, O., Duerksen, D. R., Hill, I., Crowe, S. E., Brown, A. R., Pracaccini, N. J., Wonderly, B. A., Hartley, P., Oreci, J., Bennett, N., Horvath, K., Burk, M., Fasano, A. "Detection of celiac disease in primary care: a multicenter case-finding study in North America." *Am J Gastroenterol.* 2007: 102(7): 1454–1460.

Catassi, C., Fabiani, E., Iacono, G., D'Agate, C., Francavilla, R., Biagi, F., Volta, U., Accomando, S., Picareli, A., De Vitis, I., Pianelli, G., Gesuita, R., Carle, F., Mandolesi, A., Bearzi, I., Fasano, A. "A prospective double-blind, placebo-controlled trial to establish a safe gluten threshold for patients with celiac disease." *Am J Clin Nutr.* 2007: 85(1): 160–166.

Catassi, C. "Where is celiac disease coming from and why?" *J Pediatr Gastroenterol Nutr.* 2005: 40(3): 279–282.

Catassi, C., Fasano, A. "New developments in childhood celiac disease." *Curr Gastroenterol Rep.* 2002: 4(3): 238–243.

Cavell, B., Stenhammer, L., Ascher, H., Danielsson, L., Dannaeus, A., Lindberg, T., Lindquist, B. "Increasing incidence of childhood coeliac disease in Sweden: Results of a national study." *ActaPaediatr.* 1992: 81(8): 589–592.

Collin, P., Kaukinen, K., Vogelsang, H., Korponay-Szabo, I., Sommer, R., Schreier, E., Volta, U., Granito, A., Veronesi, L., Mascart, F., Ocmant, A., Ivarsson, A., Lagerqvist, C., Burgin-Wolff, A., Hadziselimovic, F., Furlano, R. I., Sidler, M. A., Mulder, C. J., Goerres, M. S., Mearin, M. L., Ninaber, M. K., Gudmand-Hoyer, E., Fabiani, E., Catassi, C., Tidlund, H., Alainentalo, L., Maki, M. "Antiendomysial and antihuman recombinant tissue transglutaminase antibodies in the diagnosis of celiac disease: a biopsy-proven European multicentre study." *Eur J Gastroenterol Hepatol.* 2005: 17(1): 85–91.

Collin, P., Kaukinen, K., Välimäki, M., Salmi, J. "Endocrinological Disorders and Celiac Disease." *Endocrine Reviews.* 2002: 23(4): 464–483.

Coury, D. L., Ashwood, P., Fasano, A., Fuchs, G., Geraghty, M., Kaul, A., Mawe, G., Patterson, P., Jones, N. E. "Gastrointestinal conditions in children with autism spectrum disorder: developing a research agenda." *Pediatrics.* 2012: Suppl 2: S160–168.

de Magistris, L., Picardi, A., Siniscalco, D., Riccio, M. P., Sapone, A., Cariello, R., Abbadessa, S., Medici, N., Lammers, K. M., Schiraldi, C., Iardino, P., Marotta, R., Tolone, C., Fasano, A., Pascotto, A., Bravaccio, C. "Antibodies against food antigens in patients with autistic spectrum disorders." *Biomed Res Int.* 2013: 729349.

Denery-Papini, S., Bodinier, M., Pineau, F., Triballeau, S., Tranquet,

O., Adel-Patient, K., Moneret-Vautrin, D. A., Bakan, B., Marion, D., Mothes, T., Mameri, H., Kasarda, D. "Immunoglobulin-E-binding epitopes of wheat allergens in patients with food allergy to wheat and in mice experimentally sensitized to wheat proteins." *Clin Exp Allergy.* 2011: 41(10): 1478–1492.

Drago, S. El Asmar, R., Di Pierro, M., Grazia Clemente, M., Tripathi, A., Sapone, A., Thakar, M., Iacono, G., Carroccio, A., D'Agate, C., Not, T., Zampini, L., Catassi, C., Fasano, A. "Gliadin, zonulin and gut permeability: Effects on celiac and non-celiac intestinal mucosa and intestinal cell lines." *Scand J Gastroenterol.* 2006: 41(4): 408–419.

Dowd, B., Walker-Smith, J. "Samuel Gee, Aretaeus, and the coeliac affection." *Br Med J.* 1974: 2(5909): 45–457.

Fasano, A., Catassi, C. Clinical Practice. "Celiac disease." *N Engl J Med.* 2012: 367(25): 2419–2426.

Fasano, A. "Novel therapeutic/integrative approaches for celiac disease and dermatitis herpetiformis." *Clin Dev Immunol.* 2012: 959061.

Fasano, A. "Intestinal permeability and its regulation by zonulin: diagnostic and therapeutic implications." *Biochim Biophys Acta.* 2012: 10(10): 1096–1000.

Fasano, A. "Zonulin, regulation of tight junctions, and autoimmune diseases." *Ann N Y Adac Sci.* 2012: 1258: 25–33.

Fasano, A. "Neurologic and psychiatric manifestations of celiac disease and gluten sensitivity." *Psychiatr Q.* 2012: 83(1): 91–102.

Fasano, A. "Leaky gut and autoimmune diseases." *Clin Rev Allergy Immunol.* 2012: 42(1): 71–78.

Fasano, A., Catassi C. "Early feeding practices and their impact on development of celiac disease." *Nestle Nurtr Workshop Ser Pediatr Program.* 2011: 68: 201–209.

Fasano, A. "Zonulin and its regulation of intestinal barrier function: the biological door to inflammation, autoimmunity, and cancer." *Physiol Rev.* 2011. 91(1): 151–175.

Fasano, A. "Should we screen for celiac disease? Yes." *BMJ.* 2009: 17: 339: b3592.

Fasano, A. "Surprises from celiac disease." *Sci Am.* 2009: 301(2): 54–61.

Fasano, A. "Physiological, pathological, and therapeutic implications of zonulin-mediated intestinal barrier modulation: living life on the edge of the wall." *Am J Pathol.* 2008: 173(5): 1243–1252.

Fasano, A. "Systemic autoimmune disorders in celiac disease." *Curr Opin Gastroenterol.* 2006: 22(6): 674–679.

Fasano, A., Shea-Donohue, T. "Mechanisms of disease: the role of intestinal barrier function in the pathogenesis of gastrointestinal autoimmune diseases." *Nat Clin Pract Gastroenterol Hepatol.* 2005: 2(9): 416–422.

Fasano, A. "Celiac disease–how to handle a clinical chameleon." *N Engl J Med.* 2003: 348(25): 2568–2570.

Fasano, A., Berti, I., Gerarduzzi, T., Not, T., Colletti, R. B., Drago, S., Elitsur, Y., Green, P. H., Guandalini, S., Hill, I. D., Pietzak, M., Ventura, A., Thorpe, M., Kryszak, D., Fornaroli, F., Wasserman, S. S., Murray, J. A., Horvath, K. "Prevalence of celiac disease in at-risk and not-at-risk groups in the United States: a large multicenter study." *Arch Intern Med.* 2003: 163(3): 286–292.

Folstein, S., Rutter, M. "Infantile autism: a genetic study of 21 twin pairs." *Journal of Child Psychology and Psychiatry.* 1977: 18(4): 297–321.

Franco, G., Franco, F. "Bernadino Ramazzini: The father of occupational medicine." *Am J Public Health.* 2001: 91(9): 1382.

Gilbert, A., Kruizinga, A. G., Neuhold, S., Houben, G. F., Canela, M. A., Fasano, A., Catassi, C. "Might gluten traces in wheat substitutes pose a risk in patients with celiac disease? A population-based probabilistic approach to risk estimation." *Am J Clin Nutr.* 2013: 98(2): 511.

Gadewar, S., Fasano, A. "Celiac disease: is the atypical really typical? Summary of the recent National Institutes of Health Consensus Conference and latest advances." *Curr Gastroenterol Rep.* 2005: 7(6): 455–461.

Gee, S. J. "On the coeliac affection. St Bartholomew's Hospital Report." 1888: 24: 17–20.

Gelfond, D., Fasano, A. "Celiac disease in the pediatric population." *Pediatr Ann.* 2006: 41(4): 408–419.

Goldberg, D., Kryszak D., Fasano, A., Green, P. H. "Screening for celiac disease in family members: is follow-up testing necessary?" *Dig Dis Sci.* 2007: 52(4): 1082–1086.

Green, P. H. "The many faces of celiac disease: Clinical presentation of celiac disease in the adult population." *Gastroenterology.* 2005: 128(4)

Suppl 1: S74–S78.

Green, P. H. "Trends in the presentation of celiac disease." *Am J Med,* 2006: 119(4).

Harris, K. M., Fasano, A., Mann, D. L. "Monocytes differentiated with IL-15 support Th17 and Th1 responses to wheat gliadin: implications for celiac disease." *Clin Immunol.* 2010: 135(3): 430–439.

Hill, I. D., Dirks, M. H., Liptak, G. S., Colletti, R. B., Fasano, A., Guandalini, S., Hoffenberg, E. F., Horvath, K., Murray, J. A., Pivor, M., Seidman, E. G. "Guideline for the diagnosis and treatment of celiac disease in children: recommendations of the North American Society for Pediatric Gastroenterology, Hepatology and Nutrition." *J Pediatr Gastroneterol Nutr.* 2005: 40(1): 1–19.

Hollon, J. R., Cureton, P. A., Martin, M. L., Puppa, E. L., Fasano, A. "Trace gluten contamination may play a role in mucosal and clinical recovery in a subgroup of diet-adherent non-responsive celiac disease patients." *BMC Gastroentrol.* 2013: 13(40).

Ivarsson, A. "The Swedish epidemic of coeliac disease explored using an epidemiological approach—some lessons to be learnt." *Best Pract Res Clin Gastroenterol.* 2005: 19(3): 425–40.

Jackson, J., Eaton, W., Cascella, N., Fasano, A., Warfel, D., Feldman, S., Richardson, C., Vyas, G., Linthicum, J., Santora, D., Warren, K. R., Carpenter, W. T., Kelly, D. L. "A gluten-free diet in people with schizophrenia and anti-tissue transglutaminase or anti-gliadin antibodies." *Schizophr Res.* 2012: 140(1–2): 362–363.

Joslin, C. L., Bradley, J. E., Christensen, T. A. "Banana therapy in the diarrheal diseases of infants and children." *Pediatrics.* 1938: 12(1): 66–70.

Kasarda, D. D. "Can an increase in celiac disease be attributed to an increase in the gluten content of wheat as a consequence of wheat breeding?" *J Agric Food Chem.* 2013: 61(6):1155–1159.

Kasarda, D. D., Dupont, F. M., Vensel, W. H., Altenbach, S. B., Lopez, R., Tanaka, C. K., Hurkman, W. J. "Surface-associated proteins of wheat starch granules: suitability of wheat starch for celiac patients." *J Agric Food Chem.* 2008: 56(21): 10292–10302.

Kasarda, D. D. "Triticum moncoccum and celiac disease." *Scand J Gastroenterol.* 2007: 42(9): 1141–1142.

Kognoff, M., Rostom, A., Murray, J. "American Gastroenterological Association (AGA) Institute Technical Review on the Diagnosis and Management of Celiac Disease." *Gastroenterology.* 2006: 131(6): 1981–2002.

Kudlien, F. "Aretaeus of Cappadocia." *Dictionary of Scientific Biography* 1. New York: Charles Scribner's Sons. 1970: 234–235.

Lammers, K. M., Khandelwal, S., Chaudhry, F., Kryszak, D., Puppa, E. L., Casolaro, V., Fasano, A. "Identification of a novel immunodulatory gliadin peptide that causes interleukin-8 release in a chemokine receptor CXCR-3 dependent manner only in patients with celiac disease." *Immunology.* 2011: 132(3): 432–440.

Lammers, K. M., Lu, R., Brownley, J., Lu, B., Gerard, C., Thomas, K., Rallabhandi, P., Shea-Donohue, T., Tamiz, A., Alkan, S., Netzel-Arnett, S., Antalis, T., Vogel, S. N., Fasano, A. "Gliadin induces an increase in intestinal permeability and zonulin release by binding to the chemokine receptor CXCR3." *Gastroenterology.* 2008: 135(1): 194–204.

Lionetti, E., Castellaneta, S., Pulvirenti, A., Tonutti, E., Francavilla, R., Fasano, A., Catassi, C., Italian Working Group of Weaning and Celiac Disease Risk. "Prevalence and natural history of potential celiac disease in at-family-risk infants prospectively investigated from birth." *J Pediatr.* 2012: 161(5): 908–914.

Lionetti, E., Catassi, C. "New clues in celiac disease epidemiology, pathogenesis, clinical manifestations, and treatment." *Int Rev Immunol.* 2011: 30(4): 219–231.

Ludviggson, J. F., Leffler, D. A., Bai, J. C., Biagi, F., Fasano, A., Green, P. H., Hadjivassiliou, M., Kaukinen, K., Kelly, C. P., Leonard, J. N., Lundin, K. E., Murray, J. A., Sanders, D. S., Walker, M. M., Zingone, F., Ciacci, C. "The Oslo definitions for coeliac disease and related terms." *Gut.* 2013: 62(1): 43–52.

Ludviggson, J. F., Fasano, A. "Timing of introduction of gluten and celiac disease risk." *Ann Nutr Metab.* 2012: Suppl 2: 22–29.

Ludviggson, J., Zugna, D., Richiardi, L., Akre, O., Stephansson, O. "A nationwide population-based study to determine whether coeliac disease is associated with infertility." *Gut.* 2010: 59: 1471–1475.

Millward, C., Ferriter, M., Calver, S. J., Connell-Jones, G. G. "Gluten and casein-free diets for autism spectrum disorder." *Cochrane Summaries.* Published online: January 21, 2009. http://summaries.cochrane.org.

Reilly, N. R., Fasano, A., Green, P. H. "Presentation of celiac disease."

Gastrointest Endosc Clin N Am. 2012: 22(4): 613–621.

Rossi, F., Bellini, G., Tolone, C., Luongo, L., Mancusi, S., Papparella, A., Sturgeon, G., Fasano, A., Nobili, B., Perrone, L., Maione, S., del Giudice, E. M. "The cannabinoid receptor type 2 Q63R variant increases the risk of celiac disease: implication for a novel molecular biomarker and future therapeutic intervention." *Pharmacol Res.* 2012: 66(1): 88–94.

Samaroo, D., Dickerson, F., Kasarda, D. D., Green, P. H., Briani, C., Yolken, R. H., Alaedini, A. "Novel immune response to gluten in individuals with schizophrenia." *Schizophr Res.* 2010: 118(1–3): 248–255.

Sapone, A., Bai, J. C., Ciacci, C., Dolinsek, J., Green, P. H., Hadjivassiliou, M., Kaukinen, K., Rostami, K., Sanders, D. S., Schumann, M., Ullrich, R., Villalta, D., Volta, U., Catassi, C., Fasano, A. "Spectrum of gluten-related disorders: consensus on new nomenclature and classification." *BMC Med.* 2012: 10(13).

Sapone, A., Lammers, K. M., Casolaro, V., Cammarota, M., Giuliano, M. T., De Rosa, M., Stefanile, R., Mazzarella, G., Tolone, C., Russo, M. I., Esposito, P., Ferraraccio, F., Carteni, M., Riegler, G., de Magistris, L., Fasano, A. "Divergence of gut permeability and mucosal gene expression in two gluten-associated conditions: celiac disease and gluten sensitivity." *BMC Med.* 2012: 9: 9–23.

Sapone, A., Lammers, K. M., Mazzarella, G., Mikhailenko, I., Caretni, M., Casolaro, V., Fasano, A. "Differential mucosal IL-17 expression in two gliadin-induced disorders: gluten sensitivity and the autoimmune enteropathy celiac disease." *Int Arch Allergy Immunol.* 2010: 152(1): 75–80.

Sellitto, M., Bai, G., Serena, G., Fricke, W. F., Sturgeon, C., Gajer, P., White, J. R., Koenig, S. S., Sakamoto, J., Boothe, D., Gicquelais, R., Kryszak, D., Puppa, E., Catassi, C., Ravel, J., Fasano, A. "Proof of concept of microbiome-metabolome analysis and delayed gluten exposure on celiac disease autoimmunity in genetically at-risk infants." *PLoS One.* 2012: 7(3): e33387.

Thomas, K. E., Sapone, A., Fasano, A., Vogel, S. N. "Gliadin stimulation of murine macrophage inflammatory gene expression and intestinal permeability are MyD88-dependent: role of the innate immune response in celiac disease." *J Immunol.* 2006: 176(4): 2512–2521.

Tripathi, A., Lammers, K. M., Goldblum, S., Shea-Donohue, T., Netzel-Arnett, S., Buzza, M. S., Antalis, T. M., Vogel, S. N., Zhao, A. "Identification of human zonulin, a physiological modulator of tight junctions as prehaptoglobin-2." *Proc Natl Acad Sci U S A.* 2009: 106(39): 16799–16804.

Tye-Din, J. A., Stewart, J. A., Dromey, J. A., Beissbarth, T., van Heel, D. A., Tatham, A., Henderson, K., Mannering, S. I., Gianfrani, C., Jewell, D. P., Hill, A. V. S., McCluskey, J., Rossjohn, J., Anderson, R. "Comprehensive, quantitative mapping of T cell epitopes in gluten in celiac disease." *Sci. Transl. Med.* 2010: 2(41): 41–51.

van Berge-Henegounen, G. P., Mulder, C. J. "Pioneer in the gluten free diet: Willem Karel Dicke 1905-1962, over 50 years of gluten free diet." *Gut.* 1993: 34(11): 1473–1475.

Zawahir, S., Safta, A., Fasano, A. "Pediatric celiac disease." *Curr Opin Pediatr.* 2009: 21(5): 655–660.

Zuidmeer, L., Goldhahn, K., Rona, R. J., Gislason, D., Madsen, C., Summers, C., Sodergren, E., Dahlstrom, J., Lindner, T., Sigurdardottir, S. T., McBride, D., Keil, T. "The prevalence of plant food allergies: a systematic review." *J Allergy Clin Immunol.* 2008: 121(5): 1210–1218.

OTHER REFERENCES

FALCPA

http://www.fda.gov/Food/GuidanceRegulation/GuidanceDocuments-RegulatoryInformation/Allergens/ucm106890.htm

Healthy Hunger-Free Kids Act of 2010

http://www.fns.usda.gov/cnd/governance/Legislation/CNR_2010.htm

National Human Genome Research Institute, National Institutes of Health

http://www.genome.gov/

National School Lunch Act

http://www.fns.usda.gov/nslp/history_5#nationalweekest

National School Lunch Program

http://www.fns.usda.gov/nslp/national-school-lunch-program

University of Georgia, Department of Crop and Soil Sciences

http://ses.library.usyd.edu.au/bitstream/2123/3389/1/O25.pdf

U.S. Department of Education Office of Civil Rights

http://www2.ed.gov/about/offices/list/ocr/504faq.html

Fact Sheet on Section 504 of the Rehabilitation Act

http://www.hhs.gov/ocr/civilrights/resources/factsheets/504.pdf

National Human Genome Research Institute, National Institutes of Health

http://www.genome.gov/

Resources

U.S. CELIAC CENTERS AND PROGRAMS

East Coast
eet
Alfred I duPont Hospital for Children
Pediatric GI Division
Wilmington, DE
http://www.nemours.org/service/medical/gastroenterology.html?location
=naidhc

Beth Israel Deaconess Medical Center, Celiac Center*
Boston, MA
www.CeliacNow.org

Boston Children's Hospital Celiac Disease Program*
Boston, MA
http://www.childrenshospital.org/centers-and-services/celiac-disease-
program

Center for Celiac Research, Massachusetts General Hospital*
Boston, MA
www.celiaccenter.org

The Celiac Center at Paoli Hospital
Paoli, PA
www.mainlinehealth.org/paoliceliac

The Celiac Disease Center at Columbia University
New York, NY
www.celiacdiseasecenter.columbia.edu

The Jefferson Celiac Center at Thomas Jefferson University Hospital
Philadelphia, PA
www.jeffersonhospital.org/

Kogan Celiac Center at the Barnabas Health Ambulatory Care Center
Livingston, NJ
www.barnabashealth.org/services/celiac/index.html

Midwest/South

The Celiac Center at the University of Tennessee Medical Center
Knoxville, TN
www.utmedicalcenter.org/

Center for Digestive Diseases at the University of Iowa Hospitals
and Clinics
Iowa City, IA
www.uihealthcare.org/CeliacDisease/

Children's Hospital of Wisconsin
Bonnie Mechanic Celiac Disease Clinic
Milwaukee, WI
http://www.nemours.org/service/medical/gastroenterology.html?location
=naidhc

Digestive Health Center at the University of Virginia Health System
Charlottesville, VA
www.uvahealth.com/services/digestive-health

Mayo Clinic in Minnesota
Rochester, MN
www.mayoclinic.org/celiac-disease

Nationwide Children's Hospital
Columbus, OH
www.nationwidechildrens.org

The University of Chicago Celiac Disease Center
Chicago, IL
www.cureceliacdisease.org

West Coast

The Celiac Disease Clinic at Rady Children's Hospital
San Diego, CA
www.rchsd.org

Children's Hospital Colorado
Aurora, CO
www.childrenscolorado.org

Division of Gastroenterology and Nutrition at the Children's Hospital,
Los Angeles
Los Angeles, CA
www.chla.org/

Stanford Celiac Sprue Management Clinic
Palo Alto, CA
www.stanfordhospital.com/clinicsmedservices/clinics/gastroenterology/
celiacsprue

University of Colorado Hospital
Anschutz Medical Campus
Aurora, CO
www.uch.edu/conditions/digestive-liver-pancreas/celiac-sprue-disease/

Wm. K. Warren Medical Research Center for Celiac Disease at the University of California, San Diego
La Jolla, CA
http://celiaccenter.ucsd.edu/

* Special thanks to these three New England organizations for providing resources. Known as the Celiac Program at Harvard Medical School, the doctors, dietitians, and other staff members of these three groups are working together to advance research, raise awareness, and improve patient care for people with celiac disease and other gluten-related disorders.

NATIONAL CELIAC ORGANIZATIONS AND SUPPORT GROUPS

Academy of Nutrition and Dietetics (formerly American Dietetic Association)
www.eatright.org
www.eatright.org/search.aspx?search=celiac+disease

American Celiac Disease Alliance
www.americanceliac.org

American Gastroenterological Association
www.gastro.org
www.gastro.org/patient-center/digestive-conditions/celiac-disease

Celiac Sprue Association
www.csaceliacs.org

Canadian Celiac Association
www.celiac.ca

Celiac Disease Foundation
www.celiac.org

Children's Digestive Health and Nutrition Foundation
www.cdhnf.org

Gluten Intolerance Group of North America
www.gluten.net

National Foundation for Celiac Awareness
www.celiaccentral.org

National Institute of Diabetes and Digestive and Kidney Diseases
www.niddk.nih.gov

National Institute of Health Celiac Disease Awareness Campaign
www.celiac.nih.gov

North American Society for the Study of Celiac Disease
www.nasscd.org

North American Society for Pediatric Gastroenterology, Hepatology, and
Nutrition (Gastrokids)
www.gastrokids.com

Raising Our Celiac Kids (R.O.C.K.)
www.celiackids.com

Glossary

Amino acids nitrogen-containing compounds that serve as the building blocks of protein.

Amylase inhibitors molecules that block alpha amylase, a protein that breaks down starches in foods during digestion. Alpha amylase inhibitors are commonly referred to as "starch blockers."

Anaphylactic shock/anaphylaxis a life-threatening allergic reaction. Anaphylaxis involves the whole body; symptoms develop within seconds or minutes. These include abdominal pain, high-pitched breathing sounds, anxiety, chest tightness, cough, diarrhea, difficulty breathing and swallowing, dizziness, hives, nasal congestion, nausea or vomiting, palpitations, skin redness, slurred speech, swelling of the face or tongue, unconsciousness, and wheezing.

- **Food-dependent exercise-induced anaphylaxis (FDEIA)** anaphylaxis caused by the combination of eating a food one is allergic to and engaging in physical activity shortly afterward.
- **Wheat dependent exercise-induced anaphylaxis (WDEIA)** anaphylaxis that occurs when a person who is allergic to wheat eats the substance and then engages in physical activity.

Adaptive immune system cells and other tissues that become activated when foreign substances are able to overcome the body's innate immune system. Once activated, the adaptive immune system creates cellular mechanisms for eliminating the foreign invaders.

Anemia any condition in which the blood is unable to deliver adequate oxygen to the body.

Antibodies large proteins produced by the immune system when the body is invaded by foreign substances. Antibodies protect the body by deactivating the foreign intruders.

Antigen a foreign substance that triggers an allergic reaction in the body.

Antigen-presenting cells a group of cells that processes antigens in the body and "presents" them to cells that are involved in triggering the body's immune response.

Anti-gliadin antibodies (AGA) antibodies produced by the body when a person with celiac disease consumes gluten-containing foods.

Atopic dermatitis a disease that causes itchy and inflamed skin that often begins in infancy.

Attention deficit hyperactivity disorder (ADHD) a behavioral syndrome, typically diagnosed in childhood, characterized by inattentiveness and other behaviors that interfere with performance at school, at work, and in social situations.

Atypical unusual; not typical.

Autoantibodies proteins, produced by the immune system, that target the body's own healthy tissues.

Autoimmune disorder a disorder in which the body launches an abnormal, defensive immune response to its own healthy tissues.

Autism Spectrum Disorder (ASD) an umbrella term for a group of developmental brain disorders, including autistic disorder, pervasive development disorder, and Asperger's syndrome.

B cells white blood cells that are part of the body's immune system. Each B cell makes a specific antibody that blocks a specific foreign invader, such as a virus.

Baker's asthma a type of asthma caused by breathing in flour dust and other substances found in bakeries. Symptoms include coughing, shortness of breath, wheezing, and chest tightness.

Banana baby a member of a group of pediatric patients diagnosed with celiac disease in the U.S. in the 1930s who were fed on a diet developed by Dr. Sidney Haas that consisted primarily of bananas.

Basal cell a type of cell found in the deep layers of the skin.

Basophils white blood cells involved in immune reactions. Basal cells produce chemicals such as histamine.

Biomarker a measurable physical characteristic that is used to detect the presence or severity of disease or infection.

Biopsy a procedure in which a small sample of fluid or tissue is removed from the body and examined under a microscope. It is often used to diagnose disease.

Case finding the act of finding people who have contracted a particular disease or infection.

Casein a protein found in milk.

Celiac disease a genetic disorder in which most people suffer a variety of symptoms, both gastrointestinal and extraintestinal, after eating foods that contain gluten. In people with celiac disease, gluten triggers the immune system to produce chemicals that can damage the intestinal tract. Some individuals experience "silent celiac disease."

Cholera an infection of the small intestine that causes diarrhea, vomiting, cramps, and dehydration.

Cohort a group of people, such as those people undergoing treatment as part of a research study.

Comorbidities when two or more diseases or disorders occur in a person at the same time.

Crohn's disease a chronic condition that causes inflammation of the gastrointestinal tract. Common symptoms include persistent diarrhea, rectal bleeding, abdominal cramps, and constipation.

Cross-contamination when bacteria, allergens, or other substances in one food are inadvertently transferred to another food, thereby contaminating it. Common causes of cross-contamination are cutting boards and knives not cleaned between uses with different foods.

Cystic fibrosis a chronic disease caused by a genetic defect that makes the body produce abnormally thick, sticky mucus that clogs the lungs and inter-feres with digestion.

Cytokines a group of chemicals involved in the body's immune response. In people with celiac disease, ingestion of gluten triggers production of cyto-kines that attack the intestines and cause damage and illness.

Dermatitis herpetiformis a chronic disease characterized by an extremely itchy rash appearing as bumps and blisters or, less frequently, scratch marks. Although the cause of the disease is unknown, dermatitis herpetiformis has been linked to celiac disease.

Diagnostic algorithm a step-by-step procedure used to diagnose disease.

Double-blind study an experimental method in which both the participants in a study and the scientists conducting it do not know which participants are being treated by a particular method. That is, both scientists and participants are "blinded."

Embryogenesis the development of an embryo.

Endorphins substances released by the brain that relieve pain and stress.

Endoscopy a medical procedure in which a long thin tube with a camera attached to the end is threaded into a person's body, allowing doctors to see internal organs on a screen attached to the camera.

Endoymysial Antibodies (EMA) in people with celiac disease, antibodies generated in response to eating gluten-containing foods.

Enteropathy disease of the intestinal tract.

Enzyme linked immunosorbent assay (ELISA) a test used to detect presence of specific substances, such as viruses or allergens, in a blood sample. It is often used as a diagnostic tool.

Enzymes proteins that serve as catalysts in the body by launching chemical reactions, such as digestion.

Epidemiology the study of the causes of diseases and how they spread throughout different populations.

Epstein-Barr virus the virus that causes mononucleosis.

Extraintestinal located or occurring outside of the intestine.

Food Allergen Labeling and Consumer Protection Act of 2004 (FALCPA) an amendment to the Federal Food, Drug, and Cosmetic Act that requires food labels to list ingredients that are major food allergens or proteins from major food allergens. For example, "contains wheat, milk, egg, and soy" or "ingredients: enriched flour (wheat flour)."

Gliadin a component of the protein found in gluten-containing foods.

Gliadorphin a substance produced during the digestion of gluten.

Glutamine an amino acid found in large amounts in gliadins.

Gluten a protein found in wheat, with similar proteins found in barley (secalin) and rye (hordein). Gluten is made up of different subproteins, including gliadin. Use of term "gluten" often includes barley and rye proteins.

Gluten ataxia a neurological condition triggered by consuming gluten (in people with celiac disease). Antibodies to gluten damage the area of the brain responsible for gross motor skills, such as walking. This damage potentially can cause loss of coordination and even significant, progressive disability in some cases.

Gluten challenge a test to see how the body reacts to gluten. It involves following a gluten-free diet for a certain period and then eating gluten and undergoing blood tests that measure the body's response.

Gluten-free containing no gluten.

Gluten-free diet an eating plan that does not contain any gluten.

Glutenin the major protein found in wheat flour.

Gluten prolamins protein components of gluten; gliadins and glutenins.

Gluten-related disorders conditions caused by an adverse reaction to gluten or wheat, such as celiac disease, gluten sensitivity, and wheat allergy.

Gluten sensitivity or non-celiac gluten sensitivity a reaction to consuming foods containing gluten. Symptoms can include diarrhea and bloating, fatigue, "foggy mind," depression, joint pain, and anemia. Symptoms caused by gluten sensitivity are often less severe than symptoms associated with celiac disease, but this is not always the case.

Hashimoto's thyroiditis a condition caused by inflammation of the thyroid gland. The inflammation occurs when the body's immune system attacks and damages the thyroid. Hashimoto's thyroiditis causes low blood levels of thyroid hormone (hypothyroidism).

Histamine a chemical released by the immune system when the body is exposed to an allergen. Histamines cause inflammation and many other allergy symptoms.

Histological the microscopic structure of tissue.

Hordein a protein found in rye.

Human Leukocyte Antigen (HLA) proteins that help the immune system distinguish between the body's own proteins and proteins made by foreign invaders, such as viruses.

HLA-DQ2 and HLA-DQ8 the two main genes associated with celiac disease. Experts believe that a person must inherit a copy of at least one of the genes to get the disease.

Humoral being a part of the immune system that involves antibodies and bodily fluids.

Immune system cells and other tissues that protect the body against invasion by foreign substances, such as viruses and bacteria.

Immunoglobulin A (IgA) circulating antibodies that can reach the mucosal interfaces, including the gut, and be secreted in body fluids like those found in the intestine. IgA protects the body against invasion through the mouth, eyes, and other entrances to the body.

Immunoglobulin E (IgE) a type of antibody that is the cause of allergy symptoms.

Immunoglobulin G (IgG) the most common type of antibody. IgG plays a key role in defending the body against infection by foreign invaders, such as viruses.

Immunology study of the immune system.

Inflammatory bowel disease a condition characterized by chronic inflammation in the gastrointestinal tract. The two main forms of the immune-mediated disorder are Crohn's disease and colitis.

Innate immune system cells and other tissues that serve as the immune system's first line of defense. They are always ready and available to fight foreign invaders, such as viruses.

Intestinal permeability also known as "leaky gut," a condition in which the intestinal barrier that keeps potentially harmful substances at bay is not functioning properly. Many autoimmune disorders, including celiac disease, are characterized by increased gut permeability.

Irritable Bowel Syndrome (IBS) a group of symptoms, including abdominal pain and discomfort, caused by changes in the workings of the gastrointestinal tract.

Kwashiorkor a type of malnutrition caused by consuming inadequate amounts of protein and calories.

Lyme disease a disease caused by bacteria that is transmitted to people through tick bites. Symptoms include fever, headache, fatigue, and a skin rash. Left untreated, the disease can also affect the joints, heart, and nervous system.

Lymphoma any type of cancer that originates in the lymph nodes and other lymph tissue.

Lysine an essential amino acid that has to be obtained through food, because the body cannot make it.

Macrophages white blood cells that play a role in the immune system.

Malabsorption difficulty absorbing nutrients from food.

Manioc another name for cassava, which is the starch used to make tapioca.

Marasmus starvation, caused by not consuming enough calories.

Mast cells white blood cells involved in the immune system's reaction to allergens. Mast cells produce chemicals such as histamine.

Microbes microorganisms, such as bacteria.

Microbiome the community of microbes in the gut.

Microbiota microorganisms living in a particular part of the body, such as the intestine; also known as flora.

Morbidity rate the incidence of disease in a group.

Mortality rate the number of deaths in a group.

Mucosal involving the mucous membrane.

Natural selection the process in nature whereby people and other organisms who are healthiest tend to survive and produce more healthy offspring than those who are less healthy.

Neurological involving the nerves and nervous system.

Osteopenia low bone mineral density.

Osteoporosis a condition in which the bones become brittle and porous.

Pathogenesis the origin and development of a disease.

Pathology the study of disease.

Peptide a compound containing two or more amino acids, which are the building blocks of protein.

Peripheral neuropathy damage to the peripheral nervous system, which is the network of nerves that transmits signals from the brain and spinal cord to all of the other parts of the body.

Persistent parasthesia a tingling sensation of the skin.

Placebo a sham treatment, such as an inactive pill, given to people who do not know it is not really a viable treatment. Placebos are often used in research to see whether people improve after its use because they believe they have been legitimately treated. This phenomenon is known as the "placebo effect."

Prevalence the total number of people in a certain group who are affected by a disease at a particular time.

Prolamin a class of simple proteins found in grains including wheat, barley, and rye.

Proline an amino acid found in large amounts in gliadins.

Pylorus the valve that divides the stomach from the small intestine.

Refractory celiac disease a rare condition in which there is an absence of long-term improvement in symptoms of celiac disease on the gluten-free diet.

Schizophrenia a severe mental disorder characterized by hallucinations and loss of touch with reality.

Secalin a protein found in barley.

Sensitivity the statistical measurement of the percentage of people who are correctly diagnosed as having a particular condition; also known as true positive rate.

Serological pertaining to the study of blood serums.

Silent celiac disease also called "asymptomatic celiac disease," this occurs when an individual does not have major symptoms but has been diagnosed with celiac disease through blood tests and endoscopy; often occurs in conjunction with testing for other conditions.

Specificity the statistical measurement of the percentage of people who are correctly diagnosed as not having a certain condition; also known as true negative rate.

Subcutaneous located right under the skin.

Subjects when discussing medical research, the participants in a study.

T-cells white blood cells that play a key role in triggering the body's immune response to foreign invaders, such as viruses.

33-mer peptide a peptide with thirty-three amino acids that is thought to trigger the body's response to gluten in people with celiac disease.

Thyroid Stimulating Hormone (TSH) a hormone responsible for stimulating the workings of the thyroid gland.

Tight junctions formed from specific proteins, these regulate the passages of substances in and out of the intestine and affect intestinal permeability.

Tissue transglutaminase (tTG) an enzyme normally present in the intestines. In people with celiac disease, the immune system produces antibodies that attack the enzyme.

Urticaria an itchy skin rash characterized by pale red, raised bumps.

Visco-elasticity a material's ability to remain sticky, thick, and elastic when under stress, and still maintain its shape.

Villi fingerlike projections that line the inside of the intestine.

Watson's capsule a device developed in the 1960s that was once widely used to diagnose celiac disease. A child would swallow the capsule, which was the size of an olive pit. It was attached to a long tube that was threaded to the intestine, where it was used to trap a small tissue sample that could be examined under a microscope.

Wheat allergy an allergy to foods containing wheat.

Xylose a sugar found in plants.

Zonulin a protein that acts as the gatekeeper between the lining of the intestine and the substances inside the intestine.

Zot zonula occludens toxin, a cholera protein that can regulate tight junctions and affect intestinal permeability.

Index

World-renowned pediatric gastroenterologist and research scientist Alessio Fasano is founder and director of the Center for Celiac Research at Massachusetts General Hospital, the first research and treatment center for celiac disease, wheat allergy, and gluten sensitivity in the U.S. Dr. Fasano created the Center in 1996 to advance the treatment, research, and awareness of celiac disease; his research established the prevalence of the autoimmune disorder as one in 133 in 2003. A national and international keynote speaker, he is also widely sought by national and international media and has been featured in hundreds of outlets including *The New York Times, The Wall Street Journal,* NPR, CNN, *Bloomberg News, USA Today, Los Angeles Times, Huffington Post, Good Morning America, VOGUE,* and numerous health-related websites and magazines. Trained in Naples, Italy, Dr. Fasano is visiting professor at Harvard Medical School and chief of the Division of Pediatric Gastroenterology and Nutrition at MassGeneral Hospital *for* Children.

Nationally award-winning higher education writer and editor Susie Flaherty is director of communications for the Center for Celiac Research at Massachusetts General Hospital. The former speechwriter to university presidents and international bank executives has led a wide variety of marketing and strategic communications projects, including a stint as senior editor at the University of Maryland. Her current work at the Center for Celiac Research includes promoting Dr. Fasano's research into the causes, treatment, and prevention of celiac disease and other autoimmune disorders. A member of the National Association of Science Writers, Susie is also an accomplished singer and songwriter.

CPSIA information can be obtained
at www.ICGtesting.com
Printed in the USA
BVOW08s2205040418
512450BV00023B/1000/P

9 781681 620510

W9-DBK-265

Bible Workbook

VOLUME 2
New Testament

Catherine B. Walker

MA in Biblical Education, Doctor of Religious Education

MOODY PUBLISHERS

CHICAGO

ACKNOWLEDGMENTS

I wish to express my great indebtedness to those who assisted in compiling this work, especially Miss Sara Petty, and my sister, Mrs. Kenneth Strachan, both of whom taught Bible in high schools. I am most grateful to Dr. Robert C. McQuilkin, and the Rev. Frank Sells for permission to make use of some of their helpful Bible notes and outlines. The splendid maps are the work of the Rev. Byron M. Wilkinson. To the great host of Bible teachers and authors who directly or indirectly have contributed to this book by their contribution to my own Christian life and Bible knowledge, I give my deep appreciation.

BIBLE WORKBOOKS

Volume 1—Old Testament
(A chronological study)

Volume 2—New Testament
(A brief study of all the books)

✦✦✦✦✦✦✦

Copyright © 1943, 1944 by
Catherine B. Walker

Revised edition
Copyright © 1952

All rights reserved. No part of this book may be reproduced in any form without permission in writing from the publisher, except in the case of brief quotations embodied in critical articles or reviews.

All Scripture quotations are taken from the King James Version.

Cover and interior design: Erik M. Peterson
Cover engraving, "The Descent of the Spirit" (1891) by Gustave Dore. Public domain.

ISBN-13: 978-0-8024-0752-8

We hope you enjoy this book from Moody Publishers. Our goal is to provide high-quality, thought-provoking books and products that connect truth to your real needs and challenges. For more information on other books and products written and produced from a biblical perspective, go to www.moodypublishers. com or write to:

Moody Publishers
820 N. LaSalle Boulevard
Chicago, IL 60610

67 69 70 68

Printed in the United States of America

NOTE TO THE TEACHER

Although this workbook was originally planned for high school Bible classes meeting every day for a semester, it has found a wider use by various age groups in churches and colleges and by individuals desiring direction in their personal Bible study. The workbook was first produced as a method of giving notes and assignment questions quickly, thereby leaving more valuable classroom time for explanations, discussions, and student participation. The workbook may be placed in a regulation size binder. Separate pages can be handed in when completed. Other notes, assigned papers, and themes can be placed throughout the notebook.

This is in no sense a textbook. It is hoped that no one will make the completion of the workbook a goal in itself but that the questions and notes may stimulate and guide each student in searching and knowing the Bible. The questions do not cover all the important points in any chapter. It is hoped, however, in the course of the study that all the main New Testament teachings will be brought out.

Most schools give about half the semester to the life of Christ in the Gospels and the rest of the semester to Acts and the Epistles. Three or four chapters a day are usually assigned. In order to cover all the main incidents in the life of Christ special emphasis has been chosen in each gospel. Studying Mark first, in four or five lessons, as a short survey of Christ's life has proved a good start for students unfamiliar with the Bible. The main miracles and chief characters then become familiar. Matthew is more easily understood after having had this simple introduction to Christ through Mark. Matthew is studied with emphasis on the teachings of Christ. Students should become familiar with all unfamiliar terms. Places mentioned should be located on the map. In Luke the parables and new stories are especially noted. The more intimate revelation of Jesus given in John's gospel should prove a personal blessing to each student. Students should become familiar with the content of the simple chronological outline of Christ's life as drawn from the four gospels that has been included in this edition.

The Acts and the Epistles are taken in the order they appear in the Bible. The missionary message in Acts and the Christian life teachings in the epistles have been kept in mind. Since time prohibits the complete study of each epistle, a limited number of chapters have been selected for study. Several teachers assign the Revelation as parallel reading giving a brief preview at the time of the assignment and a discussion of the book after it has been read.

It is my prayer that all who use this book will be guided by it into a deeper, more personal, knowledge of the living Word, the Lord Jesus Christ, as well as the written Word, the Bible. It is the teacher's wonderful privilege to bring from the Scripture its vital, interesting message for personal living. Students sometimes come from a Bible course saying, "Yes, we learn the facts all right, but that Book is too dull and boring for me." That teacher had failed to take advantage of a most wonderful privilege. The Book that was written to give men life should be taught in a way that presents real life to men. May students come from your class with the appreciation expressed in these comments: "Bible is the most interesting course I've ever had." "I surely have learned to love the Bible. I read it every day, now." "Studying Bible has not only cleared up questions that have always puzzled me but it has helped me so much in my everyday living." "It was through that Bible course that I became a Christian. I wouldn't have missed it for anything."

Catherine B. Walker

FROM MALACHI TO MATTHEW

Be able to explain each emphasized term as it is connected with this period.

The period from the close of Malachi until the opening of the New Testament is known as the **"400 Silent Years,"** because the events of this time are not recorded in the Bible. Other books describe this period as one in which momentous historical events took place. Great empires rose and fell and many battles were fought.

The **Persians** were ruling the world at the close of the Old Testament and continued in power for another hundred years. The Jews enjoyed religious freedom under this tolerant Persian rule. The Jewish high priest was given some civil power along with his religious duties. Palestine, however, suffered much from the constant warfare between Egypt and Persia.

The **Greek** rule of Palestine began in 333 BC when Alexander the Great conquered the land. At his death the empire was broken up and divided among his four generals, Egypt going to Ptolemy, and Syria going to Seleucus. Palestine was again in the midst of struggle, first falling under the rule of the Ptolemies, the Greek kings of Egypt, and later taken by the Syrians. While under the rule of Egypt, a great many Jews were moved to Egypt and enjoyed the privileges of the Greek population there. In 285 BC the Jews in Alexandria, Egypt, made a translation of their Hebrew Old Testament into the Greek language. This translation, called the **Septuagint** (LXX), or Bible of the Seventy, is famous as the one in use in Palestine during the time of Christ. Jesus and His disciples often quoted from it.

Syria took Palestine in 198 BC The division of the land into Galilee, Samaria, Judea, Trachonitis, and Perea was made at this time. At first, the Jews were allowed to live as usual with their own laws, under the council and high priest. Then **Antiochus Ephiphanes,** the eighth king in the Seleucid line of Syrian kings, decided to abolish the Jewish religion and establish Greek idolatry. Terrible times followed. Antiochus plundered Jerusalem, desecrated the temple, and enslaved many of the people. On December 25, 168 BC, he offered a pig on the great altar of the temple and then erected a heathen altar to Jupiter. Temple worship and all Jewish rites and ceremonies were forbidden. The people were even compelled to eat swine's flesh.

These horrible practices of Antiochus Ephiphanes could not be tolerated. Loyal Jews had to revolt. Matthias, a priest of strong convictions and righteousness, led this movement. He did little more than gather together other Jews who determined to free the nation by overthrowing this monster, Antiochus, and establishing again the sacred worship at the temple. Matthias was the first of this family of liberators called the **Maccabees.** He was succeeded by his son, Judas Maccabeus, who was assisted by four brothers of whom Simon is the best known. They regained possession of Jerusalem, purified the temple, and again established the daily sacrifices. Trouble continued, however, until in 142 BC the Maccabees gained national independence. The high priest had both civil and religious power similar to that of a king. Civil war between two brothers who desired this influential position of high priest was ended when the Romans conquered Palestine.

The **Roman** control of the land began when Pompey conquered Palestine in 63 BC Hyrcanus was given the position he desired, that of high priest. In 47 BC Julius Caesar made Antipater ruler of Judea and his son, Herod, governor of Galilee. After the disorder in Judea following the murder of Caesar, Herod fled to Rome where he received the appointment to become king of the Jews. On his return he married Mariamne, the beautiful granddaughter of the former high priest, Hyrcanus, hoping by this to gain the good will of the people. Herod was so brutal, cunning, and cold-blooded that he committed crimes of unspeakable cruelty, even murdering his wife and two sons. Later in an attempt to kill Christ, he slew the children of Bethlehem. To gain the favor of the people he rebuilt their temple. It was to this magnificent temple of Herod's that Christ came many times.

The New Testament opens with the Roman Empire ruling the world, Caesar Augustus as its emperor, and with Herod as King of the Jews in Palestine.

INTRODUCTION TO THE NEW TESTAMENT

I. CONTENTS: 27 books.

II. DIVISIONS AND BOOKS IN EACH DIVISION: (Learn the names of these books in order)
Gospels (4)–Matthew, Mark, Luke, John
History (1)–Acts
Pauline Epistles (14)–Romans, 1 and 2 Corinthians, Galatians, Ephesians, Philippians, Colossians, 1 and 2 Thessalonians, 1 and 2 Timothy, Titus, Philemon, Hebrews
General Epistles (7)–James, 1 and 2 Peter, 1, 2, and 3 John, Jude
Prophecy (1)–Revelation

III. AUTHORS: Eight men:
1. Matthew wrote 1 book . . . . . . Gospel of Matthew
2. Mark wrote 1 book . . . . Gospel of Mark
3. Luke wrote 2 books . . . . Gospel of Luke and Acts
4. John wrote 5 books . . . . Gospel of John, 1, 2, 3 John, Revelation
5. Paul wrote 13 or 14 books . . . (Listed above)
6. James wrote 1 book . . . . James
7. Peter wrote 2 books . . . . 1 and 2 Peter
8. Jude wrote 1 book . . . . Jude

IV. DATE: The New Testament was written between AD 50 and 100.

V. ORIGINAL LANGUAGE: Greek.

VI. TYPES OF LITERATURE:
(By each type place the name of a New Testament book in which you think that style of writing could be found.)

1. Biography _____
2. Poetry _____
3. History_____
4. Letters _____
5. Sermons _____
6. Prophecy_____

VII. THEME: Christ
Christ is the theme and central character of the Old Testament as well as the New Testament. The Old Testament continually promises "Christ will come." The New Testament says "Christ has come." The Old Testament tells of God's preparing and preserving a people through whom the Savior would come. The Jews were given many beautiful types or pictures of the life and work of Jesus. Besides this there are many definite prophecies telling both of Christ's first coming—as a Savior to die; and of His second coming—as King to reign. First Peter 1:10–11, clearly tells us this. *(Read and mark this passage.)*

VIII. OUTLINE OF THE LIFE OF CHRIST as found by harmonizing the four gospels. (Learn the main divisions.) The stories from each are needed in order to give the complete account. Many of the following events are told in several other gospels besides the one listed. No one knows the exact order of all the happenings or the time covered by each.

1. **Thirty years of preparation**

   Ancestry, birth, flight to Egypt, in the temple at twelve. Matt. 1:1–2:23, Luke 1:1–2:52

2. **Year of Obscurity—Beginning of Public Ministry**

   (First ministry in Perea, Galilee, Judea, and Samaria)

   a. Baptism and temptation. Luke 3:1–4:13
   b. First disciples and first miracle. John 1:19–2:12
   c. Early Judean ministry. Temple cleansed, Nicodemus. John 2:13–3:36
   d. Samaritan ministry. John 4:1–42

3. **Year of Popularity—Galilean Ministry**

   a. Beginning. Nobleman's son. John 4:1–54; Nazareth, Capernaum. Luke 4:16–31
   b. First preaching tour. Mark 1:16–45
   c. Growing hostility of scribes and Pharisees. Mark 2:1–3:6
   d. Twelve disciples chosen. Mark 3:13–19
   e. Sermon on the Mount. Matt. 5:1–7:29
   f. Second preaching tour. Luke 7:36–8:3
   g. A day of teaching. Matt. 12:22–13:53
   h. A day of miracles. Matt. 8:18–9:34
   i. Third preaching tour. Mark 6:1–29
   j. Crisis at Capernaum. Five thousand fed. Matt. 14:13–15:20
   k. In various northern regions. Mark 7:24–8:26
   l. Jesus with apostles. Discussion, transfiguration. Matt. 16:13–17:23
   m. In Capernaum again. Discussions. Matt. 17:24–18:35

4. **Year of Opposition**
   Later Judean Ministry

   a. On way to Jerusalem. Luke 9:51–62
   b. In Jerusalem. John 7:11–10:21
   c. In Judea. Luke 10:1–13:21

   Later Perean Ministry

   d. Withdrawal from Jerusalem. Luke 13:22–17:10; John 11:1–54
   e. Last journey to Jerusalem by way of Samaria and Galilee. Luke 17:11–18:14
   f. In Perea. Matt. 19:1–20:28
   g. Going toward Jerusalem. Luke 18:35–19:28; John 11:55–12:11

   Closing Events of Jesus' Ministry

   The Passion Week. Trial. Crucifixion. (see page 38)
   The Forty Days. Resurrection. Ascension. (see page 39)

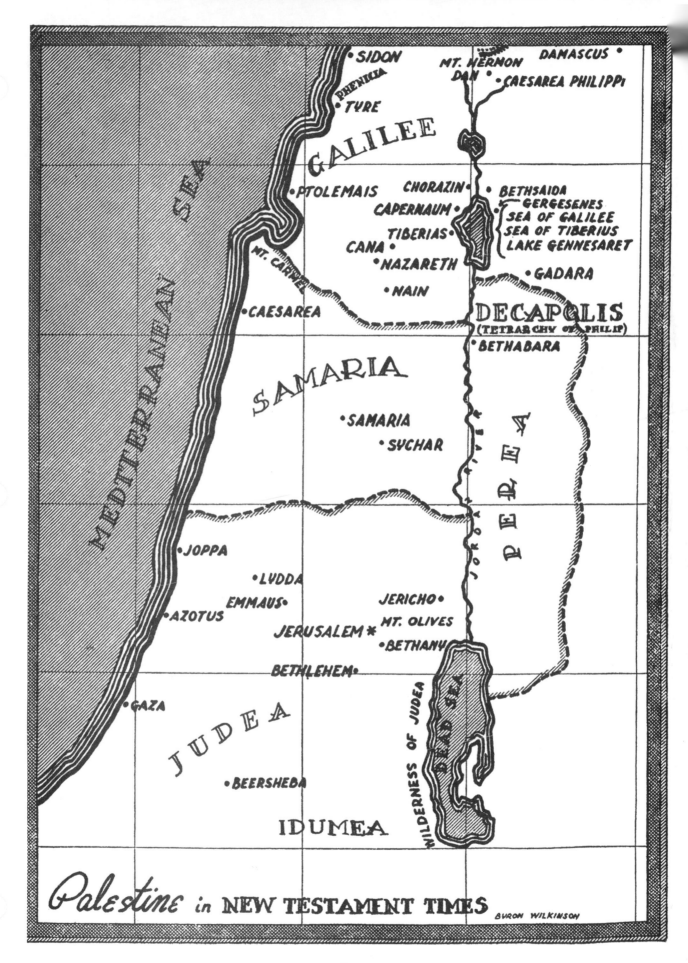

Palestine in NEW TESTAMENT TIMES

BYRON WILKINSON

THE FOUR GOSPELS

Matthew—Mark—Luke—John

"Gospel" (good story or God's story) is the English translation of the word meaning "glad tidings" or "good news."

"The first four books of the New Testament are called biography because they tell the life of Christ. Each biographer presents a different picture of the same person—Christ. Each gospel was evidently written with a distinct class of readers in mind and the four gave distinct pictures of Christ."

Matthew wrote to the Jews—presenting Christ as _____ (Zech. 9:9).

Mark wrote to the Romans—presenting Christ as _____ (Isa. 42:1).

Luke wrote to the Greeks—presenting Christ as_____ (Zech. 6:12).

John wrote to the world—presenting Christ as _____ (Isa. 40:9).

Matthew
Mark
Luke
} **EMPHASIZE THE *WORKS* OF CHRIST**

These are called Synoptic Gospels. "Synoptic" means "to see or look together."

John **EMPHASIZES THE *WORDS* OF CHRIST**

TERMS DEFINED

1. **Pharisees:** A powerful religious and political group among the Jews. Politically they looked forward to a glorious future for their nation. Religiously they stressed outward forms more than inward righteousness. They not only followed closely the Mosaic law of purity but were strict in keeping the great host of man-made regulations which had been added. They believed in the resurrection of the dead. Jesus exposed their hypocrisy and self-righteousness. They in turn violently hated Jesus.
2. **Sadducees:** A small wealthy influential sect of Jews, who opposed the Pharisees. They did not believe in the resurrection, angels, or spirits. They also were bitter enemies of Christ.
3. **Scribes:** These men copied and interpreted the Scripture, worshipping the mere letter of the law. They were usually Pharisees. They are also called "lawyers."
4. **Herodians:** Jewish political party that supported Herod and Rome.
5. **Zealots:** A religious, political party of Jews who opposed Roman aggression.
6. **Samaritans:** A mixed race, descendants of Jews and Gentiles brought in by the Assyrian king during Israel's captivity. Samaritans were despised by the Jews.
7. **Sanhedrin:** Supreme council of the Jews composed of 71 members–Pharisees and Sadducees.
8. **Synagogue:** Jewish place of worship and schooling in the Scriptures.
9. **Levites:** Men of the tribe of Levi. They took care of the temple.
10. **Publicans:** Tax collectors employed by the Roman government. Many of them greatly oppressed the people, using extortion and graft. Jews who were publicans were hated by other Jews.
11. **Centurion:** Captain of a hundred men.
12. **Disciple:** Any follower of Christ.
13. **Apostle:** A sent one, a messenger. The name is especially applied to the chosen twelve.

> *"We are writing a gospel; a chapter each day,*
> *By the deeds that we do; by the words that we say.*
> *People read what we write, whether faithless or true.*
> *Say! What is the gospel according to YOU?"*
> —Bishop McIntyre

MARK

AUTHOR: John Mark. Many believed that Mark was influenced a great deal by Peter. Read these verses on Mark: Act 12:25, 13:13. Compare Acts 15:26–40 with what Paul later says about Mark in Colossians 4:10–11 and 2 Timothy 4:11. It is significant that **Mark,** the unfaithful missionary and servant of God, later made faithful by the grace of God, should be chosen to write the gospel of the obedient servant.

PEOPLE TO WHOM WRITTEN: The Romans in particular.

THEME: Jesus, the Servant.

KEY VERSE: Mark 10:45, "For even the Son of man came not to be ministered unto, but to minister, and to give his life a ransom for many."

CHARACTERISTICS:

1. It is the gospel of **rapid-fire action.** The word "straightway" occurs 40 times in Mark.
2. **Miracles** are more emphasized in Mark than in any other gospel. Little attention is given to the words of Christ but much to His **works.**
3. It is the **briefest** of the Gospels, having only 16 chapters.
4. Mark is filled with **descriptive details.**
5. The **public life** of our Lord is stressed.
6. Christ is called **"Master"** frequently in **Mark.**
7. Christ's seasons of retirement and prayer are prominent.
8. There are very **few references to the Old Testament** in Mark. The Roman people would be unfamiliar with the sacred writings of the Jews.
9. There are only about 24 verses given in Mark which could not be found in some form in either Matthew or Luke.

THINGS FOR YOU TO DO:

1. *Read the entire book, watching for the parts which seem to help you to know Jesus better. Watch for verses which would help a Christian become a better servant of God.*
2. *Memorize Mark 10:45 and Mark 8:35–38.*
3. *As you read, list the miracles found in **Mark**.*
4. *As you read, identify the outstanding characters mentioned.*
5. *Learn from Mark 11–16 the happenings of the last week of Jesus' life. (Study pages 38, 39)*
   Why is this week called the "Passion" Week?_____
   Approximately one-third of all four gospels is given over to the last week of our Lord's life. Man is born to live, and his death is incidental. With the Lord Jesus, it was different. He was born to die.

MIRACLES:

Purposes of Miracles:

1. To show that Jesus was God, doing the works of God.
2. To help people in need.

Kinds of Miracles—Miracles show Jesus' control over:

1. Death—raised the dead;
2. Hell—cast out demons;
3. Disease—healed the sick;
4. Nature—showed power over the **forces** of nature (such as miracles connected with food, fish, the sea, etc.).

Inner Spiritual Meaning: The outward physical miracle is a sign of a deeper spiritual miracle Jesus performs. Cleansing the leper is an outward sign of a greater thing that Christ does when He cleanses a sinner. Stilling the tempest is no greater than the miracle God performs even today when He stills the heart of a worried, anxious person.

List in order the miracles you find in Mark. By each tell the kind of miracle it is:

Chapter	Miracle	Kind
1.	_____	_____
2.	_____	_____
3.	_____	_____
4.	_____	_____
5.	_____	_____
6.	_____	_____
7.	_____	_____
8.	_____	_____
9.	_____	_____
10.	_____	_____
11.	_____	_____

Be able to tell any one of these miracles in an interesting fashion.

CHARACTERS:

Give the outstanding event connected with each of the following in the book of Mark:

1. **John the Baptist** _____

2. **Simon Peter** _____

3. **Andrew** _____

4. **James, son of Zebedee** _____

5. **John, son of Zebedee** _____

6. **Levi** *(compare Mark 2:14 with Matt. 9:9)* _____

7. **Titus** _____

8. **Herod** _____

9. **Herodias** _____

10. **Simon, the leper** _____

11. **Judas Iscariot** _____

12. **Pilate** _____

13. **Barabbas** _____

14. **Simon of Cyrene** _____

15. **Joseph of Arimathea** _____

16. **Mary Magdalene** _____

MATTHEW

Renan, the French sceptic, called Matthew the most important book of Christendom;
the most important book that has ever been written.

AUTHOR: Matthew, also called "Levi." One of the twelve apostles. A hated tax collector living at or near Capernaum. Luther called him "the best tax gatherer, as he brought in to God and the Saviour human toll."

PEOPLE TO WHOM WRITTEN: Matthew was written especially to the Jews to prove that Jesus of Nazareth was their long-expected Messiah, repeatedly promised in the Old Testament Scriptures. Its message, however, is for all people as well as for the Jews.

THEME: Jesus, the King.

KEY VERSE: Matthew 2:2, "Saying, Where is he that is born King of the Jews? for we have seen his star in the east, and are come to worship him."

OUTLINE:

The King's Coming . . . . Matthew 1–4
The King Presented. . . . . Matthew 5–16
The King Rejected . . . . Matthew 17–25
The King Crucified and Risen . . . . Matthew 26–28

CHARACTERISTICS:

1. Written **topically** rather than in the order in which the events happened. Matthew systematically groups things of the same kind together.
2. **Old Testament quotations** are frequently used. "It has been estimated that no less than 90 allusions, references, and verbal quotations from the Old Testament are contained in Matthew."
3. The **rejection** of Christ is more prominent in Matthew than in the other gospels.
4. Five great sermons of our Lord are recorded in Matthew.
   1. Sermon on the Mount . . . . Matthew 5–7
   2. Sermon at the sending out of the twelve apostles . . . . . Matthew 10
   3. Seven parables of the kingdom . . . . Matthew 13
   4. The seven terrible woes . . . . Matthew 23
   5. The Olivet Discourse . . . . Matthew 24–25
5. Emphasizes the **final rewards and punishments.** Matthew often mentions "judgment," "hell," "fire," "hypocrite," and "woe."
6. Presents Christ as **King of the Jews.** Matthew speaks of the kingdom in general some 54 times. "The Kingdom of Heaven" occurs 33 times in Matthew and in none of the other gospels.

THINGS FOR YOU TO DO:

1. *Read the gospel according to Matthew as assigned.*
2. *Answer all the questions. Use your own words. Do not quote verses unless the question asks for that.*
3. *Especially notice the teachings of Christ. Also notice and be familiar with any characters and miracles not already studied in Mark.*
4. *Memorize Matt. 2:2, 5:1–12, 6:33, 16:16, 22:36–40, 24:44, 28:19–20, if assigned. Matthew has frequently been called the "Genesis of the New Testament," for it lays the foundation for the New Testament.*

QUESTIONS ON MATTHEW:

List the main idea of the quotations from the Old Testament in Matthew 1 and 2:

1:23 _____

2:6 _____

2:15 _____

2:18 _____

2:23 _____

List the names and titles given Jesus in Matthew 1 and 2:

_____

_____

_____

ANCESTRY AND BIRTH OF THE KING

MATTHEW 1

1. Matthew begins with the family line through whom Joseph, Christ's foster father, came. In your mind does this link the Old Testament to the New? _____
2. Of how many ancestors mentioned in verses 2 to 16 have you heard? _____
    Name them. _____
3. The line of Christ begins in Matthew with which of His ancestors? (1:2) _____
4. Who is the first king in the line of Jesus' ancestors? (1:6) _____
5. To whom did the angel appear? _____
6. *Find the words of the angel concerning the birth of Jesus (1:20).* "For that which is conceived in her is of the _____ "
7. What does the name Jesus mean? (1:21) "Thou shalt call His name Jesus: for _____ "
8. What does Immanuel mean? _____

RECEPTION OF THE KING

MATTHEW 2

1. Who was king in Judea at the time of the birth of Christ? _____
2. Whom were the wise men seeking? (2:2) _____
3. What question did Herod ask the chief priests and scribes? _____
4. What did they answer? _____
5. Why did the wise men not return and tell Herod? _____
6. To what country was Jesus taken? _____
7. How many **years** before had the wise men first seen the star? (2:16) _____
8. After whose death did Joseph bring Mary and the Child back to Palestine? _____
9. Satan has made many attempts to keep Jesus from being able to die on the cross and save us from sin. What did Satan do in this chapter to try to spoil this plan? (2:16) _____
10. In what city was Jesus reared? (2:23) _____

THE HERALDING AND BAPTISM OF THE KING

MATTHEW 3

1. Who is the forerunner of Jesus? _____
2. Where did John preach? _____
3. What did John preach? _____

4. What did John wear? _____
5. What did John eat? _____
6. To whom did John refer when he said, "He that cometh after me is mightier than I"?_____
7. The true God is a Trinity, one God yet three persons. How were each of the persons of the Godhead manifested at the baptism?
   God the Father _____
   God the Son_____
   God the Holy Spirit _____
8. What were the Father's words concerning His Son? (3:17) _____
   _____

THE TEMPTATION OF THE KING AND THE BEGINNING OF HIS GALILEAN MINISTRY
MATTHEW 4

1. What was the first temptation of Jesus? _____
   _____
   *Give Jesus' answer:*_____
   _____

2. What was the second temptation? _____
   _____
   *Give Jesus' answer:*_____
   _____

3. What was the third temptation? _____
   *Give Jesus' answer:*_____
   _____

4. *Name the first four disciples that Jesus called. (4:18, 21)*_____
   _____

FOUNDATION PRINCIPLES OF THE KINGDOM—(SERMON ON THE MOUNT)
MATTHEW 5, 6, 7

What are the three famous passages found in the Sermon on the Mount called?
1. (5:1–12) _____
2. (6:9–15) _____
3. (7:12)_____
4. These verses beginning with: "Blessed" are called beatitudes. "Blessed" means "happy."
   Quote your favorite beatitude _____
5. What does Jesus say to do when one is persecuted for righteousness' sake? _____
   _____
6. To what two things does Christ compare His followers? (5:13–14) _____
   _____
7. How does Christ show His approval of the Old Testament? (5:17–18) _____
   _____
8. How can one easily be guilty of breaking the command "Thou shalt not kill"? *Quote 1 John 3:15a:*
   _____
   _____
9. What does Christ say concerning the person who calls another, "Thou fool"? _____
   _____

10. What should one do when he comes to offer gifts and remembers that his brother has something against him? (5:23–24) _____

_____

11. What does Christ teach about divorce? (5:31–32) _____

_____

12. What does Christ teach about swearing? (5:34) _____

_____

13. What does Christ say as to whom we should love? (5:43–47) _____

_____

14. What does Christ say about "doing our alms" (giving money to the poor)? (6:1–4) *Put the thought of the verses in your own words.* _____

_____

_____

15. How should one pray? (6:5–7) _____

_____

_____

16. After Christ had given the "disciples' prayer," what clause does He explain more fully? (6:14–15) _____

_____

17. Where should one lay up treasure? (6:19) _____

18. Why can one not serve both God and Satan? (6:24) _____

_____

_____

19. *List a number of the reasons Christ gives for a Christian not worrying. (6:25–34)* _____

_____

_____

_____

Said the Robin to the Sparrow, "I should really like to know
Why these anxious human beings rush about and worry so."
Said the Sparrow to the Robin, "Friend, I think that it must be
That they have no Heavenly Father such as cares for you and me."

20. Why should one not criticize and judge another? (7:1–5) _____

21. *Give some facts which should encourage one to pray. (7:7–11)* _____

_____

22. What are the two gates, and where does each lead? (7:13–14) _____

_____

23. To what two kinds of trees are people compared? (7:17) _____

24. What is the only test we can have to tell whether others are Christians, or others know whether we are Christians? (7:20) _____

25. Where did the wise man build, and where did the foolish man build, and with what result? (7:24–27)

_____

_____

_____

_____

MIRACLES SHOWING THE KING'S POWER

MATTHEW 8, 9

1. *List the five miracles in chapter 8:*
   1. _____
   2. _____
   3. _____
   4. _____
   5. _____

2. *List the five miracles in chapter 9:*
   1. _____
   2. _____
   3. _____
   4. _____
   5. _____

   *(The last **two** are found only in **Matthew's** gospel.)*

THE AMBASSADORS OF THE KING

MATTHEW 10

1. Learn the names of the twelve apostles:
   Their address is 52 Mab St.

5 Js	2 Ps	M	A	B	S	T
John	Peter	Matthew	Andrew	Bartholomew	Simon	Thomas
James	Philip	(Levi)		(Nathanael)		
James, son of Alpheus						
Judas, son of James (Thaddaeus)						
Judas Iscariot						

   (This arrangement of the apostles taken from "Bible Story," by Mrs. Adelaide Knoedler, is used by permission.)

2. Most of the instructions given in this chapter were for that particular journey that the apostles took. But there are some statements that could be applied to all Christians. *Give one verse which applied to them but not to all whom Christ sends out* _____

   _____

   _____

   Give one verse from Matthew 10 which always would be good instruction _____

   _____

   _____

RESPONSE TO THE KINGDOM PREACHING

MATTHEW 11, 12

1. When John the Baptist had doubts as to whether Jesus was the Messiah, what did Christ tell John's disciples to tell him? (11:2–5) _____

   _____

   _____

2. Why will it be worse for Bethsaida or Capernaum in the judgment day than for Tyre, Sidon, or Sodom? (11:20–24) _____

   _____

3. To whom has God seen fit to reveal spiritual truths? (11:25)_____

4. Whom did Christ heal on the Sabbath day? (12:9–14)_____

5. What argument did Jesus use to show them it was right to do deeds of kindness on the Sabbath day? (12:10–12)_____ ____

_____

_____

6. How did the Pharisees explain Christ's ability to cast out devils?_____

_____

7. After reading the entire passage what would you say was the unpardonable sin? (12:22–32)_____

_____

8. From what source come good or bad words? (12:34–35) _____

9. How do you know Jesus believed Jonah was in the fish? (12:39–41) _____

_____

_____

THE SEVEN GREAT PARABLES OF THE KINGDOM
MATTHEW 13

"A parable is an earthly story with a heavenly meaning."

1. Six of these parables fall into groups of two each:
    1. The wheat and tares, and the dragnet—teach the mixture of good and evil in the kingdom.
    2. The mustard seed, and the leaven—teach the growth aspect of the kingdom.
    3. The hid treasure and the pearl of great price—teach the value of the kingdom.
2. The first four parables were spoken to the multitude by the sea. They are:
    1. (13:1–23) _____ _____
    2. (13:24–30) __ _____
    3. (13:31–32)_____ ____ _____
    4. (13:33–35) _____ _____
3. The last three were spoken to the disciples in the house. They are:
    5. (13:44)_____ _____ _____
    6. (13:45–46) _____ _____ _____
    7. (13:47–52) __ _____
4. *Tell what Jesus says the different kinds of soil represent in the parable of the Sower. (13:18–23) Also look again at Mark 4:1–20.*

    Seeds that fell by the wayside and the birds came and devoured them: _____

    _____

    Seeds that fell upon rocky places and when the sun was risen the tender plants were scorched and withered: _____

    _____

    Seeds that fell among thorns and were choked: _____

    _____

    Seeds that fell on good ground and brought in an excellent crop: _____

    _____

REJECTION OF THE KING'S FORERUNNER
MATTHEW 14

1. Why had John the Baptist been cast in prison? _____

_____

_____

2. For what did the dancing daughter of Herodias ask Herod when he promised her whatsoever she would ask? _____

3. What two outstanding miracles are recorded in this chapter?
   1. _____
   2. _____

(The feeding of five thousand is the only miracle recorded in all four gospels. It marks a peak in Christ's popularity.)

ATTITUDES TOWARD THE KING'S MINISTRY, CLIMAXING IN PETER'S CONFESSION
MATTHEW 15, 16

1. What did Christ tell the Pharisees it was that defiled a man? (15:11) _____

2. What does Christ say are some of the things that come out of the human heart? (15:19) _____
_____
_____

3. Why did Jesus cast the evil spirit out of the daughter of a woman of the coast of Tyre and Sidon (a Syrophenician)?_____

4. How many thousand did Christ feed the second time? (15:32–38) _____

5. How many baskets were left over? _____

6. Who did men say Jesus was? _____
_____

7. Who did Peter say that Jesus was? (16:14–16)_____
   (Matt. 16:16 is called the Great Confession. Learn it.)

8. To what events do you think Christ is referring in 16:21? _____
_____

THE GLORY OF THE KING, THE TRANSFIGURATION
MATTHEW 17

1. What three disciples were present at the transfiguration?_____
_____

2. What two Old Testament characters were there? _____

3. What did the voice from heaven say? (17:5) _____
_____

4. To what was Christ referring in 17:22–23? _____
_____

5. How did Jesus get the half-shekel or temple tax? _____
_____
_____

TEACHINGS OF THE KING ON HUMILITY AND FORGIVENESS
MATTHEW 18

1. Who did Christ say would be greatest in the kingdom of heaven? (18:1–4)_____
_____

2. What truth do you think Christ wished to teach in the parable about the lost sheep? (18:11–14)
_____
_____

3. How many times should a Christian forgive? (18:21–22)_____

4. What does this really mean?_____
_____

5. *Read very carefully 18:23–35 and then tell the story of the unforgiving servant in your own words.*
   _____
   _____
   _____

6. What is the heavenly meaning of this story? _____
   _____
   _____

FINAL JOURNEY OF THE KING TOWARD JERUSALEM
MATTHEW 19, 20

1. What does Jesus teach about divorce? (19:1–12) _____
   _____
   _____

2. What was Christ's attitude toward little children?_____
   _____

3. Did the rich young ruler really love his neighbor as himself? (19:16–22) _____
   How do you know? _____
   _____

4. *Be able to tell the story of the laborers in the vineyard. (20:1–16)*
5. *Notice Christ's words concerning His coming death and resurrection. (20:17–19)*
6. What request did the mother of the sons of Zebedee, James and John, make of Jesus?
   _____

7. What question did Jesus ask of the two blind men in Jericho, a question He asks of us each time we pray? (20:29–34) _____
   _____

IN JERUSALEM, PREPARING FOR DEATH
MATTHEW 21, 22, 23

PASSION WEEK BEGINS.

1. What did the multitudes cry out as Christ made His entry into Jerusalem? _____
   _____

2. What did Christ do when He went into the temple? (21:12–14)_____
   _____

3. What fruit tree did Jesus curse?_____
   Why?_____

4. *Tell the story of the two sons. (21:28–31)* _____
   _____
   _____
   _____

   (This may mean that the Jews who promised to do God's will failed but the Gentile publicans and sinners who never professed to follow God now are doing God's will.)

5. *Tell the story of the wicked husbandman. (21:33–43)* _____
   _____
   _____
   _____
   _____
   _____

If God is the householder, who are the servants and the son which were sent? _____

_____

Why did the Pharisees not like this story? _____

_____

6. In the parable of the marriage feast how did the invited guests respond to the invitation to come?

_____

What invitation of Christ's can you think of that is often unheeded today? _____

_____

7. What did the Pharisees and Herodians ask Jesus? _____

8. How did Jesus answer? (22:21) _____

_____

9. What did the Sadducees ask Jesus? _____

_____

10. What did the Sadducees believe about the resurrection? (21:23) _____

11. How did Jesus answer them? (22:29–30) _____

12. *Memorize Matthew 22:36–40.* _____

13. List any eight things Jesus said about the Pharisees. (23:4–7, 23–24, 27, etc.) _____

_____

_____

_____

14. How did Jesus feel toward Jerusalem? (23:37) _____

_____

_____

THE OLIVET DISCOURSE OF THE KING

MATTHEW 24, 25

These chapters record a talk given on the Mount of Olives in regard to the future. The parables in the chapters are to show believers how to act in view of these coming events.

1. What do you think is the application to us today of the parable of the ten virgins? _____

_____

2. What do you think is the application to us today of the parable of the talents? _____

_____

_____

THE KING TRIUMPHS IN DEATH AND RESURRECTION

MATTHEW 26, 27, 28

MATTHEW 26

1. During what feast season was Jesus to be betrayed and crucified? _____

2. What loving deed was to be told wherever the gospel was preached? _____

_____

3. How much silver did Judas receive for betraying Christ? _____

4. At the last supper how did Jesus show who would betray him? _____

_____

5. At the last supper what two foods or elements did Jesus offer to His disciples as a memorial?

   _____

6. After the supper where did they go? (26:30) _____

7. Who did Jesus say would deny Him three times? (26:33–35) _____

8. When Jesus went to pray, which disciples did He take with Him? (26:37) _____

   _____

9. What did Jesus pray in the garden? (26:39) _____

   _____

10. What did Peter, James, and John do while Jesus prayed? _____

11. How was Judas to show which of the men was Jesus? _____

12. Why do you think Jesus did not call for the twelve legions of angels to help? (26:53–54)

   _____

   _____

13. Before whom was He first brought for trial? _____

    (The assembly or council mentioned here and later is known as the Sanhedrin.)

14. What important question did the high priest ask Jesus? (26:63) _____

   _____

15. What claim of Jesus made the people think He was worthy of death? (26:64–66) _____

   _____

   _____

16. How did the people insult Jesus? (26:67–68) _____

   _____

   _____

17. How do we know Peter was sorry for three times denying that he knew Christ? (26:74–75)

   _____

MATTHEW 27

1. To what Roman ruler did the Sanhedrin send Jesus for trial? _____

2. What did Judas do with the money he had received for betraying Christ? _____

   _____

3. How did Judas die? (27:5) _____

4. What did the chief priests buy with the money Judas returned? _____

   _____

5. What question did Pilate ask Jesus? (27:11) _____

6. How did Jesus' behavior surprise Pilate? (27:12–14) _____

   _____

7. Why had they arrested Christ? (27:18) _____

8. Which prisoner did the people ask the governor to release at the Passover season? _____

9. Why did Pilate's wife not want Pilate to harm Jesus? (27:19) _____

   _____

10. Did washing his hands make Pilate innocent of Christ's blood? _____

11. How did the governor's soldiers mock and abuse Jesus? _____

   _____

12. Who helped carry Christ's cross? (27:32) _____

13. What place was Christ crucified? (27:33) _____

    (Golgotha is the Hebrew word and Calvary the Latin word, both meaning "the skull.")

14. What stupefying drink did Jesus refuse to take? _____

15. What became of Christ's clothes? _____
_____

16. What inscription was written over the cross? _____
_____

17. Who was crucified with Christ? _____

18. What jeering remarks did the passersby make? _____
_____
_____

19. For how many hours was there darkness? _____

20. What did Jesus cry out when God turned away from Him while He was taking the sins of man upon Himself? _____
_____

21. What happened to the veil in the temple when Christ died? (27:51) *Read Hebrews 10:19–20.*
_____

22. What did the centurion on duty say of this one who had died? _____
_____

23. Who asked for the body of Jesus? (27:57–58) _____

24. Where was Jesus buried? _____

25. Why did the chief priests want a watch placed over the tomb? _____
_____
_____

MATTHEW 28

1. Which is the first day of the week? _____

2. Who rolled the stone away from Christ's tomb? _____

3. What did the angel say to the women? _____
_____
_____
_____

4. The chief priests bribed the watchers of the tomb to tell what tale? _____
_____
_____

5. What is the last great command of Christ to His disciples? (28:19) _____
_____
_____

6. What is Christ's last great promise? _____
_____

LUKE

AUTHOR: Luke, the "beloved physician"; wrote under the influence of Paul, his friend.

PEOPLE TO WHOM WRITTEN: Primarily to the Greeks, who were Gentiles.

THEME: Jesus, the Son of Man. (Read Heb. 4:15.)

KEY VERSE: Luke 19:10, "For the Son of man is come to seek and to save that which was lost."

PURPOSE: Written to a friend (1:1–4 and Acts 1:1) named_____ to give an authentic report of the life of Jesus.

CHARACTERISTICS:

1. The **universality** of the gospel, its being for all men everywhere, is shown in Luke.
2. Luke is the gospel of **glad acceptance,** just the opposite of Matthew which is the gospel of sad rejection.
3. The **humanity** of Jesus as the perfect Son of Man is emphasized.
4. It is the most **literary and logical** of the Gospels. Luke's grace of style is simply magnificent. Renan was right when he called Luke "the most beautiful book in the world."
5. More **pictures** have been painted from Luke than from any of the other gospels. Artists revel in this book.
6. **Miracles of healing** and mercy are prominent.
7. **Angels** are mentioned often in Luke.
8. The **parables** are emphasized more than the miracles.
9. The **prayer life** of Christ is more prominent in Luke than in other gospels.
10. The dignity of **womanhood** is especially recognized in Luke.
11. The **social life** of Jesus is recorded. Luke tells us of Jesus' presence as a dinner guest at least six times.
12. Luke contains five great **"Holy Songs."** It is the "Gospel of Song." *(In the blank place the name of the person giving the song.)*
    1. "Ave Maria" (Hail Mary) of_____ Luke 1:42–45.
    2. "Magnificat" (Magnifies) of _____ Luke 1:46–55.
    3. "Benedictus" (Blessed) of _____ Luke 1:68–79.
    4. "Gloria in Excelsis" (Glory in the highest) of the _____ Luke 2:14
    5. "Nunc Dimittis" (Now let us depart) of _____ Luke 2:29–32.

THINGS FOR YOU TO DO:

1. *Read the entire gospel according to Luke, as assigned. Especially notice the parables.*
2. *Memorize Luke 19:10.*
3. *Review the Outline of the Life of Christ, page 6.*
4. *As you read, watch for the characters and places listed below and identify them.*
5. *Be able to tell in class the new incidents and parables given in Luke. Answer questions.*

PEOPLE IN LUKE: *(Identify each)*

1. Zacharias _____
2. Elisabeth _____
3. Gabriel _____
4. Mary (of Nazareth) _____
5. Simeon _____
6. Anna _____
7. Mary (of Bethany) _____
8. Martha _____

23

9. Simon, the Pharisee _____

10. Lazarus _____

11. Zacchaeus _____

12. Cleopas _____

13. Theophilus _____

PLACES IN LUKE:

(Tell what event or events of importance in Luke happened at each of the following places. Locate each place on the map, page 7.)

1. Nazareth _____

_____

2. Bethlehem _____

_____

3. Capernaum (headquarters for Galilean ministry) (4:31–44) _____

_____

4. Lake of Gennesaret (Sea of Galilee) _____

_____

5. Nain _____

6. Jericho _____

7. Bethany _____

_____

8. Jerusalem _____

_____

9. Mount of Olives _____

10. Emmaus _____

QUESTIONS ON STORIES TOLD ONLY IN LUKE:

Birth of John the Baptist promised to Zacharias (1:5–25)

1. What was Zacharias doing in the temple when the angel spoke to him? _____

_____

2. What did the angel promise him? _____

3. What was to happen to Zacharias for not believing the words of Gabriel, the angel? _____

_____

4. Who was Elisabeth? _____

Angel's visit to Mary (1:26–38)

1. What was the angel's name? _____

2. Where was Mary living? _____

3. What did the angel tell Mary? _____

_____

4. By what names would the child be called? (1:31) _____

(1:32) _____ (1:35) _____

24

Mary's visit to Elisabeth (1:39–56)

1. What relation was Elisabeth to Mary? (1:36)_____

2. *Quote the verse you consider to be the loveliest in Mary's song, the Magnificat. (1:46–55)* _____
   _____
   _____
   _____

3. How long did Mary stay?_____

Birth of John the Baptist

1. By what name did the neighbors and cousins want to call the baby boy?_____

2. When was Zacharias again able to speak?_____
   _____

3. *Quote the verse you consider the best in Zacharias' song of praise. (1:68–79)* _____
   _____
   _____

Birth of Jesus (2:1–7)

1. Who ruled the world at this time? (2:1) _____

2. Why were Joseph and Mary in Bethlehem?_____
   _____

3. Why was Jesus placed in a manger rather than a bed?_____
   _____

Visit of the shepherds (2:8–20)

1. How did the shepherds know the Savior had been born? _____
   _____

2. What city is called "the city of David"? _____

Jesus presented at the temple (2:22–38)

1. What offering did they bring for a sacrifice? (2:24) _____
   _____

2. What man had been shown that before his death he would see the Christ? _____

3. What prophetess also recognized this baby as the promised Redeemer?_____

Visit to Jerusalem at twelve years of age (2:41–52)

1. Why was Jesus in Jerusalem with His parents?_____
   _____

2. What did His parents find Him doing in the temple? _____
   _____

3. What did Jesus call His "Father's house"?_____

Jesus in the synagogue in Nazareth (4:16–30)

1. From which book did Jesus read in the synagogue? _____

2. How did Jesus explain the meaning of the passage He quoted from Isaiah 61:1–2? _____
   _____
   _____

3. When Jesus spoke well of Gentiles, the widow in Sidon, and the leper in Syria, what did the Jews of Nazareth do?_____
   _____

4. What city did Jesus choose for His headquarters for His Galilean ministry? (4:31)_____
   _____

Raising of the widow's son to life (7:11–17)

1. In what city was the funeral? _____

2. What did Jesus say to the mother? _____

   _____

3. What did Jesus say to the son? _____

Anointing of Jesus and the parable of the two debtors (7:36–50)

1. What did the sinful woman do to Jesus? _____

   _____

   _____

2. What story did Jesus tell Simon, the Pharisee? _____

   _____

   _____

   _____

3. How had Simon failed to be even courteous to Jesus? (7:44–46) _____

   _____

   _____

4. Who loved Jesus the most? _____

The parable of the good Samaritan (10:25–37)

1. Who asked "who is my neighbor"? _____

2. Where was the man traveling when beaten and robbed? _____

3. What three people passed that way? _____

   _____

4. Which proved himself a neighbor to the needy man? _____

5. What kind things did the Samaritan do? _____

Visit with Martha and Mary (10:38–42)

1. Of what did Jesus disapprove in Martha? _____

   _____

2. What did Jesus appreciate in Mary? _____

   _____

Parable of the friend at midnight (11:5–10)

1. What did he ask from his friend? _____

2. Why did his friend give it to him? _____
   (Importunity means persistent urging.)

3. From this parable what is taught about prayer? _____

   _____

Parable of the rich fool (12:16–21)

1. What did the rich man do? _____

   _____

2. How was he a fool? _____

   _____

Woman healed on the Sabbath (13:10–17)

1. How long had the woman been sick? _____

2. Why did the ruler of the synagogue object to Christ's healing her? _____

   _____

3. Why did Jesus mention about loosing an ox or an ass? _____
_____
_____

Parable of the ambitious guest (14:1–15)
1. Where was Jesus when He told the story? (14:1)_____
_____
2. Where should one sit when coming to a wedding?_____
_____
3. Why?_____
_____
_____

Luke 15 has three parables of lost things:

Parable of lost sheep (15:3–7)
1. How many sheep were lost?_____
2. How many sheep were safe? _____
3. What does this story teach us of God? _____
_____

Parable of the lost coin (15:8–10)
1. How does this story show the love of God for the lost?_____
_____
_____

Parable of the lost son, the prodigal son (15:11–32)
1. Who left home? _____
2. Why did he return? _____
_____
3. How did his father receive him? _____
_____
4. How did the elder brother feel about this welcome?_____
_____
5. What is the "heavenly meaning" of this parable? _____
_____

Parable of the unjust steward (16:1–13)
1. How did the steward who was to be fired make friends? _____
_____
_____
2. Did his lord or employer commend him for his honesty or for his wise shrewdness? _____

The rich man and Lazarus (16:19–31)
1. Who was Lazarus? _____
2. Where did the rich man go after death? _____
3. Why could Lazarus not bring water to the rich man in torment?_____
_____
4. If a person will not believe the Bible (writings of Moses and the prophets), would they believe the warnings of one who returned from the dead? _____

Ten lepers healed (17:11–19)

1. How many of the ten thanked Jesus for the healing? _____
2. What was his nationality? _____

Parable of the unjust judge (18:1–8)

1. Who asked the judge for help? _____
2. Why did the judge decide to give her justice? _____
   _____
3. What does this teach about prayer? (18:1, 7) _____
   _____

Parable of the Pharisee and publican (18:9–14)

1. How did the Pharisee pray? _____
   _____
2. How did the publican pray? _____
   _____
3. With which prayer was God pleased? _____

Visit to Zacchaeus (19:1–10)

1. Describe Zacchaeus's occupation, wealth, and appearance: _____
   _____
   _____
2. Where was he when Jesus saw him? _____
3. What did Zacchaeus do which showed he had really received salvation? _____
   _____

Parable of the ten pounds (19:11–27)

1. Before the nobleman went away what did he give to the ten servants? _____
   _____
2. When the nobleman returned, with which servants was he pleased? _____
   _____

Jesus before Herod and Pilate (23:4–16)

After Jesus had been tried by the Jewish Sanhedrin and brought before Pilate, Luke tells us that Pilate sent Him to the Galilean governor, Herod, who was then in Jerusalem.

1. Why did Pilate send Jesus to Herod? _____
   _____
2. What did Herod hope Jesus would do? _____
3. What did Pilate say of Jesus' innocence? (23:14) _____
   _____
4. What did Herod say? (23:15) _____

Jesus' walk to the village of Emmaus (24:13–35)

1. Whom did Jesus join on the way to Emmaus? _____
2. Why were these believers so sad? _____
   _____

3. Of what did Christ talk as they walked along? (24:25–27)_____

_____

_____

4. When did they recognize Jesus? _____

5. After Jesus vanished what did they do?_____

_____

The commission of the disciples (24:36–49)

1. What was to be preached among all nations? _____

_____

2. Where was the preaching to begin?_____

3. Before the disciples went forth, what were they to receive? _____

_____

Ascension into heaven (24:50–53)

1. From what place did Jesus ascend? _____

2. What was He doing as He left them? _____

3. What did His disciples do when their Master departed?_____

_____

JOHN

AUTHOR: John, the beloved disciple. He was one of the three in the "inner circle." He appears to have been the youngest apostle. He is the author of five New Testament books, this gospel, 1, 2, and 3 John, and Revelation.

PEOPLE TO WHOM WRITTEN: To the world. The word "world" occurs more frequently in the gospel of John than in all of the other gospels combined.

THEME: Jesus Christ is the Eternal Son of God. This gospel is filled with personal interviews and miracles which are designed to emphasize Christ's deity and life-giving power.

KEY VERSE: John 20:31, "But these are written, that ye might believe that Jesus is the Christ, the Son of God; and that believing ye might have life through his name."

OUTLINE: One of the best outlines is based on John 16:28.
1. "I came forth from the Father" 1:1–18
2. "I am come into the world" . . . . 1:19–12th chapter
3. "Again I leave the world" 13–19
4. "I go to the Father" 20–21

CHARACTERISTICS:
1. Written in **simple style.**
2. Christ's early **ministry in Judea** is stressed.
3. John emphasized the **deity** of Jesus, that Jesus is God, proving it in many ways. Some of them are:
   a. Christ is called God in John 1:1; 1:18
   b. He does what only God can do 1:3; 5:21–22
   c. He received worship as God would receive worship 5:23; 20:28
   d. He claims God as His Father 5:17; 14:9
   e. Jesus was supernatural in His eternal existence, resurrection, and ascension . . 1:1; 3:13
4. The **eight miracles** or signs stress the power of Christ.
5. The **temple** and **feasts** are mentioned often. From other gospels one might think that the public life of Christ lasted only a year or so. Because of John's mention of three or four Passover feasts, historians have fixed the length of Christ's public ministry at three years.
6. Several **private interviews** and **public talks** are told only in John's gospel.

THINGS FOR YOU TO DO:
1. *Read the gospel according to John as assigned.*
2. *As you read, mark in your Bible the best verses telling one how to receive everlasting life.*
3. *Answer the questions on the chapters read each day.*
   Over half the things told in John are not told elsewhere. The questions are chiefly on these points.
4. *As you read John, see how each chapter fulfills John's purpose given in John 20:31.*
   Think of these three questions:
   a. What does the chapter tell as to who Jesus is?
   b. What does it show about faith or believing?
   c. What does it show about life?
5. *As you read, complete the lists of miracles and of the "I am" statements of Jesus.*
6. *Memorize John 1:12, 3:3, 3:16, 3:36, 14:1–3, 20:31.*

MIRACLES:

There are eight miracles called "signs" in John. Six are recorded only in this book.

List the miracles and where they are found and check the two you have already studied.

Miracle	Chapter	Check
_____	_____	_____
_____	_____	_____
_____	_____	_____
_____	_____	_____
_____	_____	_____
_____	_____	_____
_____	_____	_____
_____	_____	_____

Of what are these miracles signs? _____

_____

THE "I AM" STATEMENTS:

List, as you read, the different important things Jesus says He is when He begins "I am." Watch for these. Tell where they are found:

Statement	Reference
_____	_____
_____	_____
_____	_____
_____	_____
_____	_____
_____	_____
_____	_____

QUESTIONS ON JOHN:

"I came forth from the Father" (1:1–18)

JOHN 1

1. What other book in the Bible opens with the words "in the beginning"? _____

2. Who is the one called "the Word"? (Study 1:14) _____

3. *List the names and titles given to Jesus in chapter 1:*

   _____
   _____
   _____
   _____
   _____
   _____

"I am come into the world" (1:19–12)

4. Whom did Andrew bring to Jesus? (1:37–42) _____

5. What did Christ say to Peter? _____

   _____

6. Whom did Philip bring to Jesus? (1:43–51)_____

1. What did Jesus say to Nathanael? _____

_____

JOHN 2

1. What was the first miracle Jesus performed? (2:11)_____

_____

2. In what town did it happen? _____

3. What was a great result of this miracle? (2:11) _____

_____

4. What historical Jewish event did the Passover feast celebrate? (Exodus 12) _____

_____

_____

5. What did Jesus do to cleanse the temple?_____

_____

_____

(This cleansing of the temple was at the beginning of Jesus' public life. At the end the same thing was repeated.)

6. What did Jesus mean when He said "Destroy this temple, and in three days I will raise it up"? (2:19–22) _____

_____

JOHN 3

1. Who was Nicodemus? (3:1)_____

2. When did he come to see Jesus? _____

3. What did Jesus say was his great need? (3:3, 7)_____

_____

4. In what way was Moses' lifting up the serpent in the wilderness like Christ's being lifted up on the cross? (3:14–15) Compare with Numbers 21:5–9. _____

_____

_____

5. What verse sums up the whole story of salvation? _____

6. What two classes of people are there? (3:36)_____

_____

JOHN 4

1. In what country was Jacob's well? (4:3–6) _____

2. How did the Jews feel toward the Samaritans? (4:9)_____

_____

3. What did Jesus offer the Samaritan woman?_____

4. What did Jesus ask her to do that showed up the sin in her life? (4:16–19)_____

_____

5. Who did Jesus finally tell the woman that He was? (4:25–26) _____

_____

6. How did this woman show she was a good witness to what she knew of Jesus? (4:29, 39–40)

_____

_____

7. Where was the nobleman's sick son? _____

8. How did Jesus heal the son? _____
_____

9. What was interesting about the hour the son began to get well? _____

JOHN 5

1. Where did many of the sick in Jerusalem stay? _____

2. How long had the impotent (helpless) man been sick? _____

3. What are some of the things Jesus said that showed He was equal with God:

   5:17–18 _____

   5:21 _____

   5:22 _____

   5:23 _____

   5:26 _____

   5:27 _____

JOHN 6

1. After having been fed by Jesus, what did the 5,000 want to do? (6:15)_____
_____

2. That night why were the disciples afraid? _____
_____

3. What were the main thoughts of Jesus' talk to the people on the following day?_____
_____
_____
_____

JOHN 7

1. To what feast in Jerusalem did Jesus come? _____

2. What did Jesus say to the crowd on the last day of the feast? (7:37–39) _____
_____
_____
_____

JOHN 8

1. To whom did Jesus show mercy and forgiveness?

2. Who is a servant of sin? (8:32–34) _____
_____

3. Who can free sin's servant? (8:36)_____

4. What claim of Jesus made the Jews want to stone Him? (8:56–59)_____
_____
_____

JOHN 9

1. Why was this man born blind? (9:2–3) _____
_____

2. How did Jesus heal the blind man? (9:6–7) _____

_____

3. Why did some Pharisees think Jesus, who had healed the man, could not be God? _____

_____

4. Why were the man's parents afraid to speak what they knew? (9:20–22) _____

_____

5. Did the blind man believe that Jesus was of God? (9:32–38) _____

JOHN 10

1. From this chapter list several ways in which Jesus is like a shepherd. (Notice especially 10:4, 10–11, 14) _____

_____

_____

_____

_____

_____

2. In what way is Jesus like a door? _____

_____

JOHN 11

1. Who was the brother of Mary and Martha? _____

2. Why do you think Jesus waited so long to come when Lazarus was so sick? (11:15) _____

_____

3. What words did both Martha and Mary say when they saw Jesus? (11:21, 32) _____

_____

4. How long had Lazarus been in the grave? (11:17, 39) _____

5. Where is the shortest verse in the Bible found? _____

6. What effect did the resurrection of Lazarus have on many people? (11:45) _____

7. What effect did it have on the Pharisees? (11:47–48, 53)

JOHN 12

1. How did Mary show her love for Jesus? _____

_____

2. Why did Judas object to this gift? (12:4–6) _____

3. Why would the chief priests want to put Lazarus to death too? (12:10–11) _____

4. Why is the day Jesus rode a young ass into Jerusalem called "Palm Sunday"? (12:13)

_____

"Again I leave the world" (13–19)

JOHN 13

1. What two lessons did Jesus want to teach the disciples by washing their feet? (13:12–16) _____

_____

_____

_____

2. Which disciple in the upper room got up and left the presence of Jesus?_____

3. What new commandment did Jesus give His disciples that last night? (13:34–35)_____
_____

JOHN 14

1. What verses and subjects discussed in John 14 make it one of the best loved chapters of the Bible?
_____
_____
_____
_____
_____
_____

2. In whose name do we offer prayer? (14:14)_____

3. Who is the "Comforter" Jesus promised to send? (14:16–17, 26)_____

JOHN 15

1. Who is the husbandman (farmer or caretaker)?_____

2. Who is the vine?_____

3. Who are the branches? _____

4. Why should a follower of Christ not expect to receive better treatment than He did?
(15:19–20)_____

JOHN 16

1. *Name three or four things the chapter says about the Holy Spirit. (16:7–15)*_____
_____
_____
_____

JOHN 17

1. For whom did Jesus pray? (17:6–26) _____
_____
_____

JOHN 18

1. Who betrayed Jesus? _____

2. What happened to Malchus? _____

3. Why did the Jews not put Jesus to death? (18:31)_____

JOHN 19

1. How did Pilate and the soldiers mistreat Jesus?_____
_____
_____
_____

2. Why did the Jews think Jesus should die? (19:7) _____
_____
_____

3. Was Jesus the Son of God?_____

4. How did the soldiers unknowingly fulfill an Old Testament prophecy concerning the clothes of Jesus? (19:23–24) _____

_____

_____

5. Whom did Jesus tell John to take care of as though she were his mother?_____

6. How did the soldiers fulfill the Old Testament prophecy that not a bone would be broken? (19:32–37)

_____

7. Who helped Joseph of Arimathea bury Jesus? _____

"I GO TO THE FATHER" (20–21)

JOHN 20

1. John never mentions his own name in his book. Who do you think ran with Peter to the empty tomb?_____

2. What did John believe when he saw the empty sepulchre? (20:8) _____

_____

3. Who was the first to see Jesus on this first Easter Sunday morning? _____

4. What happened that Sunday evening? (20:19–23) _____

_____

_____

5. What disciple beside Judas was not present? _____

6. One week later what did Thomas say when he saw Jesus? _____

_____

JOHN 21

1. In this last miracle of the book what did the discouraged fishermen have to do to get the 153 great fish?_____

2. With whom did Jesus talk after they had eaten? _____

3. How many times did Jesus ask "Lovest thou me"? _____

4. Are all the things Jesus did recorded in the Bible? (20:30, 21:25) _____

    *Think back over this book and list several reasons why the gospel of John is one of the best loved books in the Bible.*_____

_____

_____

_____

_____

QUOTATIONS FROM JOHN'S GOSPEL:

Give the "who said," the "when," or the "to whom" of the following quotations:

1. "Behold the Lamb of God."

_____

2. "They have no wine."

_____

3. "Take these things hence; make not my Father's house an house of merchandise."

_____

4. "Ye must be born again."

_____

5. "If thou knewest the gift of God, and who it is that saith to thee, Give me to drink; thou wouldest have asked of him, and he would have given thee living water."

    _____

6. "Go thy way; thy son liveth."

    _____

7. "There is a lad here, which hath five barley loaves, and two small fishes; but what are they among so many?"

    _____

8. "He that is without sin among you, let him first cast a stone at her."

    _____

9. "A man that is called Jesus made clay, and anointed mine eyes."

    _____

10. "Lord, if thou hadst been here, my brother had not died."

    _____

11. "Why was not this ointment sold for three hundred pence, and given to the poor?"

    _____

12. "Hosanna: Blessed is the King of Israel that cometh in the name of the Lord."

    _____

13. "Thou shalt never wash my feet."

    _____

14. "Verily, verily, I say unto you, that one of you shall betray me."

    _____

15. "The cock shall not crow, till thou hast denied me thrice."

    _____

16. "I pray not that thou shouldest take them out of the world, but that thou shouldest keep them from the evil."

    _____

17. "Art thou the King of the Jews?"

    _____

18. "Not this man, but Barabbas."

    _____

19. "Behold, I bring him forth to you, that ye may know that I find no fault in him."

    _____

20. "What I have written I have written."

    _____

21. "Let us not rend it, but cast lots for it, whose it shall be."

    _____

22. "Woman, behold thy son!"

    _____

23. "Sir, if thou have borne him hence, tell me where thou hast laid him, and I will take him away."

    _____

24. "Reach hither thy hand, and thrust it into my side: and be not faithless, but believing."

    _____

25. "Lovest thou me?"

    _____

THE PASSION WEEK

Especially for use the week preceding Easter

The week of Christ's life in which he was crucified is called "Passion Week." "Passion" means "suffering." This most important week of all history covers events which have changed the world.

The scene of most of the happenings was in Jerusalem, but Jesus probably retired each evening to Bethany, a village about a mile from the outskirts of Jerusalem.

SATURDAY night: Matt.: 26:6–13, Mark 14:3–9, John 11:55–12:11.

Jesus was anointed in Bethany by Mary.

SUNDAY—DAY OF POPULARITY: Matt. 21:1–11, Mark 11:1–11, Luke 19:29–44, John 12:12–19.

Jesus enters Jerusalem in triumph.

MONDAY—DAY OF AUTHORITY: Matt. 21:12–19, Mark 11:12–19, Luke 19:45–48.

Jesus cursed the barren fig tree and cleansed the temple.

TUESDAY—DAY OF CONFLICT: Matt. 21:20–26:16, Mark 11:20–14:11, Luke 20:1–22:6, John 12:20–50.

Jesus taught in the temple and on the Mount of Olives.

WEDNESDAY—DAY OF REST: No record.

Jesus probably spent a day of rest with His friends at Bethany.

THURSDAY—DAY OF FELLOWSHIP: Matt. 26:17–35, Mark 14:12–31, Luke 22:7–38, John 13:1–17:26.

Last supper followed by Jesus' arrest in Gethsemane about midnight.

FRIDAY—DAY OF SUFFERING: Matt. 26:36–27:61, Mark 14:32–15:47, Luke 22:39–23:56, John 18:1–19:42.

Trial: Jewish and Roman.

About sunrise Jesus was officially condemned by Caiaphas and the Jewish Sanhedrin.

Sanhedrin took Jesus to the Roman governor, Pilate, about 6 a.m.

Pilate sent Jesus to Herod.

Herod returned Jesus to Pilate who released Barabbas and delivered Jesus to be crucified.

Jesus was crowned with thorns and mocked.

Judas committed suicide.

Crucifixion: About 9 a.m.

Simon of Cyrene helped Jesus take the cross to Calvary.

Jesus refused the stupefying drink.

1. Jesus said (Luke 23:34) _____

    _____

Soldiers parted Jesus' garments.

Jews mocked Jesus.

One of the two thieves repented and believed.

2. Jesus said (Luke 23:43) _____

    _____

3. Jesus said (John 19:26–27) _____

    _____

Darkness lasted from 12 to 3 p.m.

4. Jesus said (Matt. 27:46) _____

_____

5. Jesus said (John 19:28) _____

6. Jesus said (John 19:30) _____

_____

7. Jesus said (Luke 23:46) _____

_____

Jesus died.

The veil in the temple was torn from top to bottom.

The earth quaked and graves opened.

Jesus' side was pierced.

Burial:

Jesus was buried in the tomb of Joseph of Arimathea.

SATURDAY—Day of Silence: Matt. 27:62–66.

Guards were placed at the tomb.

SUNDAY—Day of Triumph: Matt. 28:1–15, Mark 16:1–14, Luke 24:1–43, John 20:1–25.

Jesus victoriously arose from the dead.

THE FORTY DAYS

From the Resurrection Until the Ascension

Jesus appeared:

On the day of His resurrection

1. To Mary Magdalene at the tomb. John 20:14–18
2. To the other women. Matt. 28:8–10
3. To Peter. Luke 24:34, 1 Cor. 15:5
4. To two disciples on the road to Emmaus. Luke 24:13–31
5. To ten apostles in upper room in Jerusalem, Thomas being absent. Luke 24:36–43, John 20:19–25

Eight days later

6. To the eleven apostles. Thomas being present. John 20:26–29

In Galilee

7. To seven apostles by the Sea of Galilee. John 21:1–23
8. To about 500 on hillside in Galilee. 1 Cor. 15:6

At Jerusalem and Bethany

9. To James, brother of Jesus. 1 Cor. 15:7
10. To the eleven apostles in Jerusalem. Matt. 28:16–20, Mark 16:14–20, Luke 24:44–53, Acts 1:3–12

ACTS

TITLE: The Acts of the Apostles, or The Acts of the Holy Spirit.

AUTHOR: Luke, the beloved physician; at times a companion of Paul.

PEOPLE TO WHOM WRITTEN: To Theophilus, the Gentile, to whom the gospel of Luke was addressed.

PURPOSE: To write a history of the beginning and growth of the church.

KEY VERSE: (The last recorded words of Jesus.) Acts 1:8 "But ye shall receive power, after that the Holy Ghost is come upon you: and ye shall be witnesses unto me both in Jerusalem, and in all Judaea, and in Samaria, and unto the uttermost part of the earth."

OUTLINE:

    I.   Home missions . . . . Acts 1–12

        The witness to the Jews in Jerusalem, Judea, and Samaria. Outstanding leader—Peter.

        Important city—Jerusalem.

    II. Foreign missions . . . . Acts 13–28

        The witness to the Gentiles, to the "uttermost *parts!*"

        Outstanding leader—Paul.

        Important cities—Antioch, Ephesus, and Rome.

THINGS FOR YOU TO DO:

1. *Read all of the Acts.*
2. *Answer the questions and fill in the outline. Use your own words. Do not quote verses unless the question asks for that.*
3. *Be able to locate on the map, page 7, the places mentioned in Acts 1–12.*
4. *Draw Paul's first and second journeys on the map, page 47, and Paul's third and fourth on the map, page 53.*
5. *Memorize Acts 1:8, 4:12, 16:31.*
6. *Make a report on the life of at least one great missionary.*
7. *If assigned by the teacher, make reports on certain cities and characters, using reference materials.*

QUESTIONS ON ACTS:

HOME MISSIONS—ACTS 1–12

ACTS 1

1. For how many days after the resurrection was Jesus seen on earth? (1:3)_____
2. Why were the disciples not to depart from Jerusalem? (1:4–5)_____
   _____
3. In what order are the places mentioned to which the disciples were to go as witnesses?
   _____
4. What did the two men in white say about Jesus' returning to earth again? _____
   _____
   _____
5. About how many all together were in the upper room? (1:15) _____
6. Who was chosen to take Judas' place?_____

ACTS 2

1. On what day did the Holy Spirit come? _____

2. What three outward things happened to show that the Holy Spirit had come? (2:2–4)

    _____

    _____

3. Why did those in Jerusalem marvel? (2:7–8) _____

4. Who stood up to explain what had happened?_____

5. What connection did Christ (whom these Jews crucified) have with the strange happenings among the believers in Jerusalem at Pentecost? (2:32–36) _____

    _____

6. What words did Peter have for those who were sorry they had crucified Jesus? (2:37–40)

    _____

    _____

7. As the result of Peter's sermon how many people became believers? _____

8. *List the things you find the early church doing. (2:42–47)*_____

    _____

    _____

    _____

ACTS 3

1. Who asked for alms (money) at the gate called Beautiful of the temple? _____

2. How long had the man been lame? (3:2, 4:22) _____

3. What did Peter say to him? _____

    _____

    _____

    _____

4. How did Peter explain the lame man's being healed? (3:12–16) _____

    _____

    _____

ACTS 4

1. What did the Sadducees do to Peter and John when they heard them giving the resurrected Jesus the glory for the healing of the lame man? (4:1–3) _____

    _____

2. How many believed after hearing this second sermon of Peter's? (4:4) _____

    _____

3. In the morning what did the Sanhedrin ask them? (4:7)_____

    _____

4. What did Peter, who was filled with the Holy Ghost, reply? (4:10)_____

    _____

    _____

    _____

5. What other wonderful statement about the name of Jesus did Peter make? (4:12) _____

    _____

    _____

    _____

6. What did the Sanhedrin command these apostles not to do? _____

    _____

7. After this experience what is the main thing for which the Christian company prayed? (4:23–31) _____

8. What did Barnabas do? (4:36–37) _____

9. Why do you think the Christians shared their possessions? _____

10. How is this alike or different from communism today? _____

ACTS 5

1. What evil thing did Ananias and Sapphira do? _____

2. What was their punishment? _____

3. What effect did this have on the church? (5:11) _____

4. What is said of the growth of the early church? (5:14) _____

5. What power had the apostles been given? (5:12–16) _____

6. What did the Sadducees do to the apostles? _____

7. When the council met the next morning why could the guards not bring the apostles from the prison? _____

8. Where were the apostles found fearlessly preaching? _____

9. When reminded that the council had commanded them not to preach about Jesus what did the apostles say? (5:29) _____

10. What argument did Gamaliel use that kept the Sanhedrin from slaying the apostles? (5:36–39, especially verses 38–39) _____

11. How did the apostles feel about their imprisonment and beating? (5:40–42) _____

ACTS 6

1. How many men did the brethren choose to take over the church business of serving tables, looking after the widows, etc.? _____

2. What were the twelve apostles to do? (6:2, 4) _____

3. How is Stephen, one of these deacons, described? (6:8, 10) _____

4. How did Stephen look when all manner of false witnesses spoke against him? (6:15) _____
_____

ACTS 7

1. After reviewing Israel's history before the council what strong accusation did Stephen make? (7:51–52) _____
_____
_____

2. When Stephen looked up into heaven what did he say he saw? _____

3. On casting him out of the city how did they kill Stephen? _____

4. At whose feet were the witnesses' clothes laid? _____

5. What was Stephen's last prayer? _____
_____

6. Who else had prayed such a forgiving prayer? (Luke 23:34) _____

7. The name Stephen means "crown." Why would he receive a crown in glory? (Rev. 2:10) _____
_____

ACTS 8

1. What was the result of the persecution in Jerusalem? (8:1–4) _____
_____

2. What deacon preached in Samaria? _____

3. Who in Samaria was rebuked by Philip for offering to buy the power of the Holy Ghost?
_____

4. Whom did Philip see in a chariot near Gaza? _____
_____

5. Of whom did the verses speak which the Ethiopian read in Isaiah 53:7–8? (8:30–35)
_____

6. After the Ethiopian had been baptized what happened to Philip? (8:39–40) _____
_____

ACTS 9

1. Why was Saul going to Damascus? _____
_____

2. What did he see near Damascus? _____
_____

3. What did Saul say when he realized his mistake in persecuting the Christians? (9:6)
_____

4. How long was Saul blind? _____
_____

5. What believer in Damascus visiting Saul, caused him to receive his sight and baptized him? _____
_____
_____

6. After Saul was converted, how did the Jews in Damascus treat him? (9:20–25) _____
_____
_____

7. Who in Jerusalem welcomed Saul into the fellowship of the believers there? _____

8. When the Grecians were about to slay Saul where did the brethren send him? _____
_____This was Saul's own birthplace.

9. What miracle did Peter perform at Lydda? _____

_____

_____

10. What were some of Dorcas's good works? (9:36, 39) _____

_____

11. Why did Peter go from Lydda to Joppa? _____

_____

12. Later with whom did Peter stay at Joppa? (9:43) _____

ACTS 10

1. *Describe Cornelius. (10:1–2, 22)* _____

_____

_____

2. Where did Cornelius live? _____

3. What did Peter see in his vision on the house top in Joppa? _____

_____

_____

_____

_____

4. What did God tell Peter about unclean animals? (10:15)_____

_____

5. Also, what people did the Jews consider unclean? (10:28)_____

6. What Gentile in Caesarea did Peter now willingly visit? _____

7. After Peter preached Christ to the household of Cornelius what amazing thing happened?
    (10:44, 46) _____

_____

8. Did Peter expect God to do this for the Gentiles? (10:45) _____

ACTS 11

1. What great experience did Peter explain to the Jewish brethren in Jerusalem? (11:1–18)

_____

_____

2. Who was sent to strengthen the believers in Antioch? (11:22)_____

3. Whom did Barnabas bring from Tarsus to help him in the church at Antioch? _____

4. Where were the disciples first called Christians? _____

5. The church in Antioch sent relief to the brethren in what place? _____

ACTS 12

1. What king began to persecute the church? _____

2. Who was the first of the twelve apostles to be killed as a martyr? _____

3. When Herod saw this pleased the Jews, what other apostle was imprisoned? _____

4. What did the church do when Peter was in such danger?_____

5. *Tell fully how their prayers were miraculously answered. (12:7–10)*_____

_____

_____

_____

_____

6. In whose house did Peter find the believers gathered together praying? _____

_____

7. What girl answered the door? _____

8. Why did Herod suffer a loathsome death? (12:21–23) _____

_____

FOREIGN MISSIONS—ACTS 13–28

Introduction to Paul's Life

Birth:

A. Probably born about the same time as Jesus.

B. In Tarsus, capital of the province of Cilicia, in Asia Minor.

Family:

A. Jews from the tribe of Benjamin.

(Saul may have been named for King Saul.)

B. Roman citizenship—Paul was free born.

This citizenship meant he could never be crucified or scourged and could appeal to Rome for justice.

Education:

A. In Tarsus he would receive the benefits of Greek culture. Tarsus was a famous university town and commercial center.

B. At Jerusalem under Gamaliel he received the finest Jewish training and became an outstanding Pharisee.

Conversion:

On the road to Damascus about AD 36

Trips:

A. To Cyprus and Asia Minor . . . . First journey

B. To Europe . . . . Second journey

C. To Asia Minor and Europe (especially Ephesus) . . . . Third journey

D. To Rome . . . . Fourth journey

Writings:

Thirteen or fourteen important New Testament epistles.

Imprisonments:

A. Arrested and imprisoned in Jerusalem.

B. Held as prisoner in Caesarea for two years.

C. Taken to Rome where he remained in jail for two years.

D. Temporarily released.

E. In the Roman inner prison he died a martyr under Nero.

PAUL'S FIRST MISSIONARY JOURNEY AND RESULTING CHURCH CONFERENCE

ACTS 13–15:35

"Turned the Jewish world upside down"

Beneath the following names of places and subjects write an interesting summary of what the Bible says took place. Trace Paul's first journey on the map, page 47.

A. Saul's companions:

_____and John Mark.

B. Send out from the church_____

C. At Salamis on island of Cyprus_____

_____

D. Paphos on island of Cyprus (13:6–12)

_____

_____

_____

_____

E. Perga in Asia Minor (13:13)

_____

F. Antioch in Pisidia in Asia Minor (13:14–50)

Paul preached Christ in the synagogue on the Sabbath. (13:14–41)

What else happened? (13:42–50) _____

_____

_____

_____

G. Iconium (13:51–14:5)

_____

_____

_____

_____

H. Lystra (14:8–20)

_____

_____

_____

_____

_____

I. Derbe (14:20–21)

_____

J. Back to Lystra, Iconium, Antioch, Perga (14:21–25)

_____

_____

K. Sailed from Attalia in Asia Minor back home to _____ in Syria. (14:25–28)

_____

_____

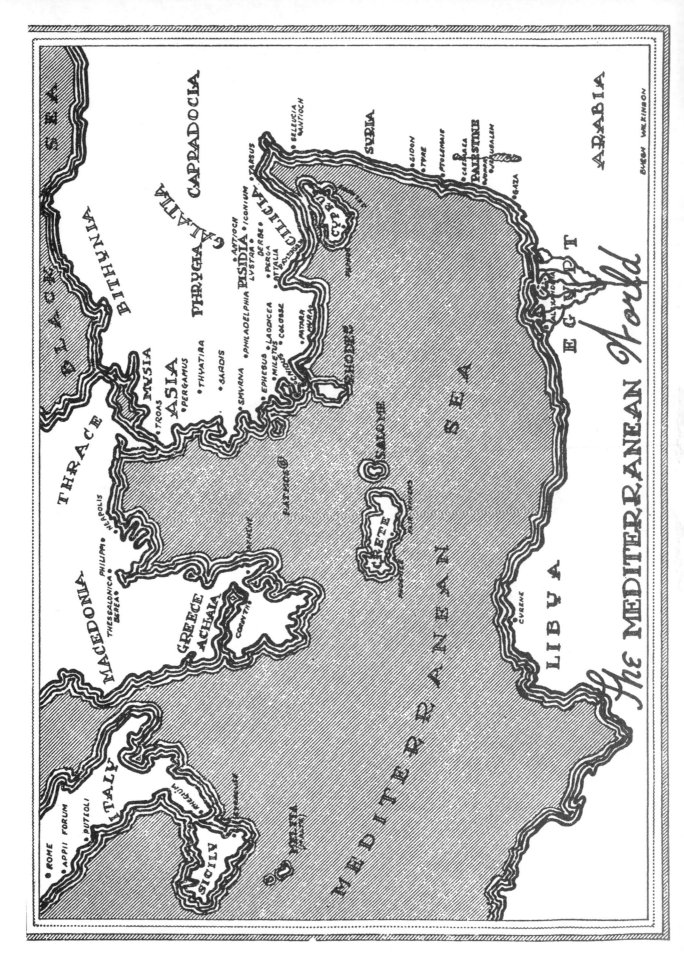

The Mediterranean World

L. CHURCH COUNCIL IN JERUSALEM ABOUT AD 50: (15:1–36)

Question discussed: Must one become a Jew before becoming a Christian? (15:5–6)

_____said God had sent the Holy Spirit to Gentiles. (15:7–11)

_____and_____spoke of wonders God worked among the Gentiles. (15:2)

_____thought the Gentiles should not be troubled by Jewish laws but should not off end the Jewish believers. They wrote_____to the Gentiles stating this. (15:13–31)

PAUL'S SECOND MISSIONARY JOURNEY–ACTS 15:36–18:22

"Turned the Roman world upside down."

Trace Paul's second journey on the map, page 47.

A. Paul's companions (15:37–40)

1. _____

What happened to Barnabas? _____

_____

Which do you think was right, Paul or Barnabas? _____

2. _____(16:1–3)

3. _____(the author of the book joins the party when he uses "we".) (16:10)

B. Purpose (15:36)

_____

_____

C. From Antioch in Syria by land to the churches in Syria and Cilicia.

D. Lystra (16:1–3)

_____

_____

E. Forbidden by Holy Ghost to go to Asia or Bithynia.

F. Troas (16:8–10)

_____

_____

_____

How has Paul's journey into Europe affected us? *(Think!)*

_____

_____

G. Philippi (having come by boat from Troas to Neapolis)

1. First European convert (16:12–15)

_____

_____

_____

_____

2. Possessed girl restored (16:16–19)

_____

_____

_____

3. In jail at Philippi (16:20–40)

_____

_____

_____

_____

_____

_____

_____

_____

H. Thessalonica (17:1–9)

_____

_____

_____

_____

_____

_____

_____

I. Berea (17:10–14)

_____

_____

_____

_____

J. Athens (17:15–34)

_____

_____

_____

_____

_____

_____

_____

K. Corinth (18:1–17)

_____

_____

_____

_____

_____

_____

_____

L. By boat to Ephesus in Asia Minor (18:18–21)

_____

_____

_____

M. Caesarea, Jerusalem, Antioch in Syria.
   Letters written on second journey: 1 and 2 Thessalonians were written by Paul from Corinth to the church at Thessalonica.

PAUL'S THIRD MISSIONARY JOURNEY–ACTS 18:23––21:17

"Turned the Greek world upside down."

Trace Paul's third journey on the map, page 53.

A. Again revisited the Asia Minor churches (18:23)

B. At Ephesus
Holy Ghost came (19:1–7)

_____
_____
_____
_____

In synagogue (19:8)

_____
_____

In school of Tyrannus (19:9–10)

_____
_____
_____

Paul's miracles (19:11–17)

_____
_____
_____

Signs of the true turning to Christ from idols (19:18–27)

_____
_____
_____
_____
_____

Uprising concerning Diana (19:23–41)

_____
_____
_____
_____
_____
_____
_____

C. Revisited and encouraged churches in Macedonia and also in Southern Greece and returned to Philippi in Macedonia.
Companions (20:4)   S_____, A_____,
S_____, G_____, T_____,
T_____, T_____,

D. Troas (20:6–12)

_____
_____

_____
_____
_____
_____

E. Melitus (met elders from Ephesus) (20:17–38)

_____
_____
_____
_____
_____

F. Landed at Tyre (21:3–6)

_____
_____
_____
_____

G. Ptolemais by sea (21:7)

_____

H. Caesarea by sea (21:8–16)

_____
_____
_____
_____
_____

I. Jerusalem

Letters written on third journey: 1 and 2 Corinthians, Galatians, Romans.

PAUL'S FOURTH JOURNEY, FROM JERUSALEM TO ROME

ACTS 21:18–28:31

Trace Paul's fourth journey on the map, page 53.

A. ARRESTED IN JERUSALEM

1. What false report was given about Paul? (21:28–29) _____
   _____

2. How was Paul rescued? (21:31–32)_____
   _____

3. What language did Paul use in asking the chief captain if he could speak to the people?
   _____

4. What language did Paul use as he spoke to the Jews in Jerusalem? (21:40–22:2)
   _____

5. *Give a number of important facts about Paul's life that are brought out in Paul's defense before the multitude. (22:1–21)*_____
   _____
   _____

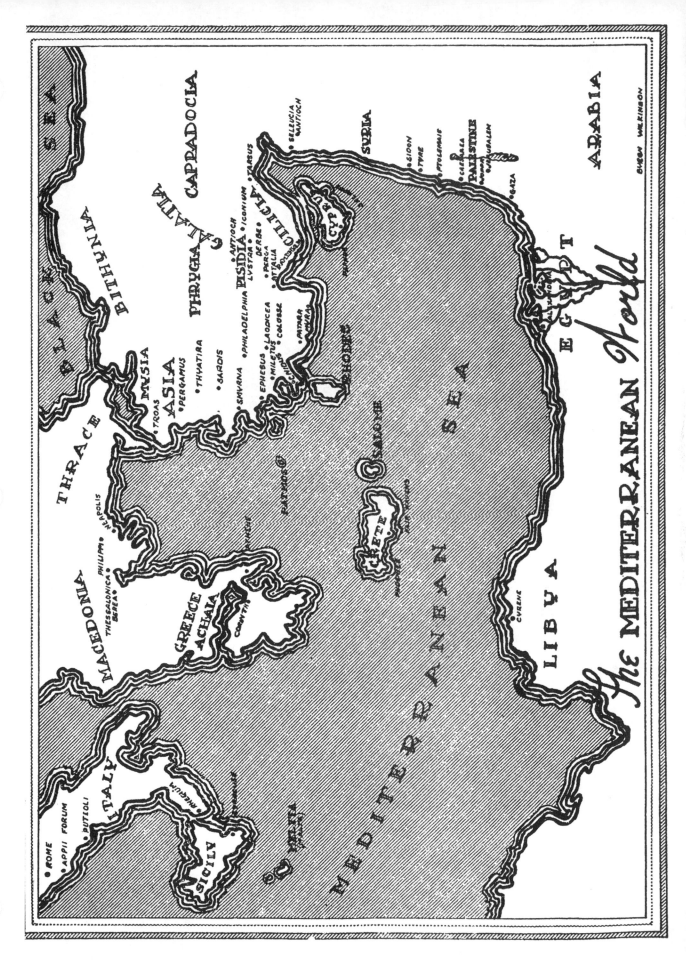

The MEDITERRANEAN World

53

6. What did the multitude do when Paul mentioned his being sent by God to the Gentiles?

_____

_____

7. How did Paul escape from being scourged? (22:24–29) _____

_____

8. On the next day when brought before the council, the Sanhedrin, what did Paul say that caused a great argument and confusion among its members? (23:6–10) _____

_____

9. What did the Lord promise Paul that night? (23:11) _____

_____

10. How many were in the band that promised not to eat or drink till they had killed Paul?

_____

11. What was their plan for killing him? (23:20–21) _____

_____

_____

12. Who told the plot to Paul and later to the chief captain? (23:16) _____

B. PRISONER IN CAESAREA

1. What governor lived in Caesarea? _____
2. Who came to Felix in Caesarea to speak against Paul? (24:1) _____

_____

3. After Paul's words of defense before Felix what privileges were given him as a prisoner? (24:10–23) _____

_____

4. After Paul spoke before Felix and his Jewish wife, Drusilla, why was Paul not released? (24:24–26) _____
5. How long was Paul a prisoner before the new governor Festus came into office? (24:27)

_____

6. To please the Jews where did Festus offer to give Paul a trial? (25:9) _____
7. Knowing a trial in Jerusalem would not bring him justice to whom did Paul appeal? (25:10–11)

_____

8. What did Festus think of Paul's innocence? (25:24–25) _____
9. Before whom did Paul next make a great speech? (25:23–26:23) _____
10. What did Agrippa say of Paul's message? (26:28) _____

11. What did Agrippa and Festus think of Paul? (26:31–32) _____

_____

_____

C. JOURNEY TO ROME

1. What centurion guarded Paul? _____
2. At which stop was Paul allowed to visit friends? _____
3. To what place was the ship going on which they set sail at Myra? (27:5–6) _____

4. At Fair Havens in Crete what suggestion or warning did Paul make? (27:8–12)_____

_____

5. In what place did the crew prefer to spend the winter? (27:12)_____

6. In trying to sail to this port what happened? (27:13–20) _____

7. What cheerful message did Paul have for those on ship? (27:22–26) _____

_____

_____

8. What did Paul say to the crew who tried to escape privately in the lifeboat? (27:30–32)

_____

9. How long were they driven by the storm? (27:27, 33)_____

10. How many were on the ship? (27:37)_____

11. How did the centurion guarding Paul save his life? (27:42–44)_____

_____

_____

12. Where did they land? (28:1) _____

(This is the same island as Malta today.)

13. What did the people of Melita think about Paul when he was bitten by the serpent? (28:1–4)

_____

14. What did they think when he did not die? (27:5–6) _____

15. What miracle of healing did Paul perform on the island?_____

_____

16. How long did they stay at Melita? (28:11)_____

17. At which places did they stop before reaching Rome?

S_____, R_____, P_____

18. How did the Christian brethren honor Paul? (28:14–15)_____

_____

19. To whom did Paul first present the gospel in Rome? (28:17)_____

20. When some did not believe to whom did Paul then present salvation? (28:28) _____

21. How long did Paul teach and preach in Rome as a prisoner in his own hired house?_____

_____

Letters written from Roman prison: Ephesians, Philippians, Colossians, Philemon.

Letters written during temporary release from prison: 1 Timothy, Titus.

Letters written during final imprisonment: 2 Timothy.

THE UNFINISHED BOOK: Acts closes abruptly. The history of the church continues on. The heroes of the church and missions have each contributed their chapter and will continue to do so till God's missionary plan for the world has been completed and Christ appears as ruler of all. Matt. 24:14

"_____

_____

_____"

THE EPISTLES

An "epistle" is a_____. The New Testament has_____epistles written to churches or individuals to teach them about Christian living.

PAULINE EPISTLES are the 13 or 14 New Testament epistles written by Paul. While in the midst of his missionary journeys or while in prison, Paul would often be concerned about the young converts in other places so he would write them the things he would have said to them if he could have been with them. Among Paul's letters are three known as pastoral epistles, namely 1 and 2 Timothy and Titus.

GENERAL EPISTLES are the other 7 letters sent to various persons and places for general use. They were written by authors other than Paul.

ROMANS (1, 2, 3, 5, 6, 7, 8, 10, 11, 12, 13)

PEOPLE TO WHOM WRITTEN: To the church at Rome, Italy, composed of Jewish and Gentile Christians. The church there was probably founded by some who had been present in Jerusalem on the day of Pentecost, or by Christians scattered by persecution of the early church.

OCCASION: Paul had not been to Rome but he greatly desired to go. Paul writes this letter to establish the Roman church and to set forth clearly the great truths of the Christian faith. Phoebe, a deaconess of Cenchreae, seaport of Corinth, was sailing for Rome, so Paul sent the letter by her. It is fitting that "the Apostle of the Gentiles should write to the capital of the Gentile world" a full explanation of salvation through Christ.

THEME: Salvation by grace through faith
1. Past—Salvation from the guilt or penalty of sin.
2. Present—Salvation from the power of sin.
3. Future—Salvation from the presence of sin.

KEY VERSE: Romans 1:16, "For I am not ashamed of the gospel of Christ: for it is the power of God unto salvation to every one that believeth; to the Jew first, and also to the Greek."

OUTLINE:

(The main divisions of this outline have been taken by permission of the author from "His Salvation," by Dr. Norman B. Harrison.)

INTRODUCTION: 1:1–17

Look at the opening verses of all of Paul's epistles and list the words most frequently used:

_____

Seek to find the Bible meaning of the following words:

Apostle _____

Gospel _____

Saints _____

Grace _____

Faith _____

I. WHAT WE ARE BY NATURE: 1:18–3:20

Complete and memorize:

"There is _____ righteous, no _____" Romans _____:_____

"For _____ have sinned, and _____"

Romans _____:_____

Are the heathen who have not heard of Christ also lost sinners? _____

Some Bible facts about the heathen are:

1. Even apart from the Bible, they have a two-fold light and are without excuse. They have the light of nature (Rom. 1:19–20), and the light of conscience. (Rom. 2:14–15)

2. All are lost (not "they will be lost if we do not preach to them," but they are already lost). (Rom. 3:23, John 3:16)

3. There is only one way to be saved—through Christ. (John 14:6, Acts 4:12)

4. They cannot believe and be saved without hearing the gospel through a preacher-human agent. (Rom. 10:14)

5. There are degrees of punishment for the unsaved. (Rom. 2:5, Rev. 20:12, Matt. 11:23–24)

6. If any man in any place at any time "hungers and thirsts after righteousness" he shall be filled. If any man seeks for the true God, the Lord will get the message of salvation to him. (Jer. 29:13)

II. HOW TO BECOME A CHRISTIAN (3:21–5:21)

A Christian is here spoken of as one who is justified. "Justified" means that a person is declared righteous by God because of his faith in Jesus.

Doing the _____ does not justify a person. (3:20, 28)

By _____ a man is justified. (3:28; 5:1)

While we were yet _____ Christ _____ for us. (5:8)

One man named _____ brought s_____ into the world and death but one man named _____ brought l_____

Memorize Romans 6:23; 10:9, 10.

III. HOW TO LIVE THE CHRISTIAN LIFE (6, 7, 8)

Reckon yourselves to be _____ to _____ but _____ to _____ (6:11)

"But, _____ yourselves unto _____

and your members as instruments of _____ unto _____." (6:13)

THE DEFEATED LIFE is described in Romans 7. What word repeated thirty-three times is characteristic of or a key to a defeated life? _____

THE TRIUMPHANT LIFE is described in Romans 8. Find four or five things in the chapter that the Spirit does to help one in the Christian life:_____

_____

_____

_____

IV. WHY ISRAEL IS SET ASIDE (9, 10, 11)

Because of _____ Israel was cast off. (11:20)

Nevertheless not all Jews rejected Jesus and the Jewish rejection was not final.

V. HOW TO SERVE GOD (12:1–15:13)

"_____ your bodies a _____ sacrifice." (12:1)

"I say . . . to every man . . . not to _____ more _____ of _____ than he ought to think."

Mark in your Bible the numerous instructions for Christians in Romans 12:9–21.

Give five definite facts about the power God has given rulers and our relationship to these governments and rulers. (13:1–7)

_____

_____

_____

_____

_____

Romans 14 and 15 discuss the Christian and Doubtful Practices.

Four rules to follow in deciding what we should do are:

1. Does it hurt my body ?
2. Does it hurt my conscience?
3. Does it hurt my testimony?
4. Does it hurt the conscience of the weaker brother?

CONCLUSION (15:14–16:27)

1 CORINTHIANS (2, 3, 6, 7, 10, 11, 12, 13, 14, 15)

PEOPLE TO WHOM WRITTEN: To the church in Corinth, Greece, which Paul had established on his second missionary journey.
Reread what happened then from your notes, page 50.

OCCASION: Paul was planning to go to Corinth but since he could not do so right away he writes. Some of the "house of Chloe" had brought Paul word that trouble had developed in the church at Corinth. Also Paul had received a letter from Corinthian Christiam1 asking Paul's opinion concerning many things.

THEME: The Christian church in a heathen community.

KEY VERSE: 1 Corinthians 10:13, "There hath no temptation taken you but such as is common to man: but God is faithful, who will not suffer you to be tempted above that ye are able; but will with the temptation also make a way to escape, that ye may be able to bear it."

OUTLINE:

1. The church and the world 1–10
2. The church as the body of Christ 11–14
3. The resurrection and the hope of the church 15–16

THINGS FOR YOU TO DO:

1. *Memorize 1 Corinthians 6:19–20.*
2. *Memorize 1 Corinthians 13, if assigned or for extra credit. (Use the word "love" in place of "charity.")*
3. *In which chapters are the following subjects discussed?*
   _____ The Christian's building of good works upon the foundation Christ.
   _____ Lawsuits, or believers going to law against one another.
   _____ Marriage
   _____ The resurrection
   _____ Women in the church
   _____ Speaking in tongues
   _____ Spiritual gifts
   _____ The Lord's Supper
   _____ Love (charity)
4. *Be able to tell the main thoughts regarding each of these subjects.*

2 CORINTHIANS (1:1–5, 5, 8, 9, 11:21–33, 12:6–10)

OCCASION: This letter was called for by the result of the first. The majority in Corinth had received the first letter and followed its instructions but there was a group in Corinth who doubted if Paul had the authority of an apostle, so Paul wrote to answer them.

THEME: Comfort and Paul's defense of his apostleship.

KEY VERSE: 2 Corinthians 12:9, "And he said unto me, my grace is sufficient for thee: for my strength is made perfect in weakness."

QUESTIONS:

1. What is one reason God comforts us in tribulation and suffering? (1:1–5) _____

    _____

2. Why is death not terrible for a child of God? (chapter 5) _____

    _____

    _____

3. II Corinthians 8 and 9 are the great New Testament chapters on giving.
    On a separate page write a good paragraph on GIVING, bringing out the main thoughts learned from these chapters.

4. *List some of the things Paul suffered which you did not read about in Acts. (11:23–33)*

    _____

    _____

    _____

    _____

    Paul mentions these to show he was truly an apostle.

5. When Paul asked for his thorn in the flesh to be removed what was God's reply? (12:6–10) _____

    _____

    _____

GALATIANS (1, 2)

PEOPLE TO WHOM WRITTEN: To the churches of Galatia, a small district in Asia Minor settled by the Gauls. Paul stopped there on both his second and third journeys.

OCCASION: Paul had heard that Judaistic teachers had come to Galatia and taught that the Jewish laws and customs were binding on the Christians as well as the Jews. Paul had taught that man was not saved by working to keep the law but through faith in Christ. The key word is "free."

THEME: Law and grace.

KEY VERSE: Galatians 2:20, "I am crucified with Christ: nevertheless I live; yet not I, but Christ liveth in me: and the life which I now live in the flesh I live by the faith of the Son of God, who loved me, and gave himself for me."

QUESTIONS:

1. After Paul's conversion where did he go? (1:17) _____

2. Why did Paul mention the Jerusalem council and the decisions there? _____

    _____

3. What verse tells us man is not justified by his works but by faith in Christ? (2:15–21)

    _____

4. *Be able to list from memory the fruits of the spirit in Gal. 5:22–23.*

EPHESIANS (1, 2, 4, 6:10–24)

PEOPLE TO WHOM WRITTEN: The church in Ephesus and the surrounding territory. Ephesus was important from the commercial, religious, and political standpoints. Next to Rome, Ephesus was the most important city visited by Paul. Paul visited Ephesus for a very short time on his second journey;

however, he had to hurry on to Jerusalem to complete a vow. (Acts 18:19–21) On the third journey, Paul stayed in and around Ephesus for a period of three years. (Acts 19–20)

THEME: What God does for us and what we should do for God.

KEY VERSES: Ephesians 2:8–9, "For by grace are ye saved through faith; and that not of yourselves: it is the gift of God: Not of works lest any man should boast."

THINGS FOR YOU TO DO:

Ephesians 1:3–14 is the longest sentence in the Bible. The subject is "Our blessings in Christ." Ephesians 2 tells what we were before we became Christians and what we are now. *On another paper make two columns listing what the chapter says about WHAT WE WERE and WHAT WE ARE.*

In Ephesians 4 choose the two commands you think you especially should be careful to obey:

1. _____

2. _____

Ephesians 6:10–24 gives the Christian's warfare and armor.

1. Who is the enemy? _____

2. The Christian should wear the girdle of _____

    the breastplate of _____

    the shoes of _____

    the shield of _____

    the helmet of _____

    the sword of _____ which is _____

PHILIPPIANS (1, 2, 4)

PEOPLE TO WHOM WRITTEN: To the church at Philippi, the city founded by Philip of Macedon, the father of Alexander the Great. Paul first visited Philippi on his second journey and there established a church. Read your summary on pages 49 and 50 of what happened.

OCCASION: Paul wrote to thank the Philippians for their gift to him; to send Epaphroditus back to them with the news that he was better after having been sick; and to settle a quarrel between two women in the Philippian church, Euodia and Syntyche.

THEME: Joy in Christ. Though written by Paul while in prison and greatly oppressed the key note of the epistle is "JOY."

KEY VERSE: Philippians 1:21, "For to me to live is Christ, and to die is gain."

THINGS FOR YOU TO DO:

Memorize Phil. 4:6 and Phil. 4:19. Answer these:

1. What is the one thing which is most important to you in life? *(Think)*_____

2. What did life mean to Paul? (1:21) _____

3. What was Paul's attitude toward death? (1:21–24) _____

    _____

    _____

4. In what ways did Christ humble himself? (2:5–8) _____
_____
_____
_____

5. In what ways will God exalt Christ? (2:9–11) _____
_____
_____

6. Instead of worrying what should one do? (4:6) _____

7. What kind of things should a Christian think about? (4:8)_____
_____
_____

8. How would believing Philippians 4:19 affect a person's life?_____
_____

COLOSSIANS (1:13–19; 3)

PEOPLE TO WHOM WRITTEN: To the church at Colosse, a town of Phrygia, in Asia Minor, 100 miles east of Ephesus. This church was neither founded or visited by Paul. The churches in Colosse met in houses since church buildings did not come into general use until the third century.

OCCASION: While in prison in Rome, Paul learned from a fellow prisoner of the conditions in the Colossian church. False teachers had taught that a life of asceticism and faithful observance of certain customs were necessary for salvation. Paul wrote that redemption was through Christ, not through a system of rules to suppress the body.

THEME: Christ is all.

KEY VERSE: Colossians 1:18, "That in all things he might have the preeminence."

THINGS FOR YOU TO DO:

Colossians tells a great deal about Christ.

List every fact mentioned about Christ in Col. 1:13–19:

_____
_____
_____
_____
_____

Colossians 3: What things are mentioned which should be put out of our lives when we are Christians? _____
_____
_____
_____

What things should be put into our lives? _____
_____
_____
_____
_____

What command is given (3:18–4:1)

to wives? _____

to husbands? _____

to children? _____

to parents? _____

to servants? _____

to masters? _____

1 THESSALONIANS (4, 5)

PEOPLE TO WHOM WRITTEN: To the church at Thessalonica. Read your summary on page 50 of what happened when Paul first visited Thessalonica on his second journey and established the church. After three weeks of preaching and teaching Paul was driven away. From there he went to Berea, to Athens, and to Corinth from which place this letter was written.

OCCASION: Timothy had returned from visiting the Thessalonian converts and reported to Paul that they were enduring persecutions bravely but were troubled about some of their number who had died. "How would they get any benefit from the Lord's coming?" Paul wrote to encourage their steadfastness and to teach them more fully about the Lord's coming. Paul said that the dead in Christ would see Him first, even before those who were living on the earth. (1 Thess. 4:16–18)

THEME: The return of Christ–the bright side.

KEY VERSES: 1 Thessalonians 1:9–10, "Ye turned to God from idols to serve the living and true God; and to wait for his Son from heaven."

THINGS FOR YOU TO DO:

Notice that the close of every chapter gives a fact about the Lord's return.

What message of comfort does Paul give the Thessalonians? (4:13–18) _____

_____

_____

In what way could the Lord's coming be compared to that of a thief? (5:1–6) _____

_____

_____

Memorize 1 Thess. 5:16–22.

2 THESSALONIANS (2, 3)

OCCASION: Paul's first letter had done much good, but some stressed the early return of the Lord to such an extent that they became very impractical—even quitting work—just waiting. They had misunderstood the editorial "we" Paul had used when he said "We which are alive and remain." Paul was speaking of the unexpectedness rather than the nearness of Christ's return. This false impression which made some of the Thessalonians quit their work was the forerunner of many false views today. In the second letter Paul showed that the coming of the Lord was not immediate in all probability. He spoke of what must take place before He returned.

THEME: The return of Christ—the dark side.

KEY VERSE: 2 Thessalonians 3:13, "Be not weary in well doing."

QUESTIONS:

1. When Christ is revealed what will happen to those who do not know God? (1:6–9) _____
_____

2. What happens to those who do know God (the saints)? (1:10) _____
_____

3. What will happen before the Lord's return? (2:3–12) _____
_____
_____
_____

4. What should Christians continue to do? (3:8–14) _____
_____

PASTORAL EPISTLES

1 TIMOTHY, 2 TIMOTHY, TITUS

These three letters are called "Pastorals" because they were written to pastors and discuss chiefly the duties of ministers. Pastorals were not written to churches but to individuals. These books add quite a bit to the history of Paul's life, for they begin where Acts ends.

1 TIMOTHY (2, 3, 4, 6)

PERSON TO WHOM WRITTEN: To young Timothy who was in charge of the church at Ephesus. He was probably from Lystra. His father was a Greek, but his mother, Eunice, and his grandmother, Lois, were Jewesses. He was brought up in the fear of the Lord, learning the Scriptures "from a babe." He was probably converted through Paul on the first missionary journey. At Lystra on the second journey he was chosen to assist Paul and he continued as Paul's coworker till the end of Paul's life, about AD 68.

OCCASION: Paul had left Timothy to strengthen the Ephesian church. Paul wrote this letter giving instruction in church organization and giving correct doctrine to counteract certain false teachers. Timothy sorely needed Paul's encouragement.

THEME: Be careful of the gospel.

KEY VERSE: 1 Timothy 3:15, "That thou mayest know how thou oughtest to behave thyself in the house of God, which is the church of the living God, the pillar and ground of the truth."

QUESTIONS:

1. What instructions for public prayer are given? (2:1–8) _____
_____
_____
_____

2. What relation are women to have to men? (2:9–15) _____
_____
_____

3. *List the qualifications for elders and deacons (3)* _____
_____
_____
_____
_____

4. In what ways should young people be an example? (4) _____
_____
_____

2 TIMOTHY (3, 4)

PERSON TO WHOM WRI'ITEN: Timothy.

PLACE OF WRITING: From Paul's final imprisonment in Rome under Nero.

OCCASION: This, Paul's last letter, was written to Timothy begging him to be faithful, though many in Asia were turning away from Paul's teaching. Also Paul wanted Timothy to hurry to Rome to visit him before winter. According to tradition, Paul was martyred before Timothy could reach him.

THEME: Be careful of the witness. Special importance is laid on the witness of the pastor against false teaching.

KEY VERSE: 2 Timothy 2:15, "Study to shew thyself approved unto God, a workman that needeth not to be ashamed, rightly dividing the word of truth."

QUESTIONS:

1. How are the last days of the age described? (3:1–9) _____
_____
_____
_____
_____

2. What do we know of Timothy's early training? (1:5, 3:15)_____
_____
_____

3. *Locate a verse showing that all the Bible is inspired of God.* _____
4. What does Paul say in his closing personal testimony? (4:7–8) _____
_____
_____
_____
_____

TITUS (2, 3)

PERSON TO WHOM WRITTEN: To Titus on the island of Crete. The Cretans were famous as bowmen, but their moral reputation was very bad. Titus was one of Paul's converts (1:4). He was a Gentile, an uncircumcised Greek. He seems to have been converted in the early years of Paul's ministry, for he was with Paul and Barnabas when they went to Jerusalem at the end of their first journey. He seems to have been a strong man physically and spiritually.

OCCASION: Paul had been with Titus in Crete, and had left him there (1:5) to minister the gospel. The Cretans were proverbially "liars, evil beasts, idle gluttons." In addition to the problems of a pastor among such people, Titus was also troubled with false teachers, especially Judaizers. (1:10)

THEME: Be careful of the life.

KEY VERSE: Titus 2:7, "In all things shewing thyself a pattern of good works: in doctrine shewing uncorruptness, gravity, sincerity."

QUESTIONS:

1. In what kind of life was the pastor Titus to instruct (2)

   Young women? _____

   _____

   Young men? _____

   _____

   Servants? _____

   _____

2. Are we saved because of our good works? (3:5) _____

3. If we are saved will we be careful to do good works? (3:8) _____

PHILEMON

PERSON TO WHOM WRITTEN: To Philemon, an elder at the church of Colosse and to the church which met in his home. He was well known, wealthy, and generous.

OCCASION: Onesimus, a slave of Philemon of Colosse, had robbed his master and fled to Rome. He came under Paul's preaching and was converted. He determined to go back to Philemon, who owned him. Paul urges Philemon to forgive Onesimus and accept him as a brother.

THEME: Christian brotherhood.

KEY VERSE: Philemon 1:17, "If thou count me therefore a partner, receive him as myself." What does Paul ask Philemon to do? (1:8–21)

HEBREWS (1, 4, 5, 9, 10:1–25, 11, 13)

AUTHOR: This epistle was not signed by Paul as were his other letters, but many Bible scholars think that Paul must have written it.

PEOPLE TO WHOM WRITTEN: To Hebrew Christians.

OCCASION: The book was written to comfort Jewish Christians undergoing persecution and to keep them from turning away from Christianity.

The problems of these Hebrew Christians were many:

1. They were severely persecuted.
2. They were no longer allowed to worship in the temple.
3. The temple worship was elaborate while the Christian worship was very simple.
4. The Christian Jews were called traitors to the Law of Moses.

THEME: Christ is better.

KEY VERSE: Hebrews 11:40, "God having provided some better thing for us."

THINGS FOR YOU TO DO:

Christ is BETTER than _____ 1:1–2

Christ is BETTER than _____ 1:4–14

Christ is BETTER than _____ 3:3

Christ is BETTER than _____ 7:26–28

In what ways does Christ differ from the Old Testament priests? (7:27 and 9:11–12)

_____

_____

_____

To what Old Testament priest is He compared? (5:5–10) _____

Christ's sacrifice is BETTER than _____ 9:13–14

How many sacrifices did Jesus offer for sin? (10:10–12) _____

The heavenly tabernacle is BETTER than _____ 9:1–11, 24

Where is the tabernacle into which Jesus has entered? (9:24) _____

Hebrews 11 is the great FAITH CHAPTER of the Bible.

How necessary is faith? (11:6) _____

_____

List ten Old Testament characters in Hebrews 11 who are mentioned for their faith:

1. _____ 6. _____
2. _____ 7. _____
3. _____ 8. _____
4. _____ 9. _____
5. _____ 10. _____

Where in Hebrews 13 is a famous benediction located?

Next Sunday notice what your pastor uses as a closing benediction.

JAMES (1–4)

AUTHOR: James, the brother of Jesus, is commonly recognized as the writer of this epistle. He was bishop of the church at Jerusalem and presided over the first Church Council at Jerusalem in AD 50. He rejected Christ for some time and was probably saved through the resurrection of Christ.

PEOPLE TO WHOM WRITTEN: To the Hebrew Christians of the "twelve tribes which are scattered abroad."

OCCASION: Written at a time when the Jewish Christians were becoming worldly. Some merely professed to believe, while others really did.

THEME: Faith works.

KEY VERSE: James 1:22, "But be ye doers of the word, and not hearers only, deceiving your own selves."

QUESTIONS:

1. What should one do who lacks wisdom? _____
2. What would show men we really believe God's words? (1:22–25) _____

_____

3. What outward works show that one has true inner religion? (1:27) _____

_____

_____

4. How are we to treat rich and poor people? (2:1–7) _____

_____

5. How is one's faith shown? (2:14–26) _____
6. What part of the body can God tame even if no man can tame it? (3) _____
7. Should a Christian try to gain the friendship of the world? (4) _____

(The "world" here may be defined as "society with God left out.")

8. What is the most important instruction for your own life you have gained from studying James?

_____

_____

AUTHOR: Simon Peter, one of the "inner circle" of three of our Lord's apostles; brother of Andrew, who introduced Peter to Jesus; a fisherman who lived at Capernaum on the shores of the Sea of Galilee; the natural spokesman of the apostles. He was the first to confess that Jesus. was the "Christ, the Son of the living God."

PEOPLE TO WHOM WRITTEN: To Christians in the northeastern part of Asia Minor.

OCCASION: The church was undergoing its first worldwide persecution. "This letter was written under the shadows of the Nero's persecution to encourage believers to bear up under their trials; to remember that CHRIST'S WORK WAS DONE THROUGH SUFFERING, and that the church should expect to endure suffering; and to caution them to be very careful to live so that they could not possibly be accused of rebellion against Rome; to honor even the cruel Emperor; to win, in those trying times, by the beauty and harmlessness of their lives."

THEME: Sufferings of pilgrims. The word "suffering" is mentioned 15 times.

KEY VERSE: 1 Peter 2:21, "Christ also suffered for us, leaving us an example, that ye should follow his steps."

THINGS FOR YOU TO DO:

To what object is Christ compared and also the Christian? (2:4–8)

Tell the instruction given to "strangers and pilgrims" from the following verses:

2:11_____

2:12_____

2:13_____

3:17 _____

3:18 _____

Look up the following verses and on another page write a paragraph on what Peter says about SUFFERING: (2:21, 2:24, 3:18, 4:1–2, 12–13)

2 PETER (1, 2:1–10, 3)

AUTHOR: Peter.

PEOPLE TO WHOM WRITTEN: To the same group addressed in Peter's first epistle. It is thought that these churches had been founded principally by Paul.

OCCASION: Peter before his death wanted to assure Christians of the truth and to impress them with the necessity of growth on the part of Christians and to keep them from falling into the pitfalls of false teaching. Peter wanted them to know that Paul and he were preaching the same gospel, and that there was no conflict between them.

THEME: True knowledge and false knowledge.

KEY VERSE: 2 Peter 3:18, "But grow in grace, and in the knowledge of our Lord and Saviour Jesus Christ."

QUESTIONS:

1. What eight things added to one's faith will make one fruitful in his knowledge of Christ? (1:5–8)

_____

_____

_____

2. How did "true knowledge" given in prophecy come? (1:21)_____

_____

3   Should we expect to find false teachers of Christianity arising? (2:1–3) _____

4.   How is the "day of the Lord" described in 2 Peter 3:10–14? _____
_____
_____

1 JOHN

AUTHOR: John, the beloved disciple.

List four things you remember about John from the Gospels:

_____
_____
_____
_____

PEOPLE TO WHOM WRITTEN: A circular letter, especially to Gentiles. No particular church is mentioned.

OCCASION: It was written that Christians who had believed might know that they have eternal life, and might live in victorious fellowship with God.

THEME: Fellowship with God through Christ.

KEY VERSE: 1 John 5:13, "These things have I written unto you that believe on the name of the Son of God; that ye may know that ye have eternal life."

THINGS FOR YOU TO DO:

1.   God is (1:5) _____. If we want to have
fellowship with Him we must (1:7) _____

2.   God is (2:29) _____. If we want to have
fellowship with Him we must (2:29) _____

3.   God is (4:8) _____. If we want to have
fellowship with Him we must (4:7) _____.

Read carefully 1 John 3:13–24 and 4:7–21 and list what seems to you to be the most striking things said about "LOVE." Do not copy verses. Express the thoughts in your own words.

_____
_____
_____
_____
_____
_____
_____

2 JOHN

AUTHOR: John, the beloved disciple.

PEOPLE TO WHOM WRITTEN: To the "elect lady" and "her children," probably a wealthy lady near Ephesus.

OCCASION: John had heard that this godly lady and her children were walking in the truth; he was expecting to make a visit to them in the near future. He warned against entertaining some false teachers who traveled about teaching anti-Christian doctrines.

THEME: The Truth. Withdraw from those who do not hold to the Truth.

3 JOHN

AUTHOR: John, the beloved apostle.

PEOPLE TO WHOM WRITTEN: Gaius. Probably a wealthy and hospitable member of the church at Corinth.

OCCASION: John was expecting soon to make a personal visit to the home of Gaius. John writes to condemn Diotrephes who refused to receive traveling preachers and to urge Gaius to entertain them.

THEME: The truth. Fellowship with those who hold the truth.
(Compare this with 2 John.)

JUDE

AUTHOR: Jude, who is commonly thought to have been the brother of Jesus.

PEOPLE TO WHOM WRITTEN: To all Christians everywhere.

OCCASION: In the church there were those who taught "Believe and do as you please," so Jude writes to urge Christians "to contend earnestly for the faith delivered to the saints."

THEME: Kept from apostasy ("apostasy" means the turning away from the truth).

THINGS FOR YOU TO DO:
How are the false, apostate teachers described? (8, 10, 12–13, 16)

_____
_____
_____
_____

Quote the benediction which closes this book:

_____
_____
_____
_____
_____
_____

REVELATION

Read as parallel reading

AUTHOR: John, the beloved disciple.

PEOPLE TO WHOM WRITTEN: The seven churches of Asia.
List their names as found in Rev. 2 and 3 and locate each place on the map, page 53.

1. _____   5. _____
2. _____   6. _____
3. _____   7. _____
4. _____

OCCASION: John was an exile on the rugged little isle of Patmos when God commanded him to write the things in this book. The churches were suffering persecution and were in danger of heresy and so needed an unveiling of the future for the benefit of the church at large.

THEME: The ultimate triumph of Christ.

OUTLINE: An outline based on Rev. 1:19 is:

1. "The things which thou hast seen" . . . . Rev. 1
   Christ, the Glorified one
2. "The things which are" . . . . Rev. 2–3
   Christ, the Head over the church
3. "The things which shall be hereafter" . . . . Rev. 4–22
   Christ, the Triumphant One

GENESIS	REVELATION
Beginning of death	"Death shall be no more."
Satan's first appearance	Satan's disappearance and doom
The curse pronounced	The curse removed, "No more curse."
Man driven from the Garden of Eden	Man welcomed to the Garden of God
Heaven and earth	New heavens and new earth
Night	"No night there"
Abraham looked for a city	The city of God
Beginning of Babylon or Babel	End of Babylon
First rest	Final rest
Judgment pronounced	Judgment executed
The face of God hidden	"We shall see His face."
The gates shut against us	The gates never shut
Satan victorious	Satan defeated
All faces wet with tears	All tears wiped away
The cherubin keeping man out	The cherubin welcoming man in
The first typical sacrificial lamb	The Lamb once slain in the midst of throne

REASONS FOR STUDYING THE BOOK:

1. Special blessing is promised to those who hear, read, and obey the prophecies (Rev. 1:3).
2. Without it, the Bible is an incomplete book, an unfinished story of redemption.
3. Revelation reaches farther into the future in detail than any other book of the Bible.
4. Christ is very prominent in the book. He is often called the "Lamb." In John's gospel He was the suffering Lamb but now He is the "Lamb on the Throne."

THINGS TO WATCH FOR:

1. *Underline the verses telling of the praise given to Christ and God.*
2. *Notice the descriptions of Christ and the names by which He is called.*

MORE TIME TO TEACH WHAT MATTERS MOST

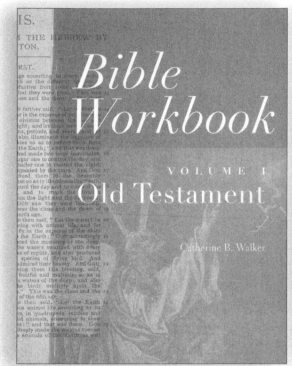

978-0-8024-0751-1

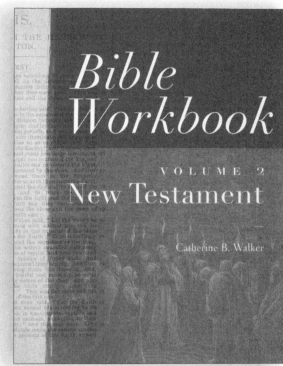

978-0-8024-0752-8

MOODY
Publishers®

*From the Word **to** Life®*

The workbooks are full of exercises, questions, and maps that ensure students have the fundamentals down before you teach. Each workbook contains thousands of fill-in-the-blank questions as well as diagrams and maps students interact with. They can be adapted for virtually any teaching setting (homeschool, Bible class, adult Sunday school).

also available as eBooks

STUDY THE BIBLE WITH PROFESSORS
FROM MOODY BIBLE INSTITUTE

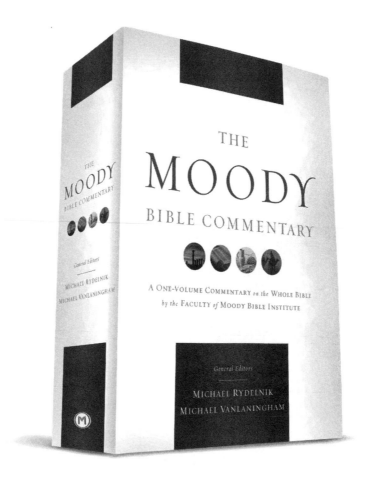

MOODY
Publishers®

From the Word to Life®

Study the Bible with a team of 30 Moody Bible Institute professors. This in-depth, user-friendly, one-volume commentary will help you better understand and apply God's written revelation to all of life. Additional study helps include maps, charts, bibliographies for further reading, and a subject and Scripture index.

978-0-8024-2867-7 | also available as an eBook

THE BEST ALLEGORY EVER WRITTEN

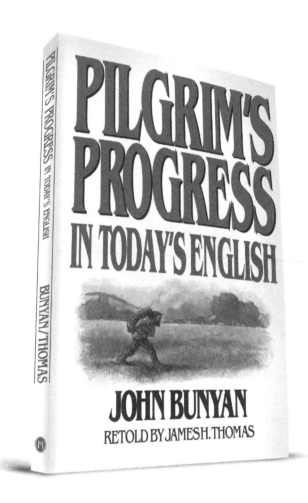

MOODY
Publishers®

From the Word to Life®

The best allegory ever written is rewritten in modern
English, making it clearer and more forceful to the
modern reader.

978-0-8024-6520-7 | also available as an eBook